Painkillers

Painkillers

HISTORY, SCIENCE, AND ISSUES

Victor B. Stolberg

The Story of a Drug
Peter L. Myers, Series Editor

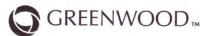

An Imprint of ABC-CLIO, LLC
Santa Barbara, California • Denver, Colorado

Library of Congress Cataloging-in-Publication Data

Names: Stolberg, Victor B.
Title: Painkillers : history, science, and issues / Victor B. Stolberg.
Other titles: Pain killers
Description: Santa Barbara, California : Greenwood, [2016] | Series: The story of a
    drug | Includes bibliographical references and index.
Identifiers: LCCN 2015047059 | ISBN 9781440835315 (hard copy : alk. paper) |
    ISBN 9781440835322 (ebook)
Subjects: LCSH: Analgesics. | Analgesics—History.
Classification: LCC RM319 .S76 2016 | DDC 615.7/83—dc23
LC record available at http://lccn.loc.gov/2015047059

ISBN: 978–1–4408–3531–5
EISBN: 978–1–4408–3532–2

20 19 18 17 16   2 3 4 5

This book is also available on the World Wide Web as an eBook.
Visit www.abc-clio.com for details.

Greenwood
An Imprint of ABC-CLIO, LLC

ABC-CLIO, LLC
130 Cremona Drive, P.O. Box 1911
Santa Barbara, California 93116-1911

This book is printed on acid-free paper ∞

Manufactured in the United States of America

I would like to dedicate this book to my immediate family, particularly my wife, Marie Rose, and our two young sons, Victor and George, for their support and tolerance during my work on this project.

Contents

Series Foreword

While many books have been written about the prevalence and perils of recreational drug use, what about the wide variety of chemicals Americans ingest to help them heal or to cope with mental and physical issues? These therapeutic drugs—whether prescription or over the counter (OTC), generic or brand name—play a critical role in both the U.S. health care system and American society at large. This series explores major classes of such drugs, examining them from a variety of perspectives, including scientific, medical, economic, legal, and cultural.

For the sake of clarity and consistency, each book in this series follows the same format.

We begin with a fictional case study bringing to life the significance of this particular class of drug. Chapter 2 provides an overview of the class as a whole, including discussion of different subtypes, as well as basic information about the conditions such drugs are meant to treat. The history and evolution of these drugs is discussed in Chapter 3. Chapter 4 explores how the drugs work in the body at a cellular level, while Chapter 5 examines the large-scale impacts of such substances on the body and how such effects can be beneficial in different situations. Dangers such as side effects, drug interactions, misuse, abuse, and overdose are highlighted in Chapter 6. Chapter 7 focuses on how this particular class of drugs is produced, distributed, and regulated by state and federal governments. Chapter 8 addresses professional and popular attitudes and beliefs about the drug, as well as representations of such drugs and their users in the media. We wrap up with a consideration of the drug's possible future, including emerging controversies and trends in research and use, in Chapter 9.

Each volume in this series also includes a glossary of terms and a collection of print and electronic resources for additional information and further study. To supplement the main text, Chapters 2 through 9 include end-of-chapter primary documents, which offer readers additional insights.

It is our hope that the books in this series will not only provide valuable information, but will also spur discussion and debate about these drugs and the many issues that surround them. For instance, are antibiotics being over-prescribed, leading to the development of drug-resistant bacteria? Should anti-psychotics, usually used to treat serious mental illnesses such as schizophrenia and bipolar disorder, be used to render inmates and elderly individuals with dementia more docile? Do schools have the right to mandate vaccination for their students, against the wishes of some parents?

As a final caveat, we wish to emphasize that the information we present in these books is no substitute for consultation with a licensed health care professional, and we do not claim to provide medical advice or guidance.

—Peter L. Myers, PhD
Emeritus member, National Addiction Studies Accreditation Commission
Past President, International Coalition for Addiction Studies Education
Editor-in-Chief Emeritus, *Journal of Ethnicity in Substance Abuse*

Preface

The title of this work might be a little misleading, as a discussion of painkillers is not simply the story of "a" drug, but rather the story of several somewhat similar but also of many other somewhat disparate drugs. There are, as you will discover in reading this work, many different drugs that are used as painkillers. This book will present an overview of opium, morphine, other opiates and opioids, and of other painkiller use and abuse from ancient times to the contemporary era; these other painkiller drugs include non-steroidal anti-inflammatory drugs and an array of many different other substances, some of which are available for sale over the counter, while others are available only with a physician's prescription, and some of which are available both ways, usually with the higher dosages of the painkiller medication requiring a prescription from a medical professional. Each painkiller drug, or at least groups of painkiller drugs, has its own somewhat unique story; thus this story is composed of many different stories.

The historical and cross-cultural background of painkiller use and abuse will be examined along with considerations of various societal approaches of how to deal with these issues. This consideration will utilize historical studies of respective painkiller drugs, principally opium and morphine, from various time periods that can be used for developing a better understanding of the historical background of such phenomena. Attention will first be concerned with the early evidence for the use of opium, including discussion of Near Eastern civilizations, particularly Egyptian and Mesopotamian, as well as those from elsewhere in the world, notably including China and India. Cross-cultural evidence of painkiller use and abuse elsewhere will also be presented. The development of morphine and other similar painkillers will briefly be reviewed. Historical studies of opiates, opioids, and other painkiller drugs, as well as those reviewing specific approaches to addressing abuse at various time periods, and other related works will be used in an attempt to provide a richer and fuller appreciation of the broad dimensions of the field. A brief review of the science of how different painkiller drugs work will also be presented along with coverage of their respective effects and applications. Attention will also be directed at some of the risks of painkiller use, their misuse, and potential overdose concerns. We will also explore issues around the production, distribution, and regulation of respective painkiller drugs. This discussion will include the early evidence of painkiller use, cross-cultural evidence, modern developments, abuse patterns, treatment approaches, policy issues, and several other additional perspectives.

This work is intended to broaden the scope of the participant's frame of reference within the area of historical and cultural foundations of addiction studies by focusing on the story of painkiller drugs, examining the pharmacological basis of their effects and applications, risks, production, distribution, and regulation, as well as reviewing some of the social dimensions of the use and abuse of painkiller drugs, and thoughts on the future of these particular type of drugs.

Acknowledgments

I would like to acknowledge my family, particularly my wife and two young sons, for their support and tolerance during this project. I would also like to thank all the staff behind the scenes at ABC-CLIO. Chiefly, I would like to heartedly thank the series editor, my good friend and colleague of nearly three decades, Dr. Peter L. Myers. His unwavering support and friendship has been a stalwart base not only for much of my career advancement, but also for my own personal growth and development. I am particularly indebted to his insightful criticisms and helpful suggestions that have contributed to the completion of the present volume.

Most importantly, I would like to acknowledge all of those individuals struggling with painkillers and other drugs of abuse. The hard work of so many individuals in recovery striving to improve their lives and health is a testament to humanity at its best.

Chapter 1

A Case Study: Misery and Relief

Not all individuals use drugs for the same reasons, nor will they all have the same experiences with the use of a particular drug whether it is or is not a painkiller or any other type of drug. Many individuals will try a particular drug, use it for a time, perhaps for only a short period of time, and then leave it alone and move on with the rest of their lives. Other individuals relate that from the very first time that they tried a particular drug, they became hooked and progressively moved through the stages to addiction. Such varied tales, and many more, are certainly true with respect to individual users of respective painkiller drugs. We will briefly examine two fictitious case studies to examine some of the types of interactions that can occur among those who come to use these painkiller drugs and the varied impacts that this practice causes in their lives.

CASE 1: MISERY

Trevor is an African American male, age 47; he is 5 feet 10 inches tall and weighs 178 pounds. Trevor's high school years were trying for him and his family; he got involved briefly with a small street gang and was smoking marijuana and drinking alcoholic beverages almost every day. Trevor was also very gifted intellectually and athletically. He was actually an outstanding young student-athlete, winning many awards and trophies. He played basketball and ran track. Trevor used to work part time as a mover while he was in his freshman year at college. One day, while moving a large leather couch, he seriously hurt his lower back. He went to see a doctor who gave him a prescription for Vicodin. Vicodin was the trade name for a combination pharmaceutical product that contained doses of both acetaminophen and hydrocodone.

Hydrocodone, of course, is a powerful opioid painkiller medication, and acetaminophen is a less potent non-steroidal anti-inflammatory drug, or NSAID, that increases the effects of the hydrocodone. Vicodin was intended to be used for relief of moderate to severe pain.

Trevor was supposed to take 2 Vicodin pills twice a day as prescribed. He was initially prescribed the formulation of Vicodin that consisted of 300 mg of acetaminophen and 5 mg of hydrocodone. However, not long after starting to use the Vicodin, Trevor felt that the 2 pills were not strong enough, so he started taking more. This should not be too surprising, as only about 50% of prescribed medications are, according to the World Health Organization (WHO), taken in accordance with directions. He soon then progressed to 3 pills twice a day, and not too long thereafter, he was taking 3 pills 3 times a day as his tolerance increased. Trevor was able to get his prescription changed to the stronger formulation of Vicodin that consisted of 500 mg of acetaminophen and 5 mg of hydrocodone. However, he was not much more satisfied with that dosage, and not long thereafter, he found another doctor who gave him a prescription for Vicodin HP, a formulation of Vicodin that consists of 600 mg of acetaminophen and 10 mg of hydrocodone. However, Trevor's pharmacist substituted the generic formulation of Vicodin, which is manufactured by Norco, and each pill consists of 325 mg of acetaminophen and 10 mg of hydrocodone. He was more than satisfied with its effects. The Vicodin did not just numb the pain in his lower back, however; he really, really liked the way it made him feel. When using the Vicodin, Trevor felt more relaxed than usual and he was less anxious about things in his life. But he was tired a lot of the time, and on some days he even had to push himself to get out of the house. In addition, he often became somewhat depressed and wondered if his life would ever get any better while having these types of feelings. Trevor dropped out of college after the beginning of his sophomore year; he would soon have been expelled for poor academic performance anyhow.

One day Trevor's Vicodin prescription ran out, and he quickly started to feel really sick. He was soon sweating profusely without engaging in any physical activity, and his whole body was in intense pain. He felt better only after he got his prescription refilled. Trevor had developed high tolerance, and he was dependent on the drug at that point. He needed to take his painkiller medication just to not feel in pain. His body started to show the wear and tear of his drug abuse. The acetaminophen in the high levels of Vicodin he had consumed over the years of abuse had caused severe deterioration to most of his vital body organs, particularly his liver.

Trevor started looking for different doctors so that he could get more Vicodin prescriptions. He would lie to the doctors and tell them that he was in horrible pain, far worse than he really was feeling. One day Trevor intentionally slammed a door on his finger and broke it. This helped him get even more pills. Another time he had a friend pull out a tooth so that he could go to a dentist whom he had heard would write painkiller prescriptions for him. When he visited his grandmother's house, he would check her medicine cabinet for any pills he could take.

Trevor had so many different prescriptions from so many different doctors that he had to go to different pharmacies to fill his Vicodin prescriptions. One day he went to a pharmacy with his mother, and the pharmacist told him that he could not fill his prescription. Their computer records indicated that Trevor had already purchased a lot of Vicodin pills in a rather brief period of time at many different pharmacies. He was embarrassed that he was caught, but he was really ashamed that his mother heard the whole thing.

Vicodin was a potent painkiller that was a combination formulation of hydrocodone bitartrate and acetaminophen. On December 9, 1988, the U.S. Food and Drug Administration (FDA) approved the marketing of Vicodin by Abbvie; it was first produced as an oral tablet composed of 500 mg of acetaminophen and 5 mg of hydrocodone bitartrate, but was on that date approved as a 750 mg acetaminophen and 7.5 mg hydrocodone bitartrate combined-formulation oral tablet. On September 23, 1996, the FDA approved the marketing of a more potent 660 mg acetaminophen and 10 mg hydrocodone bitartrate combination formulation oral tablet manufactured by Abbvie. This is the form of Vicodin that Trevor started using. In 2007, 99% of hydrocodone was consumed in the United States, and by 2012, it was the most commonly prescribed opioid in the United States. However, there were mounting concerns with Vicodin. On June 30, 2009, an FDA advisory panel voted to remove Vicodin from the market because of the high likelihood of overdose. On October 6, 2014, hydrocodone was moved from a Schedule III to a more controlled Schedule II drug.

Trevor was a very bright young man, and he well knew that he had reached the point of having a very serious drug problem. However, he was too proud to ask anyone for help. He had tried going cold turkey a few times, but as soon as the pain of the withdrawal symptoms from this painkiller arose, he picked up again, and again. He then tried to taper off his use by cutting down his daily dosage; he was able to make it for 2 days at half of his normal dose, then he went a day and a half of being clean. The second day of not using, his regular supplier showed up unannounced with a ready stash. Trevor purchased a bag of pills from his dealer, but after an hour and a half of relying on his willpower to not pick up, he gave in to the overwhelming temptation and was back to his habitual level of use. The next time that he tried to detox by tapering off his use, he made it longer because he had gotten some Xanax, which is a formulation of alprazolam, a benzodiazepine medication. Trevor found that taking 0.5 mg of alprazolam every 3 hours helped him amazingly to cope with the withdrawal symptoms. He made it a week clean from the Vicodin, but the Xanax was increasing his feelings of anxiety and also gave him some very troubling insomnia. So he stopped the Xanax and relapsed back to the Vicodin.

The next change in Trevor's drug use came when he found a bottle of OxyContin at his girlfriend's mother's house. The OxyContin pills contained the semisynthetic opioid oxycodone as their active ingredient, and Trevor discovered that these pills not only covered the pain of withdrawal, but made him feel really good. Oxycodone had thereby become his new drug of choice. As it was getting progressively more difficult for Trevor to obtain prescriptions to maintain his level of painkiller drug use, he moved into the world of illicit drug supplies. He easily found a drug dealer in his neighborhood who, for a price, would supply him with as many painkiller pills of whatever type as long as he could afford to pay for them.

While Trevor was taking the Vicodin, and when he switched over primarily to OxyContin, he was always drinking alcoholic beverages and dabbling with assorted other drugs as well. He was clearly an example of what is commonly referred to as a polydrug abuser. Since polydrug abuse is regarded as being symptomatic of various underlying social or personality disorders, its treatment can be rather complex. It is generally felt that outpatient detoxification is rarely successful for this type of drug abuser. Withdrawal from this dependence on an inpatient basis in a drug-free environment used to be the gold standard of care, but we have since come to appreciate the value of medication-assisted treatment, particularly for the phase of detoxification. The use of clonidine, for instance, is preferred by many clinicians. Methadone can be used as a substitution drug, and considerable success has also been achieved with treatment programs that use a combination formulation of buprenorphine and naloxone with these types of cases. Naloxone is often now combined with buprenorphine to help reduce the risk of the medication being misused or of being injected for the purpose of experiencing a euphoric high, since when naloxone is injected, it can cause a withdrawal syndrome in those individuals who are opiate or opioid dependent. Trevor was fortunate enough to be admitted to a residential treatment program that employed the buprenorphine and naloxone treatment strategy. However, he had signed himself in to the treatment center, and after only 3 days at the drug treatment center, he was able to sign himself out against medical advice.

It has typically been found that polydrug abuse can rarely be treated effectively with only a single treatment modality, and that effective alternatives to the drug use must be made available and reinforced. If the support system to maintain these effective alternatives is not in place, then these alternatives are unlikely to succeed in replacing the polydrug use in the abuser's life. Polydrug abuse, particularly that involving painkiller drugs, dominates and provides a coherent, even if somewhat dysfunctional, structure for the abuser's daily existence. In an ideal situation, a comprehensive polydrug abuse treatment program would include myriad components including individual and group psychotherapy, vocational rehabilitation, family system evaluation and involvement, educational enhancement, and medical care. For drug treatment programs to be successful, they must usually provide an alternative structure to the individual for living. Few treatment programs, in fact, actually provide such comprehensive services. At any rate, Trevor's limited ventures into the treatment arena certainly did not afford him these opportunities.

Trevor was clearly heavily dependent upon painkiller drugs, and his tolerance level gradually continued to rise. This created the necessity of gradually increasing his dosages, which, in turn, meant that he had to pay more and more as time went along to support his drug habit. The next major change came when, at the suggestion of his dealer, he started to use heroin. Trevor briefly tried smoking the heroin, but soon graduated to injection drug use. His dealer, again, was very willing to explain and demonstrate how to inject heroin. Neither behavior should be very surprising, as it is known that nonmedical users of prescription opioids have been shown to be nearly 8 times more likely to use heroin and also to be more than 4 times more likely to use it intravenously.

The injection transition brought Trevor into contact with an array of other heroin users. He discovered some of the local shooting galleries, usually located in one of the many abandoned houses in his urban environment. Although he had heard about the dangers of injecting drugs, the intense pleasurable feelings he experienced from shooting up with heroin easily overrode any other concerns. The Centers for Disease Control and Prevention (CDC) issued a warning alert in April 2015 that the rise in injection drug use seen across the country could result in dramatic increases in both human immunodeficiency virus (HIV) and in hepatitis C (HCV) infections. More than 1.2 million people in the United States are living with HIV; injection drug users represent about 15% of those living with HIV. It is estimated that more than 5 million people in the United States are infected with hepatitis C; among those who currently use or those who have used injection drugs, 1 in 3 young adults and 3 in 4 older adults are infected with hepatitis C. Unfortunately, there were no needle exchange programs in his city, and so obtaining clean syringes was extremely difficult for Trevor as well as rather costly. This minor barrier, of course, did little to dissuade Trevor from the path of painkiller abuse on which he was already well along. The sharing of dirty needles, of course, put Trevor at risk for a considerable assortment of health problems. Fortunately, however, he somehow, at least for now, has avoided infection with HIV or with hepatitis C.

Trevor was soon displaying recognized signs of heroin abuse. The pupils in his eyes were routinely constricted. His nose was runny most of the time, and his skin was typically flushed. He was constantly sweating, even in the winter. He exhibited dramatic changes in behavior and soon lost his job. He was staying up at night and sleeping during the day.

Trevor was able to find jobs, for a while at least, but his excessive number of unexcused absences resulted in his losing one job after another. In fact, he had 17 different jobs in 2 years; but after that, he had no luck in finding gainful employment. He could no longer provide any good work references, and the string of jobs he had raised even more perplexing questions.

Trevor then had his first major encounter with the criminal justice system. After he had lost his last job, he had started smashing windows in parked cars and grabbing anything that he might be able to sell to help support his habit, such as cell phones and GPS devices. He was soon arrested while engaging in this illicit activity and was sent to the county jail. He spent 3 months there the first time he was incarcerated, but he received no drug abuse treatment services while incarcerated and had to go through a very painful withdrawal period. It is thought that about one-third of heroin users pass through correctional facilities each year; of these, nearly three-quarters relapse to heroin use within 3 months of their release date. Trevor did not make it 3 days after his release before he was back shooting heroin in his old neighborhood.

The adverse effects of long-term heroin use eventually caught up to Trevor after a couple of years. These were bothersome, varied, and numerous. Many of his veins had collapsed from repeated administrations of heroin, and his circulatory system was far less efficient overall. He no longer had the endurance to play a game of basketball. Trevor had went through several bouts with pneumonia as his respiratory system was seriously assaulted; he was out of breath easily and often. He once experienced a bacterial infection of his heart valves, which took a couple of courses of antibiotics to get under control. From his earlier days of Vicodin and OxyContin abuse, his liver was already impaired, and the subsequent heroin use only exacerbated the extent of decreased liver functioning. Trevor experienced various systemic problems as well; particularly worrisome were the many abscesses from the repeated injections.

The next step down the slippery slope of his painkiller addiction was his first, but not his last, overdose. Trevor had scored several bags of a particularly pure heroin; he could purchase each small bag of heroin for $10, much less than he would have had to pay for the painkiller pills. The relatively high potency of this batch of heroin made it all the more dangerous. This particularly potent strain of heroin hit the drug user community hard. A series of drug overdoses resulted from the availability of this very strong and very deadly supply in his community. Trevor overdosed while using this powerful heroin, but fortunately, the first responder to the emergency call made on his behalf was a police officer who had been trained in and was equipped with Narcan, an injectable form of naloxone. Nasal administration of naloxone necessitates a 2 mg dose. Trevor had passed out in a local park after shooting up with this highly potent variant of heroin. Fortunately, another drug user observed this and called 911. The police officer injected the Narcan into Trevor and he revived. However, a friend of Trevor's had shot up next to him with some of the same batch of potent heroin, but she went into cardiac arrest. She was taken to the local hospital and put on life-support machines. The doctors continued working on her for a long time, but she never came back. It is important to recognize that for every 1 death due to opiate or opioid painkiller drugs, there are 10 admissions to treatment for drug abuse, 32 emergency room visits for misuse or abuse, 130 individuals who abuse or who are dependent upon these painkiller drugs, and 825 individuals who take prescription painkillers for nonmedical use; this totals to about 1,000 nonfatal, yet medically serious consequences for every opiate or opioid death.

Trevor survived this and many other close calls, but he continues today to fight his battle with addiction and the litany of negative consequences that has been associated with this powerful condition. For Trevor, at least, his experiences with the use and abuse of painkiller drugs has essentially been one of misery.

CASE 2: RELIEF

Mary is a red-haired, Caucasian female, age 34; she is 5 feet 6 inches tall and weighs 127 pounds. The fact that she is a natural redhead is not unimportant to this discussion. In fact, red hair color appears to reflect a genetic link to having lower pain tolerance and thus the need for higher doses of anesthesia and painkiller medications. This difference is due to the fact that redheads generally tend to have a mutation in the melanocortin-1 receptor (MC1R) gene, which not only helps make their hair red, but also makes them more sensitive to painful stimuli. The melanocortin-1 receptor is closely related to the pain receptors in the human brain.

Since she was a late adolescent, around 17 years of age, Mary has been plagued with chronic vulvar discomfort, which she described as a burning, stabbing, or stinging pain. Her first attempt to obtain medical treatment for this condition was in her mid-20s, when she went to the emergency department of her local hospital. The fact that she went to the emergency department is not too surprising, either. In fact, pain is actually the most common reason why individuals seek care in an emergency room setting. Further, most of this pain is non-trauma-related, as was the case with Mary. Unfortunately, the emergency department was unable to make a diagnosis as to what specifically was the problem, but simply referred Mary to see her gynecologist for a follow-up appointment. Whatever this condition was, it was clearly having deleterious consequences on Mary's physical, emotional, and sexual health as well as on her ability to maintain significant relationships.

Mary's gynecologist performed a routine physical examination and noted no visible findings except for some possible erythema. Mary consistently reported that her pain sensations were generalized in her genital area and that they were unprovoked from physical stimulation. If she did rub the area, such provocation usually only exacerbated her pain symptoms. Mary's gynecologist was unable to make a diagnosis, but ordered some blood work and referred Mary to another more experienced gynecologist affiliated with the teaching hospital in the nearby city. The fact that Mary had to see a couple of doctors in seeking a diagnosis is not so unusual in this kind of case. In fact, in a population-based study funded by the National Institutes of Health (NIH), 60% of the women consulted at least three doctors in seeking a diagnosis and, of this number, 40% remained undiagnosed even after three medical consultations. Since Mary was reporting such intense pain, her primary gynecologist prescribed OxyContin, which is the trade name for an oxycodone hydrochloride formulation, a short-term opioid medication. Oxycodone is considered to be a powerful and very effective painkiller drug, but one that should generally be used only for short-term treatment. On April 5, 2010, the FDA granted approval to Purdue Pharma LP to manufacture an extended-release oral formulation, available by prescription only, of oxycodone hydrochloride in 10 mg, 15 mg, 20 mg, 40 mg, 60 mg, and 80 mg tablets that were to be marketed as Oxy-Contin. Mary was prescribed the painkiller pills with the 10 mg active ingredient formulation of the drug oxycodone.

The second gynecologist had to rule out various diagnoses known to cause vulvar pain. These diagnostic exclusions included an array of potential disorders, including infectious conditions such as bacterial vaginosis, candidiasis, genital herpes, human Papillomavirus (HPV), or trichomoniasis; inflammatory conditions such as atrophic vaginitis, contact dermatitis, lichen simplex chronicus, lichen planus, or lichen sclerosus; neoplastic conditions such as Paget's disease, vulvar intraepithelial neoplasia, or squamous cell carcinoma;

and neurologic conditions such as pudendal nerve entrapment, peripheral neuropathy, sacral meningeal (Tarlov's) cysts, or spinal nerve compression. They also had to rule out other disorders including referred pain, such as that from a ruptured intervertebral disc, or scarring around the sacral nerve roots after intervertebral disc surgery, pelvic floor muscle dysfunction, or orthopedic conditions, like a labral hip tear. Vulvodynia is essentially a differential diagnosis of exclusion in which alternative diagnoses must be ruled out. This can be a long and drawn-out process with little to no relief for the pain the patient is experiencing, compounded by a diminishing sense of hope as the process drags on.

The second gynecologist conducted a thorough examination, beginning with a visual examination, and then performed a cotton-swab exam of the vulva and vaginal vestibule; this was followed by conducting a neurosensory examination, noting sensations reported, and then conducting a pelvic floor muscle exam. The next step was evaluation of Mary's pain comorbidity, considering conditions like chronic pain syndrome, chronic headaches, endometriosis, fibromyalgia, interstitial cystitis, irritable bowel syndrome, orofacial pain (e.g., TMJ), and other contributing factors, such as emotional and sexual impairment. However, after all of this, Mary was lucky because her doctor was then able to make a diagnosis. It should be noted that a recent population-based study also funded by the NIH found that only 1.4% of women seeking medical care were accurately diagnosed for this disease, generalized vulvodynia, which is also known as hyperaesthesia of the vulva, dysesthetic vulvodynia, and vulvar dysesthesia.

Generalized vulvodynia is considered to be a neuropathic pain syndrome. Neuro-selective sensory dysfunction of the pudendal nerve and autonomic small fiber neuropathy have been demonstrated, as has increased sensitivity in peripheral body regions, as well as altered neuro-adaptation in individuals with longer durations of pain. It appears that increased sensitivity in vulvar skin in those individuals with this disease leads to increased stimulation of nerve fibers and of increased release of neurotransmitters, which results in increased pain sensation signals being transmitted along the nerve fiber path to the spinal cord; this, in turn, leads to increased pain amplification stimulus being transmitted to the brain.

Vulvodynia is actually a highly under-recognized pain disorder that is now recognized to affect 1 in 4 women and adolescent girls; it has a reported 3.1% annual incidence. All ethnicities appear to be equally affected, and although all ages are affected, the incidence of the onset of symptoms appears to be between 18 and 25 years of age. In the United States alone, it is estimated that the direct economic costs of this disease are about $31 billion annually and that the indirect costs are approximately $72 billion per year.

Mary did get some relief from the intense burning sensation that she typically experienced while she was taking the oxycodone pills. However, she did not like the way the medication made her feel; the oxycodone made her extremely groggy such that she became somewhat weak and dazed and she was unsteady on her feet. Individuals have different experiences with and reactions to opioid medications; remember that Trevor liked the way the medication made him feel, but Mary certainly did not. Due to her lack of satisfaction with the oxycodone, Mary was switched to the painkiller medication Tramadol. In June 2002, the FDA granted approval to several pharmaceutical companies to manufacture 50 mg tramadol hydrochloride oral tablets, which is what Mary had started to take; these included companies such as Actavis Elizabeth, Apotex, Asta, Mallinckrodt, Mylan, Pliva, Sun Pharm Industries Inc., and Teva. However, Mary had previously seen a psychiatrist who had put her on an antidepressant medication. Unfortunately, it is known that use of even low doses of an antidepressant along with use of Tramadol can cause what is commonly referred to as the serotonin syndrome. Tramadol partially works by inhibiting the uptake at the neuronal level of serotonin and epinephrine. The increased concentrations of serotonin associated with this condition has been found to promote hypoglycemia in some individuals. In fact, such is what happened to Mary, and she had to be briefly hospitalized for hypoglycemia. At any rate, once the Tramadol was discontinued, she ceased to have any issues with hypoglycemia or the serotonin syndrome.

After the diagnosis of generalized vulvodynia was finally made, Mary's doctors began a course of individualized multi-therapy treatments. A common first-line treatment for individuals with generalized vulvodynia is the prescribing of oral pain-blocking medications. There are three major classes of pain-blocking medications used in this treatment approach. These include anticonvulsant drugs, like gabapentin, lamotrigine, or pregabalin; serotonin-norepinephrine reuptake inhibitors (SSNRIs), like duloxetine or venlafaxine; and tricyclic antidepressant drugs, like amitriptyline, desipramine, or nortriptyline. However, to help manage the burning pain symptoms while the dose of one of these long-term medications is being titrated upward, short-term opioids, like oxycodone, are typically used. Since Mary did not like the effects of the oxycodone, nor was able to take the Tramadol, consequently she was given a short-term prescription for Palladone, the trade name for a hydromorphone hydrochloride formulation. On September 24, 2004, the FDA granted approval to Purdue Pharma LP to manufacture extended release oral formulations of hydromorphone hydrochloride to be made in 12 mg, 16 mg, 24 mg, and 32 mg capsules to be marketed as Palladone. She was initially prescribed caplets with a 12 mg active ingredient dose of hydromorphone hydrochloride; but she did not experience full pain relief, and so she was switched to the 16-mg dose, which proved to be more effective for her, but she still did not like the side effects associated with opioid medication use. The first pain-blocking medication tried with Mary was the anticonvulsant gabapentin, but after a brief period of use of this medication with little relief of symptoms, she was switched to a prescription for amitriptyline, a tricyclic antidepressant medication that worked well for Mary. On September 11, 1997, the FDA granted approval to Vintage Pharms to manufacture oral formulations of amitriptyline hydrochloride to be made in 10 mg, 25 mg, 50 mg, 75 mg, 100 mg, and 150 mg tablets. Mary eventually found that the 50 mg formulation worked best for her with the fewest side effects.

Oral pain-blocking medications, like Mary's Palladone, can be used in conjunction with compounded topical painkiller formulations. These topical formulations can include anesthetic, anticonvulsant, or antidepressant ingredients. Mary eventually found that Aspercreme with Lidocaine, which is a topical pain-relieving lotion available for purchase over the counter that contains a 4% solution of lidocaine hydrochloride as its active ingredient, provided the most effective relief. The lidocaine penetrates to desensitize aggravated nerves and the Aspercreme with Lidocaine cream is marketed as an odor-free, fast-acting topical pain reliever. She had found that regular Aspercreme, which contains trolamine salicylate, an NSAID, as its active ingredient, did not provide her with adequate pain relief; nor did several other topical pain-relief formulations that she had tried.

Adjunctive individual and couples psychotherapy, particularly those based on cognitive behavioral therapy, appears to be helpful as well. Effective stress reduction and management techniques can also contribute to symptom improvement. Some women have also reported that eliminating acidic and/or high-sugar foods helped provide some pain symptom relief. Several experimental treatments are under review by researchers in this area, such as use of leukotriene receptor antagonist medication, interferon injections, enoxaparin injections, laser therapy, motor cortex stimulation, photodynamic therapy, transcutaneous electrical nerve stimulation, transcranial direct current stimulation, and sacral neuro-modulation; however, there is no generally agreed-upon consensus yet on the efficacy of any of these approaches upon generalized vulvodynia. Nevertheless, after years of painful suffering and numerous trial-and-error treatment attempts, Mary finally found that regular consumption of amitriptyline hydrochloride, along with use as needed of Aspercreme with Lidocaine, provided effective resolution of this painful condition. In a word, she found "relief."

REVIEW

The hypothetical case studies in this opening chapter illustrate just two of the possible wide range of outcomes that can be associated with the use and/ or abuse of painkiller drugs. Painkiller drugs have become a major public health concern around the world. Painkillers, particularly opiates and opioids, top the list globally of illicit drugs that cause substantial morbidity and mortality. Throughout the rest of this book, we will examine more of the history, science, and myriad issues associated with the use, misuse, and abuse of the vast array of respective drugs that fall under the category of painkillers. Next, we will explore just what are painkillers, including the different classes of drugs included under this broad heading, as well as considering some of the other approaches used to manage pain.

Chapter 2

What Are Painkillers?

Painkillers is a very broad and rather nontechnical term that covers a rather wide array of many different types of drugs, all of which have some ability to help us manage and control pain. Opiates, for better and for worse, are certainly the type of painkiller drugs with which we have, by far, had the longest historical and cultural associations. They are also one group of painkillers that we arguably have the clearest understanding of the scientific basis of their mechanism of action. Other drug classes covered under the rubric of painkillers includes opioids, non-steroidal anti-inflammatory drugs, and COX-2 inhibitors, as well as a rather broad assortment of miscellaneous other drugs that, respectively, also have painkiller properties as well as, in many cases, other therapeutically useful properties.

DIFFERENT CLASSES OF PAINKILLERS

There are many different types of drugs that are routinely used as painkillers and each has its own somewhat unique story to tell. The major classes of painkiller medications are the opiates; the opioids, both semisynthetic and synthetic variants; the non-steroidal anti-inflammatory drugs; and the COX-2 inhibitors; as well as a relatively wide array of miscellaneous other substances that are used as well due to their ability to treat pain.

Opiates

Opium and the other opiate drugs, including particularly morphine and codeine, have taken very prominent places historically and socially in forging the relationships that people have had with drugs. Opium, in particular, was perhaps the first truly effective painkiller discovered deep in the realms of pre-history. Attempting to gain an adequate understanding of painkiller drugs, without sufficient attention directed upon opium and its descendants and the complex interactions that these substances have had with humans across the broad historical expanse to today and into the future, is unlikely to be successful.

The term "opium" itself comes from the ancient Greek word for poppy juice, *opion*. Opium is basically the coagulated juice of the poppy plant, *Papaver somniferum*. *Papaver somniferum* has been widely cultivated in many different places around the world, including Afghanistan, India, Iran, Pakistan, and Turkey as well as across much of Southeast Asia and, more recently, in Latin and South America. Opium juice contains many separate alkaloid substances, including morphine, codeine, and papaverine, for example, each of which can be used medically for painkilling and other purposes. It has been suggested by some authorities in the field that the alkaloid of morphine at least is actually merely a waste product of the metabolic activity of the opium poppy that is, in fact, useless to the plant itself, and that is therefore excreted through the lactiferous system to the capsule. Strictly speaking, opiates are the alkaloid drugs that are derived from opium. These respective alkaloidal opiate drugs have been for a long time, and will no doubt continue to be well into the future, amongst our most powerful painkiller substances. The pharmacological potency and effectiveness of these opiate drugs has been both a blessing and a curse at different times and for different individuals.

Opioids

Opioids are the biochemical synthetic substances that produce effects in the body similar to those of the natural opiate drugs; they are thus, for the most part at least, highly effective painkiller drugs. The two major categories of opioid drugs are the semisynthetic opioids and the synthetic opioids. Heroin is perhaps the best known of the semisynthetic opioid drugs; other, more recently well-known examples of semisynthetic opioid drugs include oxycodone and hydrocodone. Methadone, fentanyl, and meperidine are some of the better known of the synthetic opioid drugs. The varying chemical structures of the respective semisynthetic and synthetic opioid drugs help to determine how effective they will be for particular uses, including for addressing different types of pain, as well as for other uses. Narcotic is a far broader and more general term that is derived from the Greek word for "stupor" and that is used, strictly speaking, for substances that induce sleep and include both the opiates and the opioids. However, many policy makers and criminal justice authorities have used the term "narcotic" to refer to a much broader range of drugs, including marijuana and cocaine.

Serious adverse negative consequences have been associated with the use and abuse of these opioid drugs, including phenomena such as dependence and overdose. Overdoses from methadone, for instance, kill around 5,000 people each year in the United States. It is thus 4 times more likely to result in a fatal overdose from methadone than it is from oxycodone and more than twice as likely when compared to morphine. There has also been a dramatic resurgence in the use and abuse of heroin in the last few years. In fact, fatal heroin overdoses nearly tripled from 2012 to 2015, with over 8,250 people dying from a heroin overdose each year. Victims' profiles now tend to include more white, affluent and young individuals. The price of heroin plummeted as more Mexican so-called "black tar" heroin, which is less expensive to produce and easier to transport and which can be either smoked or injected, became available. The ready availability and ease of access of heroin, and its use to suburban white young people who tend to have cellphones, cars, and private bedrooms, all helpful attributes to those wishing to procure and use the drugs, has resulted in a significant comeback with respect to the rates of heroin use and addiction.

Non-Steroidal Anti-Inflammatory Drugs (NSAIDs)

Non-steroidal anti-inflammatory drugs, or NSAIDs, and related drugs are the major category of painkiller medications that are available for purchase over the counter, although there are various prescription formulations for many of them that are available as well. At any rate, they are among the most commonly used medications. In fact, it is thought that about 30 million people use NSAIDs each day. Aspirin, also known as acetylsalicylic acid, is the first and best-known NSAID medication; it is widely used to relieve minor pains, to reduce swelling, to bring down fevers, and to prevent the occurrence of heart attacks and strokes. Most NSAIDs inhibit the cyclooxygenase, or COX, enzymes, which block the production of prostaglandins in the body; this makes them not only effective painkiller medications, but also useful due to their action of reducing inflammation in respective body tissues. Ibuprofen, or (RS)-2-(4-(2-methylproypyl)phenyl) propanoic acid, is an NSAID medication that is rather widely used for pain relief, as well as being used for helping deal with fevers and for reducing inflammations such as those caused by headache, toothache, back pain, menstrual cramps, and minor injuries. In this regard, ibuprofen is the painkiller medication most often recommended by physicians for treating joint pain.

Acetaminophen, or N-acetyl-p-aminophenol, is a synthetic non-opioid painkiller medication used to treat minor aches and pains, like those associated with the common cold, headaches, toothaches, and so forth, but is also a highly effective antipyretic, or fever reducer, that is widely used in treating infants, children, and adults. Acetaminophen is not generally considered to be an NSAID medication as it has only limited anti-inflammatory activity. Naproxen, or (+)-(S)-2-(6-methoxynaphthalen-2-yl) propanoic acid, is an anti-inflammatory drug that has both painkiller and antipyretic properties, but that is highly protein bound, which limits its widespread applicability. Several other kinds of NSAIDs are available, including drugs such as diclofenac, ketoprofen, and ketorolac.

The NSAIDs can, in fact, be separated into several different families, each of which consists of several different respective painkiller drugs. The various families of the NSAIDs include the salicylates, propionic acids, arylalkonic acids, fenamic acids, oxicams, and pyrazolidine derivatives. The salicylates family of NSAIDs includes painkiller drugs such as aspirin, amoxiprin, benorylate, choline magnesium salicylate, diflunisal, ethenzamide, faislamine, magnesium salicylate, methyl salicylate, salicyl salicylade, salicylamide, and salsalate. The propionic acids, also known as the profens, include painkiller drugs such as alminophen, benoxaprofen, carprofen, dexibuprofen, dexketoprofen, fenbufen, fenoprofen, flunoxaprofen, flurbiprofen, ibuprofen, ibuproxam, indoprofen, ketoprofen, ketorolac, loxoprofen, naproxen, oxaprozin, pirprofen, suprofen, and tiaprofenic acid. The arylalkonic acids include drugs like diclofenac, acelofenac, acemethacin, alclofenac, bromfenac, etodolac, indomethacin, nabumetone, oxametacin, proglumetacin, sulindac, and tolmetin. The fenamic acids include drugs like flufenamic acid, meclofenamic acid, mefanamic acid, and tolfenamic acid. The oxicams include painkiller drugs such as droxicam, lornoxicam, meloxicam, piroxicam, and tenoxicam. The pyrazolidine derivatives family of NSAIDs includes painkiller drugs such as ampyrone, azapropazone, clofezone, kebuzone, metamizole, mofebutazone, oxyphenbutazone, phenazone, phenylbutazone, and sulfinpyrazone. The varying chemical structures of each respective NSAID help to determine not only its specific set of therapeutic uses but also its particular set of side effects, both positive and negative.

COX-2 Inhibitors

In 1998, celecoxib, which was marketed under the trade name of Celebrex, became the first drug approved by the FDA, or the U.S. Food and Drug Administration, under the new category of COX-2 selective inhibitors. Valdecoxib was another COX-2 selective inhibitor drug that was initially granted approval for sale in the United States by the FDA on November 20,

2001. Many of the COX-2 selective inhibitors are available for sale as over-the-counter painkiller drugs, like some of the non-steroidal anti-inflammatory drugs, but they have a more specific course of action. The COX-2 selective inhibitors do not inhibit COX-1, which is regarded as a constitutive enzyme, but mainly act selectively against COX-2, which is the second type of cyclooxygenase that is considered to be an inducible enzyme. Some of the prostaglandins produced by COX-1 help to protect the inner lining of the stomach, and they are therefore necessary for maintaining a healthy constitution. Thus, if a COX-1 enzyme is blocked, although inflammation of body tissues will be reduced, some of the protective stomach lining is lost as well, which is a common and serious complication of most traditional NSAID use. However, the COX-2 selective inhibitors, like celecoxib, essentially eliminates these problems as the COX-1 enzyme is not substantially blocked. The inhibiting of inflammation and its accompanying symptoms of additional pain, swelling, tenderness, and fever, as well as the fact that they do not appear to affect blood clotting ability, make them ideal agents for treating menstrual cramps and some arthritic conditions. Unfortunately, soon after the widespread use of COX-2 selective inhibitors occurred, it was discovered that many of these particular painkiller drugs significantly increased the risk of cardiovascular events. Accordingly, some COX-2 selective inhibitors, like rofecoxib, marketed under trade names such as Vioxx or Ceoxx, and valdecoxib, marketed as Bextra, were removed from the market by the FDA, respectively, in September 2004 and April 2005. Lumiracoxib is not currently available in the United States and has been nearly withdrawn globally due to its demonstrated liver toxicity. Parecoxib is an injectable prodrug formulation, similar to valdecoxib, that is not available in the United States as the FDA failed to grant it approval, but that is marketed in the European Union under the trade name of Dynastat, which has no effect on platelet formation and thus does not promote excessive bleeding as most of the alternative NSAIDs do. Etoricoxib, which is marketed under the trade name Aroxia, is another COX-2 selective inhibitor that is sometimes used to treat osteoarthritis and rheumatoid arthritis; it is now available in about 80 countries globally, but not currently in the United States. Hopefully, novel and safer COX-2 selective inhibitors will be developed and subsequently become available in the near future.

Other Painkillers

There are many other types of drugs in addition to those discussed above that are sometimes also used as painkiller medications. Many of these drugs are used for treating pain that is typically associated with particular types of medical problems. For example, fibromyalgia is thought by many experts to be caused by excessive nerve firing. The activity of these overactive neurons can result in a condition characterized by feelings of deep, radiating chronic pain. Some drugs, such as pregabalin, like that marketed under the trade name of Lyrica, can help calm the chronic pain of fibromyalgia and thus can be considered as a painkiller medication. It can also be prescribed for the treatment of neuropathic pain like that associated with diabetic peripheral neuropathy; for post-therapeutic neuralgias; and for neuropathic pain associated with spinal cord injury. Similarly, in the United Kingdom, nabiximols, which is manufactured under the trade name of Sativex, is marketed and prescribed for the treatment of muscle spasms and for the feelings of pain associated with multiple sclerosis (MS).

There are also many other drugs that are widely used around the world as general painkiller medications. Marijuana, or cannabis, is perhaps among the best known of these, particularly marijuana that is low in delta-nine tetrahydrocannabinol (THC) but high in cannibidiol (CBD), which is thought to be effective for managing chronic pain. Although it is also possible that CBD, THC, and the hundreds of other cannabinoids in marijuana have a synergistic effect on pain relief. In a similar vein, nabilone, which is marketed in the United States, the United Kingdom, and Mexico as Cesamet and in Austria as Canemes, is a synthetic cannabinoid that is widely used as an adjunctive painkiller medication for the management of chronic neuropathic pain. Research on medical marijuana, particularly on different strains of the plant, may yield yet more treatment options for the management and control of feelings of pain and its associated conditions. For example, a recent small, short-duration, randomized crossover trial indicated that inhaled marijuana had a dose-dependent reduction in painful diabetic neuropathy for treatment refractory subjects. Medical marijuana appears to be similarly effective for treating neuropathic pain and cancer pain; it also has been reported to improve sleep problems among individuals with conditions like fibromyalgia and multiple sclerosis.

Other plants, or parts of plants at least, are regularly used ethnobotanically as painkillers elsewhere in the world by members of respective cultures, particularly by practitioners of traditional healing. In Ghana, West Africa, for example, seed preparations of *Picralima nitida*, which the Fanti call *owemba* and the Twi call *akuama* or *nwema*, are commonly used as an all-purpose painkiller medication. An extract of the stem bark of the African locust bean tree (*Parkia biglobosa*) is used in some traditional medicine preparations in the Central African Republic as it is said to have painkiller properties. Stem bark and leaf decoctions of *Trema orientalis* are used in Madagascar to manage pain in aching bones and tired muscles, as well as in venereal diseases. In Burundi, the leaves of *Mikania cordata*, which are called *nkuyumwonga* in Rundi, are sometimes used to treat chest pain, and the leafy twigs of the same plant are also used for treating fever. In Cameroon, *Ceiba pentandra*, which in Bakweri is called *wuma*, is widely used to treat chest pain and rheumatism. In Chad, the Bidejat use a root infusion of *Boscia senegalensis*, which they call *madera*, for soothing the pain of a toothache. Similarly, in Cote d'Ivoire, the rhizomes of *Aframomum danielli*, which the Beti call *esson* and the Bangwa call *besak*, are regularly chewed by individuals wishing to soothe a toothache. Leaf juice of *Drymaria cordata*, which in Comoros is called *chirovolovou* or *namara*, is applied externally as a painkiller treatment for burns, skin diseases, and snakebites. In Ethiopia, the Tigray use the plant *Solanum marginatum* to treat abdominal pain. In Kenya, the roots of *Zehneria scabra* are considered by the Maasi to be helpful for the relief of abdominal pain. In Lesotho, a root infusion of *Cleome gynandra*, which the Zulu refer to as *amazombe*, is traditionally taken for treating chest pain. The Haya of Tanzania make a decoction for treating backache by boiling the leaves of *Pappea capensis*, which they call *omulema mpango*, with those of *Vernonia brachycalyx*, which they call *mkuraijura* or *omuw*. The Hausa of Nigeria combine the seed oil of *Jatropha curcas* with that of *Ricinus communis* and the fruit of *Balaniles aegyptiaca* to apply to painful rheumatic sites. Many new painkiller drugs and other useful medications may yet be discovered if these and other types of traditional medicinal painkillers from diverse parts of the world are further studied and developed.

There are also assorted topical agents that are applied to various parts of the body, such as joints, back, shins, and so forth, for local pain relief. These include an array of creams, lotions, sprays, patches, and so forth that are typically applied to the skin; some of the brand names for these topical painkillers include Aspercreme, Arthricare, and Icy Hot; many of these products are available for sale over the counter. The simplest topical applications consist of heat or cold; ice, cold packs, and related approaches can help numb affected areas and also reduce inflammation, while heat can help relieve muscle soreness and promote healing by increasing blood flow. When medications are delivered through the skin, such as by means of salicylate skin creams, smaller doses can often be effective as they do not have to pass through the liver first. This happens to drugs, such as those administered in pill or other similar forms, that are swallowed, pass through the stomach, then enter the bloodstream and are processed in the liver, which substantially reduces the concentration of most active ingredients. Lidocaine is a local anesthetic available in several creams and patches that can be effective for the relief of minor pain. Some throat lozenges contain local anesthetics that can be effective local painkillers, providing relief from sore throats; unfortunately, these throat lozenges tend to be rather short acting, which is also exacerbated by the natural washing actions of fluids in the throat.

There are myriad counterirritants that can also be applied topically as painkillers; these include those sorts of products that contain substances such as menthol alcohol or isopropyl alcohol, like Ben Gay and assorted liniments and ointments, which essentially work by helping to distract one from the feeling of pain by creating a slight burning or cooling feeling on the surface of the skin. There are, on the other hand, also some products that consist mainly of irritants that are occasionally used as topical agents that can sometimes also work as painkillers; for example, those varied products containing capsaicin, like an over-the-counter product marketed as Zostrix, which are presently available in several ointment, gel, and transdermal patch formulations, sold in most pharmaceutical stores, and even routinely available in supermarkets and other similar business establishments. Capsaicin, also known as 8-methyl-N-vanillyl-6-nonenamide, is a phenylpropanoid compound that is a substance P deletor, and that is the main active ingredient in chili peppers; it and related substances referred to as capsaicinoids, such as dihydrocapsaicin, are produced as secondary metabolites of many varieties of hot peppers. Other natural capsaicinods include homodihydrocapsaicin, homocapsaicin, nordhydrocapsaicin, and nonivamide; they can be synthesized as well. Capsaicin products, in addition to topical ointments, include transdermal patches and nasal sprays, such as that marketed as Sinol-M. Capsaicin binds to an ion channel type vanilloid receptor that is located on pain- and heat-sensing neurons and these receptors play a critical role in transducing thermal and inflammatory pain. Capsaicin also causes membrane depolarization and activates poorly myelinated primary afferent neurons. Capsaicin products are often effective for relief of minor pains, such as those associated with arthritis or sprains and strains, as well as for reducing the symptoms of peripheral neuropathy, like that commonly associated with shingles, and other types of pain, including, perhaps, that associated with cluster headaches.

OTHER APPROACHES TO PAIN MANAGEMENT

Traditional management of pain within allopathic Western medicine typically relies upon the prescribing and taking of assorted painkiller drugs. However, use of these types of drugs may not always be the best choice for all individuals. In fact, use of some of these medications has its own respective set of risks, which can create additional health problems; very often, such an approach usually does not actually resolve the fundamental underlying condition that is, in fact, causing the pain, but merely helps to temporarily mask the symptoms. For example, lower back pain is one of the most frequent complaints among adults in this country, and the overwhelming majority of these cases is actually caused by an imbalance of the opposing muscle groups, specifically, weakened, elongated abdominal muscles and shortened lower back muscles, that produces an accentuated curvature of the lumbar portion of the spinal column and, thereby, results in the concomitant sensation of pain. Corrective exercises directed at strengthening the abdominal muscles and stretching the lower back muscles to help restore proper muscle balance are usually the best way to resolve this complaint. Unfortunately, the more typical approach employed, namely of masking the symptoms by using a painkiller product but not, in fact, resolving the underlying issue, can actually make the problem worse by delaying proper treatments.

Various other approaches have also long been used to manage pain. Applications of heat and cold have since time immemorial proven to be effective in managing and controlling pain. Heat helps to decrease muscle spasms as well as to increase blood flow and thereby promote more rapid healing throughout the body and it can be applied by various techniques including infrared and ultrasound; while applications of cold can effectively reduce swelling and can also be useful to temporarily numb affected areas of the body. Music, prayer, and laughter are but a few of the other techniques that have also been suggested and long practiced in respective cultures around the world as potentially useful approaches to deal with sensations of pain. For example, various faith-healing practices are believed by many to be efficacious for addressing feelings of pain; these include not only Christian-based systems, but also assorted metaphysical, Eastern, psychic, and occult systems of belief. There are also a myriad array of assorted injections and selected surgical procedures that are sometimes employed in painkilling efforts. At any rate, there are even many more non-pharmacological pain management approaches that can potentially be used for a more integrative care of pain. The use of most of these other approaches to pain management can substantially help lower, if not even entirely eliminate, the amount of painkiller drugs that actually need to be taken. In fact, more people these days are successfully turning to alternative and complementary forms of medicine for these and numerous other non-pharmacological approaches to pain management and control. Furthermore, feelings of pain need not always be addressed; in this vein, Sigmund Freud, famously, refused painkillers during the last days of his life, despite suffering terribly with inoperable cancer of the jaw; then, on September 21 and 22, 1939, Max Schur, Freud's personal doctor, administered sufficient doses of morphine that resulted in Freud's overdose death on September 23, 1939.

Acupuncture

Acupuncture is an ancient Chinese medical technique that involves the insertion of thin needles at specific anatomical sites on the body along what is referred to as the meridian system of 12 energy channels or pathways. Acupuncture is known to have been practiced in ancient China at least as far back as 4,500 years ago. There are more than 367 of these acupuncture points along these meridians at which needles can be inserted and then manipulated in specific ways and for specific durations of time to produce the desired therapeutic results, including painkilling. This revered practice of Chinese medicinal specialists is supposed to balance the life force, known as the complementary life forces of yin and yang, which are said to flow through the human body. Another camp of speculation that more modern medical practitioners tend to endorse suggests that the minor stimulation provided from the inserting and manipulation of these acupuncture needles might just selectively block the impulse transmission of more intense pain signals. These small acupuncture needles can readily produce a slight tingling feeling or can even make a selected part of the body feel numb, apparently, it is suggested, by changing the pain signals sent to and from the brain. This technique has long been used in the East not only as a painkiller, but also as an adjunct to surgery. It has further been speculated by some researchers that acupuncture may actually work by stimulating the release of endorphins and other neurotransmitters that, in turn, block pain messages from being delivered to the brain. Whatever the actual mechanism of action may be behind it, it is very clear from numerous clinical studies that acupuncture can be a safe and effective non-pharmacological approach for the management and control of pain.

Biofeedback

Biofeedback techniques are particular types of practices that use specialized equipment to train individuals how to consciously gain control over what are typically regarded as involuntary physiological functions, such as their blood pressure, skin temperature, sweating, heart rate, and muscle tension. The general concept behind biofeedback is based on the premise that by using the power of your mind to consciously control what is happening inside your body, you can thereby gain better control over your state of health. Electromyography (EMG), for example, uses monitors of muscular tension to teach people how to selectively and effectively relax areas of intense tension, which can clearly help to lessen or alleviate pain sensations like those associated with anxiety disorders, headaches, and back pain. Electroencephalography (EEG), also known as neurofeedback, uses instruments to measure brain wave activity and can be particularly helpful in managing conditions like seizure disorders or attention deficit hyperactivity disorder (ADHD). Galvanic skin response (GSR), also known as electrodermal activity (EDA) or skin conductance response (SCR), can be used to monitor sweating, which is typically associated with some pain conditions and with anxiety. Biofeedback devices typically provide auditory or visual feedback to help the individual learn to voluntarily gain control over their physiological processes; this approach, unfortunately, takes a good deal of practice to adequately master as well as specialized equipment that can sometimes be costly.

Chiropractic

Chiropractic techniques are based on the premise that subluxations, or dislocations, in the arrangement of the spinal column and the resulting nerve impingement that this is said to produce causes myriad health problems, including that of feeling pain. Realignment by manipulation is the major technique used by chiropractors to purportedly adjust the structural integrity of the spinal column.

Chiropractic care typically begins with the taking of a detailed health history, a physical examination, and various laboratory tests or diagnostic imaging, such as the use of X-rays to identify abnormalities in musculoskeletal structure. Treatment usually involves manual adjustments, also known as manipulation therapy, by means of varied techniques. Chiropractors may also routinely give out dietary advice, usually advocating the taking of nutritional supplements, as well as employ various types of treatment modalities, such as hot and cold compresses, infrared or ultraviolet light, traction, and ultrasound. The benefits of chiropractic care include improved mobility and decreased pain, but relief is often temporary and necessitates ongoing treatments. Chiropractors are, of course, not legally permitted to prescribe drugs, perform surgery, or practice obstetrics. Chiropractic treatment is by far the most common nonsurgical, non-pharmacological approach used for coping with back pain, particularly acute low back pain.

Massage

Massage therapy is an approach similar to chiropractic treatment that is based on manipulation of muscles and soft body tissues to alter muscular, circulatory, lymphatic, and nervous systems. The kneading, pummeling, and stroking of muscles and other tissues as practiced in massage therapy can effectively increase metabolism, enhance lymphatic drainage, and release substances back in circulation to thereby create both physical and mental relaxation.

Studies have demonstrated that massage therapy can stimulate the release of endorphins, which can raise one's threshold for pain. Massage certainly promotes relaxation and appears to provide pain relief and improved daily functioning.

Massage techniques have demonstrated efficacy in providing comfort for chronic low back pain and also usefulness in managing other types of pain. Reiki, for example, is a traditional Japanese massage technique that uses light, energy healing based on the concept of life force energy. There are actually over 100 different types of massage varieties, including acupressure, Ayurveda, shiatsu, and Swedish styles.

Exercise

Exercise, as briefly noted above, can be used to strengthen weak muscles, restore proper muscular balance, increase blood flow, stimulate immune system responses, enhance metabolic functions, and otherwise promote a healthier condition, all of which can assist in the management of pain. Tai chi, for instance, is a traditional Chinese martial art that is based on slow, gentle movements that can help ease stiffness and pain; while there are many varieties of yoga from India that people use to help achieve a mind-body balance and for relaxation. There are many other schools of corrective exercise and physical therapy that could possibly have potential uses in managing and controlling pain.

There are many benefits demonstrated from exercise for better pain management and overall health improvement. Through the use of cardiovascular, strength, and flexibility exercises, one can improve their pain threshold and thereby reduce, if not eliminate, the use of painkiller medications. Targeted exercise can strengthen the muscles around the site of an injury and can thereby take off some of the pressure, particularly efficacious with respect to many joint injuries. However, the wrong type of exercise can also reinjure the area, and therefore, professional guidance is recommended.

Hypnosis

Hypnosis involves a set of techniques intended to improve concentration, lessen the influence of distractions, and increase the responsiveness to suggestions. Unfortunately, some individuals respond better to hypnosis than others; the expectations and motivations that an individual has significantly impacts the effectiveness of hypnotherapy. Numerous hypnotherapeutic techniques are used for pain management, such as hypnoanalysis and interpersonal approaches. Hypnotic regression to the root cause of the pain problem can lead to better acceptance and possibly relief. Hypnotic techniques are designed to produce an altered state of awareness, which can make an individual more open to specific suggestions, such as feeling less pain.

Hypnosis techniques are intended to establish a psychological shift in one's state of consciousness by more focused attention such that you gain better mastery and control over your states of awareness, which includes symptoms of pain. Hypnotherapy has been shown to reduce the need for the use of pain-killers by lowering the state of anxiety that is often associated with pain.

Relaxation

Relaxation techniques, such as meditation, guided imagery, and progressive muscle relaxation, are an array of techniques that can be used to help reduce stress, which can certainly manifest as musculoskeletal tension. Relaxation techniques not only help individuals relax muscles and achieve a calm mental state, but they also help reduce the levels of stress hormones in the body.

Various meditation techniques are intended to produce a mind-body state of inner focus and concentrated awareness, which can direct attention away from pain. These include the numerous schools of yoga, mindfulness meditation, transcendental meditation, rhythmic breathing practices, autogenic training, and visualization exercises. Since most meditation techniques help to induce a state of contemplation, they also typically help lower blood pressure, slow metabolism, and reduce anxiety, all of which can help an individual become detached from their pain sensations. The primary intent of relaxation techniques is to have the individual systematically induce a physiological state that is nearly opposite that of the stress response. Several relaxation therapies have been clinically shown to reduce symptoms of pain. Mediating, for instance, appears both to increase pain tolerance and to decrease the use of painkiller medications.

Nutrition

Nutritional therapy can also be of potential assistance in pain management. Losing weight through proper nutrition and exercise can be particularly help-ful in certain types of conditions associated with excessive weight bearing, such as osteoarthritis. A mostly vegetarian diet has been suggested to be helpful for those dealing with pain associated with fibromyalgia and premenstrual symp-toms. Nutritional supplements, like chondroitin sulfate and glucosamine sul-fate, may provide some assistance for those with osteoarthritis in their knees. Herbal remedies, fish oils, and other nutritional approaches have been suggested, but additional research is necessary before an evidence-based recommendation can be made. Some have said, for instance, that ginger can reduce exercise-induced muscle pain by up to 25%. Ayurvedic medicine from India draws heavily upon herbs and other plants in its treatments, as do numerous other schools of herbal medicine, some of which have been practiced for centuries. Unfortunately, it is very difficult if not nearly impossible to control dosages with herbal medicines, which can lead to dangerous situations—particularly, as is common practice, when these are consumed alongside more traditional medicines, like painkillers.

Aromatherapy

Aromatherapy is an approach that uses scents from the essential oils of selected plants; the essential oils are the compounds that help produce a plant's fragrance. These essential oils can be inhaled; applied directly to the skin, such as by facials or body wraps; or bathed with. Essential oils of substances like chamomile, helichrysum, lavender, marjoram, peppermint, sandalwood, and wintergreen are sometimes recommended for relief of pain associated with conditions like sciatica or a pinched nerve. Essential oils appear to help provide the most relief for minor and occasional aches and pains, like that associated with too much exercise. Aromatherapy is another not-well-understood complementary technique that has been used for thousands of years by people in many different cultures around the world to manage and control feelings of pain.

Electrotherapy

Technological therapies have also been developed to help manage and control pain, such as various types of electrotherapy. These electrotherapy approaches usually utilize various devices that can be used to help control and manage pain sensations. For example, transcutaneous electrical nerve stimulation (TENS) uses safe, mild electrical signals released by small, battery-powered devices that can be attached to the skin; while spinal cord stimulation (SCS) utilizes an electrode that is implanted near the spinal cord of a patient to block pain signals by neuro-modulation. Peripheral nerve stimulation (PNS) is an approach in which an electrode is inserted through a small surgical incision and then placed on a nerve; while peripheral nerve field stimulation (PNFS) is a slightly less invasive approach in which an electrode is inserted by means of a needle under the skin. The most invasive electrotherapy approach used to treat pain is deep brain stimulation (DBS), in which electrodes are directly placed in the brain, usually in the periacueductal gray and sensory thalamus regions. Transcranial magnetic stimulation (TMS), on the other hand, is a noninvasive electrotherapy approach in which rapid cycling electromagnetic induction is used to impart electrical stimulation in order to better manage and control pain sensations.

DOCUMENT: MAJOR CATEGORIES OF PAIN TREATMENTS

About 70 million adult Americans are living with chronic pain. Treatment of pain involves, if possible, elimination of the underlying cause of the pain as well as the use of one or more strategies for relieving the pain symptoms. The accompanying table presents an overview of the various major categories of pain treatments typically utilized to manage pain. These approaches include not only various medications, such as non-opioids, opioids, and adjuvant analgesics, but also assorted other modalities and approaches, including lifestyle changes such as losing weight and regular physical activity. Effective management of pain is routinely a complex endeavor that often enlists multiple categories of pain treatments. The use of the non-medication strategies can lessen, if not sometimes even eliminate, the need for administration of painkiller drugs.

Categories of Pain Treatments

Category	Examples
Nonopioid drugs	Acetaminophen, nonsteroidal anti-inflammatory drugs
Adjuvant analgesics	Antidepressants, anticonvulsants
Opioids	Morphine, oxycodone, fentanyl, methadone, oxymorphone, hydromorphone
Rehabilitative approaches	Modalities (heat, cold, transcutaneous electrical nerve stimulation), physical therapy, occupational therapy
Psychological approaches	Cognitive behavioral therapy, specific techniques (biofeedback, hypnosis, relaxation), other psychotherapies
Injection therapies	Trigger point injections, joint injections, spinal injections
Neural blockade	Sympathetic nerve blocks, medial branch block, celiac plexus block
Implant therapies	Spinal cord stimulator, intrathecal pump
Surgical approaches	Cordotomy, neurectomy
Complementary and alternative medicine approaches	Acupuncture, chiropractic therapy, massage, nutritional approaches and nutraceuticals, energy therapies
Lifestyle changes	Weight loss, exercise

Source: Adapted from P. G. Fine and R. K. Portenoy. (2007) "Table 1, Categories of Pain Treatments." In *A clinical guide to opioid analgesia* (2nd ed.) and included in *Opioid prescribing: Clinical tools and risk management strategies*, by A. V. Anderson, P. G. Fine, and S. M. Fishman. Available online at https://mn.gov/health-licensing-boards/images/Opioid_Prescribing_Clinical_Tools_and_Risk_Management_Strategies.pdf. Used by permission of the American Academy of Pain Management.

Chapter 3

Painkillers: A Brief History

A brief history of painkillers, beginning with early evidence from antiquity for the use of opium along with cross-cultural evidence from many parts of the world, as well as a review of the development of morphine up through the modern era and our experiences with other opiates and opioids, particularly heroin and more recently drugs like hydrocodone, oxymorphone, and oxycodone, also remembering not to ignore our experience with the assorted other classes of painkillers such as the non-steroidal anti-inflammatory drugs and the COX-2 inhibitors, is essential to better understand their story.

EARLY EVIDENCE OF OPIUM

Opium was a substance well known across much of the ancient world, with its origins lying deep within the realms of antiquity. The plant itself may have originally been indigenous in or around ancient Anatolia and the neighboring fertile-crescent region. The painkiller powers of opium were legendary, and its use was somewhat common in many early societies, such as those from Mesopotamia, Egypt, and throughout the entire ancient Near East as well as throughout much of the rest of the ancient world. Opium has served as an important item of trade for millennia. Early medical practices of Greek and Roman civilizations, for instance, drew heavily upon opium's highly effective painkiller properties, many of which were attributed to various gods and goddesses. Knowledge of the potency of opium to soothe human suffering persisted through the Middle Ages, and its use has continued beyond to the modern era.

Antiquity

The opium poppy and its psychoactive properties were discovered early in the antiquity of humankind. The initial use of opium has not been determined, and it is unlikely to ever be as it "is one of the earliest medicinal plants known to mankind" (Kapoor, 1995, p. 1). The archaeological record supports the assertion that people have known of and used opium for a considerable part of our history on this planet. For example, in an archaeological excavation conducted at Kition, an ancient city that is mostly buried under the modern town of Larnaca in Cyprus, a 12th-century BC opium pipe was found. Further, there is considerable evidence for the use of opium at much earlier times. In fact, the opium poppy was being cultivated at Neolithic lake dwelling sites in Switzerland dated to the fourth millennium BC. While in the ancient Near East, it appears from considerable archaeological evidence that opium, as well as other psychoactive plants including marijuana, mandrake, datura, and water lily, were known of and used medicinally in ancient times.

Mesopotamia

Evidence from ancient Mesopotamia clearly indicates knowledge of the use of opium. The Sumerians, one of the first Mesopotamian civilizations, appear to have been rather well acquainted with opium and its major pharmacological effects. It has been said that the Sumerians in the fourth millennium BC cultivated the poppy, for which they created the ideogram *Hul Gil*, which literally meant "joy plant." The opium poppy was widely known to and used by the Sumerians of the third millennium BC, although there are those who question this assertion.

Opium continued to be used for subsequent millennia in Mesopotamia. The Assyrians, one of the peoples who succeeded the Sumerians, also widely used opium for medicinal purposes. The Assyrians referred to the juice of the poppy as *arat-pa-pal*, which, it has been speculated, may have been the etymological source for the Latin *papaver*. Assyrian medical texts noted the continued use of opium for various ailments.

Egypt and the Ancient Near East

Opium, as briefly noted above, was also well known and apparently widely used by ancient Egyptians. The Ebers papyrus is a *materia medica* written ca.

1550 BC that consists of ancient Egyptian medical prescriptions and charms. This papyrus work mentions opium and several other natural drugs. For instance, in the well-known Ebers papyrus, the goddess Isis gives opium to the god Ra to treat his headache. It recommends that opium could be used to treat many problems, such as colic in children. Wine and beer were frequently recommended vehicles for administering various pharmacological preparations included in the Ebers papyrus, many of which included opium. Opium was so common in ancient Egypt that certain regions were known for producing superior preparations of the product.

Cypriot base ring juglets shaped like the opium poppy have been found at sites across the Ancient Near East, including those along the coasts of Syria, Lebanon, and Palestine, as well as in Egypt. These vessels have been studied as evidence for the long-distance commercial trade of opium in the ancient world. There were numerous foreign imports as well as locally produced copies of these opium-shaped vessels recovered from excavation sites across the Ancient Near East and beyond. Chemical analysis of the contents of many of these Cypriot base ring juglets has confirmed that at least some of them actually contained opium.

Greece and Rome

Opium was well known elsewhere across the ancient world. The Greeks and Romans, for example, were very familiar with opium and its painkiller and associated effects. Images of opium poppy capsules were frequently used to adorn many Greco-Roman objects of everyday life, such as coins, figurines, jewelry, and vases.

The ancient Greek poet Homer mentioned the opium poppy in Book IX of *The Iliad*. The Greek philosopher Aristotle noted the hypnotic effects of the poppy. Theophrastus, a Greek philosopher who succeeded Aristotle, mentioned opium poppies frequently, noting their hypnotic effects as well as different varieties. Herakleides of Pontus noted that the Keians used the poppy for their practice of euthanasia. Diodorus Siculus, a Greek historian, reported that the women of Egypt used opium as an antidote to anger and grief.

The Roman poet Virgil, in Book I of his *Georgics*, written around 29 BC, referred to "poppies steeped in ... slumber" (Virgil, 1982, p. 59) and in Book IV of the same work he mentioned "poppies of forgetfulness" (Virgil, 1982, p. 143). In the 1st century AD, A. Cornelius Celsus, in Book II of his *De medicina* (*On Medicine*), noted that use of the poppy was good for producing sleep. Pliny the Elder, a Roman writer of the 1st century AD, noted that opium not only induced sleep, but could be fatal if taken in sufficient doses.

Marcus Aurelius, the Stoic philosopher and Roman emperor who reigned from AD 161 to AD 180, has been identified as an opium addict based on his daily dependence upon the drug.

Opium was widely used for medicinal purposes by people in many cultures across the ancient world. The ancient Greco-Romans, for example, were very well acquainted with the role of many substances, notably including opium, in the early practice of medicine. Hippocrates, the ancient Greek physician known as the father of medicine, made frequent mention of the opium poppy in his medicinal preparations, and he made a distinction between different varieties of poppies. Galen, another very prominent Greek physician, referred to opium as the strongest of drugs that numb the senses, and he recommended opium for treating many ailments (Moraes & Moraes, 2003, p. 34). Pedanius Dioscorides, another Greek-speaking physician who practiced medicine during the reign of the infamous Roman emperor Nero, mentioned opium in his five-volume 1st-century AD *De Materia Medica*.

Gods and Goddesses

The gods and goddesses of many ancient civilizations around the world were sometimes associated with the opium poppy and its medical and psycho-active properties. The ancient Minoans, for example, had a goddess of poppies, who was the patroness of healing and was depicted with three poppy capsules in her hair. The Babylonian and Assyrian goddess Nisaba was typically portrayed with opium poppies sprouting from her shoulders. Thoth, the Egyptian god of knowledge, was credited with teaching the ancient Egyptians how to prepare opium. The Greek goddess Demeter was associated not only with grain, but also with the opium poppy; and initiates to her Elusinian Mystery cult induced visions with a psychoactive drink based on barley and other ingredients. Cybele, the Phrygian mother goddess who was also worshipped by the Greeks and Romans, was often shown wearing a wreath of opium poppies as a symbol of fecundity. The Greek and Roman gods of sleep—Hypnos and Somnos, respectively—are often depicted in association with opium poppies, as are the gods of night—Nyx and Nox, respectively—and of death—Thanatos and Mors. Statues of many other deities, such as Aphrodite, Apollo, Asklepios, Demeter, Isis, Kybele, and Pluto, were often decorated with opium poppies. Ancient myths also mention the use of opium poppies by the gods and goddesses. For example, when Demeter (known as Ceres to the Romans) was depressed over the capture of her daughter Persephone (known as Proserpina to the Romans) by Hades (known as Pluto to the Romans), the lord of the underworld, she ate pop-pies to induce sleep and to soothe her grief.

Middle Ages and Beyond

The use, abuse, and concern with opium, of course, continued to be a topic of interest for some time. During the Middle Ages, opium continued to be used and abused in respective societies. For instance, Islamic physicians in 9th-century Baghdad, which was then one of the leading centers of medical knowledge, knew of and made regular therapeutic use of opium. Baghdad of the 9th century has also been noted as the place where pharmacy emerged as a separate profession from medicine. During the late 9th and early 10th centuries, al-Razi was a noted pharmacist in Baghdad who regularly recommended opium for cases of melancholy. Abu al-Qasim Khalaf bin Abbas Al-Zahrawi, known in the West as Albucasis, was a surgeon in 10th-century Moorish Spain who wrote a medical treatise called *al-Tasrif* that recommended the use of opium. Moses Maimonides, a noted 12th-century medieval Jewish scholar, wrote a treatise on the medicinal uses of opium. In India, medicinal preparations of opium for use in treating diarrhea and sexual problems are contained in works such as the 13th-century *Shodal Gadanigraha*, the 15th-century *Sharangdhar Samhita*, and the 15th-century *Bhavapra Kasha*. The 15th-century Ottoman physician Serefeddin Sabuncuoglu wrote an illustrated surgical textbook, known as *Cerrahiyyet'ul Haniyye* (*Imperial Surgery*), and an experimental medical text called *Mucerrbnami* (*The Book of Experience*), and he recommended the use of opium for treating migraines, sciatica, and other painful conditions.

Opium continued for a long time to be used in Europe as well. For example, 15th-century Italian anatomists—who, by the way, also served as executioners—used opium to sedate prisoners before performing dissections on them. In 1551, the English naturalist and physician William Turner advocated the use of the opium poppy in his well-known herbal treatise, the first one to be published in the English language. Turner noted not only some of the reputed virtues of opium, but also many of its dangers, observing that it could be harmful and could sometimes even kill. In 1682, Georg Wolfgang Wedel advised the use of opium to restore the chemical imbalances of the body that he felt caused illness. In 1753, Carl Linnaeus published his *Species Plantarum*, in which he was the first to classify the opium poppy as *Papaver somniferum*, which literally means "sleep-inducing." In 1762, Thomas Dover, an English physician, introduced his "diaphoretic powder," which contained opium along with other ingredients and which was recommended for treating gout; it rapidly became popular for many uses, due in no small measure to its opium content and thus its painkilling properties. Experimentation with opium in the 18th century contributed substantially to new developments in the emerging fields of pharmacology and physiology.

The popularity and potency of opium insured that it would continue to be used for centuries after, even if, at times, for somewhat dubious purposes. For instance, in 1625 and 1665 in response to outbreaks of plague in London, mithridatium, a purported panacea based on a complex formulation including opium, was one of the main recommended remedies. In the 18th century, opium was often used not only as a painkiller, but also "as either a nervous sedative or as a stimulant" (Loudan, 1986, p. 63). In the 1830s, a British surgeon-apothecary recommended the use of a mixture of brandy and opium to treat cholera. In the 19th century, opium was also used as a treatment for scrofula. Theriac, an opium-based purported panacea known to the ancient Greeks and Romans as an antidote to poison, continued to be used through the late 19th century. The varied medicinal uses of opium contributed to its rather widespread use and popularity. For example, in 1840, New England merchants imported 24,000 lb. of opium into the United States; customs officials took note of this commerce and soon imposed a duty on its import. Further, during the 19th century, opium poppies were grown legally in much of the United States, particularly in southern states such as Georgia, Florida, Louisiana, Virginia, Tennessee, and South Carolina. Opium was also recommended at the time for the treatment of alcoholism and numerous other medical conditions. The first *Merck's Manual*, for example, recommended the use of opium for treating alcoholics as it may "be necessary to produce sleep; to relieve the pain of the chronic gastritis and the want of appetite" (Merck & Co., 1899, p. 86).

There is actually a long history of the injecting of substances such that attribution to its initial development is highly problematic. In the 1850s, opiates were being injected to treat neuralgia. In 1869, a Dr. Allbutt recommended the injection of morphine to treat heart disease, and in 1870, he noted the rise of the abuse of hypodermic injections of morphine. In 1875, a Dr. Anderson recommended the injection of morphine to treat asthma.

The medicinal and recreational use of opium was widespread in Western societies by the 19th century. In fact, many well-known 19th-century writers, such as Samuel Taylor Coleridge, Arthur Conan Doyle, and William Wadsworth, were open public advocates for the use of opium. Perhaps the best-known book on the subject at the time was Thomas De Quincey's *Confessions of an English Opium Eater*. Popular interest in the opium eating of celebrities such as Coleridge and De Quincey fueled the Victorian-era magazine wars. Many contemporaneous artists and musicians also claimed to have obtained inspiration from opium. Several 19th-century women writers were also known as regular users of opium, such as Elizabeth Barrett Browning. It is perhaps not that surprising, then, that opium was extensively used in

19th-century Britain for serious, minor, and even imaginary ailments as well as for strictly euphoric purposes. Social responses to the growing concerns over Victorian opium eating began to formulate into the emerging view of it as a social problem. In fact, there was the social construction of opiate addiction as the result of an impaired moral faculty within 19th-century Britain.

At the same time in the United States, homeopathic doctors could rightly sneer that most cases of pain would be "controlled by the allopathic physicians with their usual remedy, opium" (Porter, 1884, p. 43). The substantial increase in U.S. opium use during the 19th century was associated with the rise of temperance movements advocating partial, if not total, abstinence to alcohol. At about the same general time, public awareness of late 19th-century chronic opium users in Britain helped in the construction of the modern concept of addiction. Although drug addiction was not generally regarded as a major problem in Victorian England, negative social responses to the use of opium arose based on issues such as attitudes of moral superiority, racism, class tensions, and emerging professionalization, particularly of medical specialists. At any rate, books on opium addiction and varied approaches to its treatment were not uncommon then, such as Dr. H. James Brown's *An Opium Cure* (1872), Dr. Edward Levinstein's *The Morbid Craving for Morphia* (1878), and Dr. Norman Kerr's *Inebriety or Narcomania* (1894).

In late 19th- and early 20th-century America, narcotic addiction became understood as a concomitant symptom to what was to be recognized as modernity. There was a widespread recognition of opium addiction as a growing social problem. Awareness of addiction to morphine and other opiates also grew during that time, as a leading American physician observed: "The morphine habit is growing at an alarming rate, and we . . . must acknowledge that we are culpable in too often giving this seductive siren until the will-power is gone" (Witherspoon, 1900, p. 1591). Nevertheless, by the 1920s, morphine was regularly being prescribed or dispensed in municipal outpatient treatment programs for heroin addicts. Narcotic addicts were then assumed, not necessarily correctly, to be primarily members of the lower classes, with members of the middle and upper classes seen as generally immune to such a pernicious habit. The reverse social situation was, in fact, the true state of affairs. Although public awareness of the issue of addiction to opiates such as opium, morphine, and heroin was growing, it was still generally regarded as less pernicious a practice than being an alcoholic.

Opium continued to be used medicinally until the modern era. For instance, opium was frequently used in combination with marijuana or other substances as ingredients in many patent medicines at the end of the 19th century. Opium and its derivatives were considered to be among the most important drugs in the medical pharmacopeia up to the early part of the 20th century. Opium still continues to be used medically in some traditional societies around the world. Further, several modern prescription drugs—at least 15, in fact—are still derived today from the opium poppy and its by-products.

CROSS-CULTURAL EVIDENCE

Opium is a drug that has long been associated by those in the Western world with the Orient. Indeed, opium was well known for centuries in Oriental lands, such as the Middle East, India, and China. However, the use of opium, even in traditional contexts, carries the risks of substantial problems, both to health and to social functioning.

Middle East

In the Middle East, which includes the area of ancient Mesopotamia, opium, of course, had a long historical presence. Medieval Islamic physicians were consequently well acquainted with the use and abuse of opium. Abu Ali al-Husayn ibn Abdullah Ibn Sin, known as Avicenna in the Latin West, was perhaps one of the most widely respected Islamic medical authorities who, like others, recommended opium for varied uses. In his famed *al-Qanum*, or *Canon of Medicine*, he mentioned that opium was the most powerful stupefacient. Avicenna himself may actually have died from an overdose of opium. Muhammad ibn Ahmad al-Biruni, another 10th- to 11th-century Islamic scholar, wrote a book on pharmacy and *materia medica*, which included assorted comments on the use of opium. Al-Biruni noted that those living in hot climates, such as in Mecca, were daily users of opium, and that they "gradually increased the dosage to the extent where it would be considered lethal" (Biruni, 1973, p. 36). At the turn of the 17th century, opium, along with coffee, aromatics, spices, minerals, porcelains, and textiles, could be found in the market of the Yemeni port of al-Mukha and elsewhere across the Middle East.

In 18th-century Iran, opium was used regularly, at least by elites, but it was almost exclusively eaten, not smoked, and consumed only in combination with other non-psychoactive substances, typically various spices like cardamom, cinnamon, cloves, or nutmeg, to ameliorate the narcotic effects. Recreational drug use, including that of opium, often appears initially among members of the upper and middle classes and then later tends to spread to other social groups, which was certainly the pattern in Iran. Later, under the Shah, drug policies were formulated in attempts to address the use and abuse of opium. Opium continues today to be widely used in modern Iran; it is typically smoked in a pipe, and use in this form has been implicated as a cancer risk factor, particularly for esophageal cancer. Subsequent studies confirmed the risk of both crude opium and of other forms of opium use being associated with higher incidence of esophageal squamous cell carcinoma. Heroin use is also reported in Iran, predominantly by urban residents. In addition, needle and syringe sharing appears to be common among Iranians who are drug dependent. Further, leakage of packets of opium in the gastrointestinal tracts of smugglers has been recognized as a problem today in Iran and elsewhere.

India

India has also had a long history with opium. In fact, Shiva, the Hindu destroyer god, is also known as Bhole Shankar, which means he that is oblivious to the world, since he is fed opium to curb his destructive urges. The soldiers of Alexander the Great, following his conquests of Persia and India around 330 BC, first introduced opium to these lands. Opium was routinely used in ancient India for its euphoric and other pharmacological effects. It served as a status commodity for treating the elite, as an aphrodisiac to bolster the resolve of soldiers, and as a medicinal palliative. Certain Mughal princes and nobles in India were known "for their fondness for opium" (Sangar, 1981, p. 204). Later Mughal rulers tried to regulate and control the sale and use of opium substances, but they met with only limited success.

In 19th-century India, opium was regularly added to tobacco to produce *madak*, which was at the time a highly popular product. Later, consumption switched mainly to *chandu*, a more potent alternative; marijuana and opium were also sometimes mixed and used together in Mughal India. Opium itself constituted an important segment of peasant agricultural production in 19th-century India. Further, many Indian growers and merchants benefited from the profits of the opium trade. In fact, during the 19th century, most opium was grown in India, which then included what is now Pakistan, Iran, and Afghanistan. In fact, opium played a role in the history of several countries neighboring India, including Sri Lanka. It is an enlightening historical lesson that British authorities were able through the 1893 to 1895 Royal Commission on Opium to garner support for a medical misconception that opium could prevent and cure malaria. This falsehood helped provide additional rationale for the British continuing their role in the lucrative opium trade.

Great Britain began its large-scale participation in the opium trade in India during the era of the East India Company, but it then took control out of private hands and placed it in a branch of their colonial government, the Opium Administration. In fact, the monopoly on the opium trade enjoyed by the East

India Company ended in 1834 when Her Majesty's Government sent Lord Napier with a commission to open opium trading. By 1919, the British Empire had 654,928 acres in India under poppy cultivation, which yielded the treasury, after expenditures, a revenue of nearly $22 million (in 1920 dollars). On the other hand, changing conditions in India also permitted the British to later withdraw from opium trafficking. Subsequent socioeconomic development in India, as it has elsewhere, led to changes in substance use and abuse.

Ethnographic accounts of opium use in contemporary India continue to be collected. For example, in the desert state of Rajasthan, the use of raw opium, which is referred to as *amal* or *doda*, is said to be rather common and appears to be well integrated into the cultural fabric of many communities not only for the medicinal relief of distress, but also recreationally in ways that promote social bonding. On the other hand, studies of opium users in urban and rural communities in Pakistan revealed considerable differences in patterns and consequences of use. In fact, there are reported to be currently in Pakistan nearly 100,000 street-based injection drug users alone, almost exclusively using heroin. Heroin, of course, is used by addicts in modern India as well.

Asia

The indigenous use of opiates, of course, continues elsewhere as well, such as in Thailand and Laos. In this regard, opium is used as part of traditional healing practices by members of several hill tribes in Thailand to treat symptoms of many illnesses. It has been speculated that the Hmong of northern Laos and Vietnam got involved in the production of opium as a source of revenue that could be used to obtain salt. Opium was also used traditionally in Malaysia for recreation and to alleviate stress and pain associated with hard labor, such as is done by fishermen working up to 18 hours a day. However, a study of matched pairs of opium and heroin addicts in Laos suggested that the life crises that accompany heroin appear to progress faster and motivate addicts to seek treatment sooner than those addicted to opium. Similarly, the open availability of opium in certain Asian cultures, such as among the Hmong of Laos, appears to be related to an earlier onset of the problems associated with drug addiction.

Opium, not surprisingly, has been used differently by various peoples in respective locales. For example, in Hong Kong, opium was generally smoked; while in Egypt, opium was invariably eaten. Nevertheless, any form of opium use can, of course, eventually lead to abuse. For instance, regular consumption of opium poppy tea infusion has been reported to lead to the formation of dependence.

Myanmar, formerly known as Burma, is one of several Southeast Asian countries whose political and economic stability has been heavily impacted by opium production and distribution. Beginning in 1852, the British began selling opium in Burma through a governmental monopoly. More recently, heroin availability and use in Myanmar has led to a different pattern of substance abuse than existed there in earlier times.

The social, economic, and political impact of opium on selected societies has been rather substantial historically. For example, the prevalence of opium use and addiction was long recognized as a problem in China. Further, the Chinese diaspora facilitated the globalization of opium. Opium smoking, of course, was a common practice among Chinese emigrants, such as those who moved to Borneo. Consequently, opium smoking spread around the globe as long as Chinese labor was relatively inexpensive and profitable. However, the average life expectancy of an opium addict was estimated to be only about 30 to 40 years.

During the 18th century, opium was certainly the chief commodity sold by the Dutch East India Company throughout Indonesia, and its use there rapidly became part of the cultural fabric of life. In Indonesia, more recent reports suggest that physical abuse of injecting drug users by police is commonplace. Social stigma is a widespread problem, particularly with respect to injection drug users.

The importation, possession, and use of opium was strictly prohibited, except for medical purposes, in Japan; this rigid approach seems to have been very effective there. The Philippine Opium Commission was so impressed with the Japanese model that its conclusions led on March 1, 1908, to the official prohibition of opium in the Philippines.

Economic analysis has been applied to many historical questions on the use and abuse of opium and other opiates. Drug abuse in West Malaysia, for instance, was found to have accompanied steps toward early global economic systems, in particular in the early 1800s, being associated with the use of opium by Chinese and Indian immigrant laborers. Continued socioeconomic development in Malaysia, as elsewhere, led to changes in substance use and abuse, particularly among adolescents. Opium, along with textiles, clearly formed the economic basis of international trade for colonial India.

Empires

Substances like opium can play a crucial role in both establishing and maintaining empires. For instance, opium was used by the Japanese to expand their imperialistic enterprise across Asia. Control of opium in late 19th-century

Japan contributed to greater political consolidation by Tokugawa and Meiji regimes; this helped them first to resist foreign imperialism, and then Meiji Japan used opium to further their own imperialistic aims, particularly in China. The Japanese annexation of Korea in 1910 also made it necessary to formulate imperialistic policies regarding control of opium and other narcotic drugs. The Japanese, including a Special Service Section of their army, purposefully distributed quantities of opium to help pacify the Chinese populace prior to and while under Japanese occupation. After colonies are established, the role of many substances sometimes tends to shift to more of an economic focus. In this regard, the opium trade was certainly used intentionally as an important source of revenue for the British Empire in India, as mentioned earlier. Further, opium as a commodity was used by the British to offset trade deficits, as by 1854, China had become, after the United States and France, the third-largest source of imports to Britain, based chiefly on tea and silk. Opium sales were used to help cover this trade imbalance. In addition, beginning in 1800, the British Levant Company began purchasing almost half of all the opium being sold out of Smyrna, Turkey, for transport and sale to Europe and the United States.

Opium and related substances have, accordingly, heavily impacted peoples living under imperial domination. Historical data, for example, has been used to confirm that in the late colonial Netherlands Indies, in what is now part of Indonesia, opium users could be economically characterized as either high-intensity or low-intensity consumers. At the end of World War II, opium smoking was declared illegal in Indonesia; but no treatment facilities were available, which helped stimulate the establishment of drug trafficking networks. Another study focused on the Japanese colonial period in Taiwan found that opium use was virtually eradicated, despite price elasticity, but due largely to the combination of strong restrictions and the ready provision of successful treatment programs.

Opium is a substance that has had a particularly significant impact on the history of several countries around the world. As discussed above, opium was known of and used for its particular effects since ancient times. Opium became a significant source of revenue for Mughal India, a fact that was recognized by Europeans such as the Portuguese, Spanish, Dutch, and British merchants, who expanded its exportation. In 1699, the Dutch East India Company imported 87 tons of opium from India for distribution in Java and the East Indies. Portuguese sailors, trading along the East China Sea around 1500, are thought to have been the first to smoke opium. The Portuguese, beginning in 1729, are actually credited as being the first Western traders to bring opium into China. In 1745, Baron Gustaaf Willem van Imhoff established the Opium Society, which was granted the sole rights to trade opium in the Dutch empire. In the early 17th century, English merchants realized that the best way for them to obtain precious spices from Indonesia was to send ships from India laden with supplies of opium and cotton. Muslim traders established commercial networks across China's northwest border to bring opium into China, even before the British penetrated China's coastal periphery. After the British colonial governmental structure was established in India, it was imperative to find a way to finance the resulting expenses of such an ambitious undertaking. The British East India Company made several failed attempts to send opium from India to China beginning in 1767, but finally succeeded in 1794; prior to this, opium had also been transported from Turkey to China by Portuguese merchants. For example, in 1767, the Portuguese imported 200 chests of opium from Turkey into Macao. At any rate, the East India Company developed the exportation of opium from India to China as part of its triangular system of trade to bring tea, silk, and other Chinese goods to Britain and thereby to the rest of the British Empire. Opium, therefore, became the cornerstone of a cohesive trade structure that enabled Britain, India, and China to pursue mutually profitable trade relations.

Indian merchants also became very adept at smuggling opium to subvert the colonial British monopoly. Smuggling has, in fact, been an important factor in supplying the demands of those interested in using opium in many places for some time. Although the British economy no doubt benefited the most from the Chinese opium trade at that time, merchants from many other nations, including the United States, also made considerable financial profits. In this regard, on an 1842 visit to Hong Kong, Commodore Kearney noted the prominent role of two American firms, Augustine Heard & Co. and Russell & Co., in opium trafficking. Similarly, an American clipper ship, the *Frolic*, was engaged in opium trafficking from 1845 to 1850; it would transport opium from India to China and return to the United States with a load of Chinese tea. In fact, in 1858, it was estimated that about one-fifth of the opium entering Shanghai was transported on American ships. Personal accounts of Americans involved in this early opium trade are also available. In fact, adventurous entrepreneurs from many nations secured handsome profits from the highly lucrative opium trade. However, in 1880 and again in 1903, the United States through treaties agreed that no American ships would be allowed to carry opium in Chinese waters and that no U.S. citizen would import, buy, or sell opium in any of the open ports of China.

China

Chinese merchants further profited heavily from their leadership of the opium-farming syndicates that were spread across 19th-century Southeast Asia. The opium trade was so substantial an economic enterprise that from the 1830s onward, it "could not be extirpated without seriously damaging world commerce" (Downs, 1968, p. 434). Japanese and Korean merchants actively engaged in the opium trade in the 19th century along China's northeast coast, such as through the port city of Tianjin. The British opium trade in Singapore and throughout much of the rest of Southeast Asia would not have been possible without the economic networks created by the shareholding partnerships run by Chinese merchants. In fact, Scottish merchants had unsuccessfully attempted to solely conduct an opium business in Hong Kong; it was profitable only after it was placed in the hands of Chinese merchants.

The Chinese experience with opium, particularly through the 19th-century Opium Wars, has its own long, complex history. It should be noted that opium was identified as a problem in China long before the involvement of the British. In 1683, Chinese Manchu soldiers conquered the island of Formosa and thereby learned of the delights of smoking opium. This method of use significantly increased the nonmedical use of opium in China. Interestingly, the ready adoption of opium smoking in China was probably facilitated by the earlier widespread use of tobacco; certainly, the evolution of the Chinese opium pipe appears to be based on tobacco pipes. Opium smoking cut across all social levels of 19th-century China. Opium smoking became so entrenched among Chinese elites that opium paraphernalia were sometimes crafted in expensive materials, such as ivory, jade, cloisonné, porcelain, and silver. Indeed, opium was appropriated into the culture of consumption of the Chinese upper classes, as characterized by the elite recreational opium consumption in Shanghai. At any rate, by the Late Imperial era in China, opium smoking was widespread throughout the populace, and efforts were made to prohibit use. In 1729, an imperial edict was issued prohibiting the importation of opium to China; nevertheless, the trade flourished. At the same time, in order to resist foreign traders, China attempted to become increasingly dependent upon domestic sources of opium. The British, notably, began selling opium in China in 1781. By 1790, 4,054 chests of opium were imported to China. In 1799, the Chinese emperor, Kia King, banned opium, making its cultivation and trade illegal; but, of course, the practices still persisted.

From 1801 to 1820, the official British figures show that their share of the opium trade each year was about 5,000 chests. However, by 1831, it had risen to 18,956 chests, and in 1836, the figure exceeded 30,000 chests. By 1838, the British were selling about 1,400 tons of opium each year in China. In 1839, the Chinese Daoguang emperor sent a special commissioner, Lin Zexu, to Canton to suppress the by-then burgeoning opium trafficking. There were about 20,000 chests of opium stored in ships outside of Canton; each chest weighed about 133 lb. and was worth, at that time, $300 each; this would have totaled around 2.66 million pounds at a value then of $6 million. The Chinese surrounded the merchants, who then surrendered their opium stockpile, which was immediately destroyed. The British retaliated with overwhelming force in what is referred to as the First Opium War (1839–1842), also known as the Anglo-Chinese War, seizing Canton and many other ports including Shanghai, which soon became the center of drug trafficking in the Far East. The war was concluded in 1843 with the Treaty of Nanking, which granted very favorable terms to the British, including an indemnity of $21 million that not only covered the value of the destroyed opium, but also the expenses of the war and compensation for destruction of the property of British subjects. This treaty also ceded the island of Hong Kong to the British. By 1845, 45,000 chests of opium were imported from India to China by the British at a total value of $34 million (or a value of $962 million today) and by 1847, it had risen to 60,000 chests at a total value of $42 million (or $1.1 billion today). Within 15 years of the Treaty of Nanking, the Second Opium War (1856–1860), also known as the Arrow War, broke out; this war was ignited in response to the boarding of the *Arrow*, flying the English flag, by Chinese officials on October 8, 1856. The Second Opium War was concluded with the Treaty of Tianjin in 1858 that granted another $3 million in indemnity and numerous other concessions, including the opening of additional treaty port to merchants, toleration of the Christian religion, and admission of opium under a specified tariff.

There were apparently a variety of places that existed in China for the consumption of opium after the formal institutionalization of the opium trade. One of the most popular types of these establishments was the *huayan guan*, or flower smoke den, where men could enjoy opium or women and other associated pleasures.

In 1906, the Qing initiated a campaign to suppress opium use in China. The date of May 22, 1907, was set for the official closing of all opium dens in China. In places such as Sichuan, representatives of the Qing central government enjoyed considerable success in controlling opium. However, in other places in China, such as in Fujian, local provincial officials were able only to somewhat suppress opium by gaining the cooperation of local elites. In 1907, the Imperial Court at Peking estimated that there were 150 million opium smokers in China.

Opium, heroin, and morphine played a highly visible role in political affairs in China during the first half of the 20th century. At that time, China continued earlier efforts to attempt to control opium. However, opium smoking was certainly still widespread in China during the early part of the 20th century. Further, in the 1920s, an absence of a centralized national authority in China allowed separate military governments to exploit opium production as a ready source of revenue. The Guomindang, for instance, resisted interference from the National Anti-Opium Association and forced it to disband just 9 days before the Japanese invasion. In addition, the Japanese engaged in opium distribution in China as part of the preparation for furthering their imperialistic ambitions there. In this regard, Koreans were extensively involved in Japanese opium production and trafficking in China from about the 1920s to 1945. At the same time, Chinese opium growers were pressured both by tax collectors and by crop destruction campaigns from the central government, but such conflicting approaches met with little success. In 1935, Chiang Kai-shek established an anti-opium campaign that had initial success but was abandoned after the Japanese invasion. Indeed, opiate addiction continued to be a problem for imperial ambitions in China long after the British left, such as it was for the Japanese in Manchuria during the 1930s and 1940s. Chinese who collaborated with the Japanese had to support the opium operations, but this cost them any hope of gaining legitimacy with the populace. The Wang Jingwei regime in Nanjing attempted to maintain some authority, but the fiscal necessity of opium revenues made this difficult. In December 1943, university students in Nanjing took the anti-opium movement to the streets by smashing opium dens and demanding tougher suppression efforts, which weakened Japanese control. In the late 1940s and early 1950s, many refugees fled civil war in China and settled in Hong Kong and elsewhere; many of those refugees who were opium smokers then became heroin abusers. In the early 1950s, the Chinese Communist Party conducted campaigns that successfully suppressed opium and related drugs. Certainly, the 19th-century large-scale British importation of opium certainly made the later state-building enterprise of modern China more difficult.

Immigration

When people with traditional belief systems immigrate or otherwise assimilate into more modern societies, they do not necessarily abandon their beliefs, some of which can influence the ways they may use and abuse opiates and opioids. Chinese male laborers who migrated around the world usually brought their customs of smoking opium with them wherever they went; they also helped spread it to other peoples, for example, to the Malays and Siamese as well as to those in Java, Sumatra, and neighboring islands. Vietnamese heroin users in Australia, more recently, have been noted to withdraw blood in an effort to treat heroin overdose in accord with their traditional beliefs about the circulatory system and causes of illness.

The history of opiate abuse, of course, is not restricted to the Orient but was a factor in the West as well, and speculations have been raised as to its role in world history. Unfortunately, we have had a long and tragic search for nonaddicting opiates and opioids. As recently as 1935, physicians could still debate whether codeine was or was not addictive.

Opium Trade

The opium trade became a major component of the business sector in several parts of Asia during the 16th and 17th centuries. Merchants from numerous countries were very active in trading opium from India throughout the lands of Southeast Asia. Once the British gained firm control of the Indian opium trade, additional markets were developed for this highly lucrative product, including along the coastal regions of China. When the Quing dynasty enacted anti-opium laws in China, some of the efforts of the opium trade were simply redirected to other regions of Southeast Asia that were less centrally governed; this strategy effectively opened up expansive new areas to the opium drug market.

This Southeast Asian opium market served as a valuable engine for colonial government revenues. For example, in 1906, taxes from sales of opium in British Malaya provided 53% of the finances for the colonial government there; likewise, opium taxes provided 20% of the finances for Siam (Thailand), and 16% for both French Indochina and the Netherlands Indies, respectively. This revenue source remained significant for some time. As late as 1927, official British figures showed that opium revenues accounted for significant percentages of total revenue in its major Far East Crown colonies. For the Straits Settlements, it accounted for 37%; 28% for Confederated Malay; 23% for British North Borneo; 18% for Sarawak; and 14% for the Federated Malay States.

During World War II, as hostilities blocked legal access to the importing of morphine and other related drugs into the United States and to the other Allies, Mexico became a major source of morphine for the legal market. At the same time, Mexico also became a source for the illegal heroin market in the United States, Canada, and the Caribbean.

As Chinese demand for opium waned, local cultivation efforts were escalated in Burma, Laos, and Thailand. Opium production in these countries reached large-scale levels by the 1950s. A succession of military and political conflicts in the region fueled the growth of opium production, particularly in

Burma (Myanmar). In fact, large-scale production of opium began in Laos during the First Indochina War (1946–1950), when French intelligence and paramilitary agencies gained the loyalty of the poppy-growing hill tribes in Laos against Communist insurgency by assisting with the marketing of their opium crop. Production then dramatically declined and then rose again during the Second Indochina War (1959–1975), mainly to provide heroin and other opiates to U.S. military personnel stationed in Vietnam. The United States tolerated the involvement of South Vietnamese political and military leaders in opium and heroin trafficking. By the 1970s, this region of Southeast Asia, which came to be referred to as the Golden Triangle, had become the largest global supplier of opium. The Golden Triangle encompasses an area of about 150,000 square miles that runs from western Myanmar up to the Hunan province of China, eastward through Laos and Thailand, and back down to southern Myanmar. By 1986, Laos was reported to be the third-largest supplier of the world's illicit opium, a position it generally held until 2005. In this regard, opium production peaked in Laos at 167 metric tons in 2000, and by 2008, it had declined to 10 metric tons.

By the late 1980s, the government of Myanmar established cease-fire agreements with several drug-trafficking insurgent groups. Thai forces repeatedly clashed with these groups, increasing political tensions in the region and resulting in a series of border closings. China provided training to drug agents from Myanmar and Laos. The United States provided substantial financial resources to Myanmar from 1970 to 1988 in order to combat this massive opium production. This specialized funding to Myanmar was withdrawn in 1988 due to mounting concerns with human rights violations. During the 1970s, international criminal justice efforts to stem the influx of heroin street trafficking focused considerably on the so-called "French connection" that was exposed in Marseilles, France, for the intricate associations that the American Mafia had with Corsican organized crime groups. It is believed that the so-called French connection was established in the 1930s by Jean Jehan, a French criminal, and that the resulting French-Italian drug syndicate supplied, up until the 1970s, about 95% of the heroin available on U.S. streets. It operated by smuggling the raw opium base from Turkey and converting it, usually in laboratories in Marseilles, into heroin; French Corsican gangsters and the Sicilian and American Mafias then smuggled it into the United States. Nevertheless, these high-profile activities did little beyond a temporary lull to put a real dent in international drug trafficking. After the dismantling of the French connection around 1972, opium trafficking and cultivation, as well as heroin and cannabis production, increased in Mexico.

By the 1990s, it was estimated that about 80% of heroin distributed in New York City, for example, had come from Myanmar. However, by the late 1990s, a coalescence of factors including political turmoil in Southeast Asia and adverse weather conditions (that is, a major regional drought), along with international pressure, particularly from the United States and China, led to a substantial decline in opium production in the Golden Triangle. Nevertheless, by 2000, Myanmar was producing about 60% of the world's heroin. At any rate, Myanmar is currently the second-largest producer of opium behind Afghanistan and opium, and related drug use remains rampant in the region. For example, the primary drug problem in Malaysia, which borders Thailand as well as Brunei, Indonesia, and Singapore, is domestic use of heroin and opium. It is estimated that between 1.1% and 1.6% of the population age 15 to 64 in Malaysia use opiate drugs each year; since injection is the most common route of drug administration there, often with unclean hypodermic needles, rates of human immunodeficiency virus (HIV) and hepatitis C infection are exceedingly high, particularly among its prison population. In fact, overland heroin trade routes like those from Myanmar to China and to India have been associated with traceable epidemics of injection drug use and of HIV infection.

The Golden Crescent of Southeast Asia, arching across portions of Afghanistan, Iran, and Pakistan, has also long served as a center of opium production. Large-scale industrial levels of opium production began in 1850 in Iran and continued to be a major source of export revenue until 1955. In the 1920s, Iran established a state-run monopoly that controlled about two-thirds of the opium production in the country. Iran has become has become the world's largest consumer of illicit opiates. By the 1950s, it was reported that 7% to 11% of the Iranian population was addicted to opium. Several bans on opium were imposed, rescinded, and then again reimposed in Iran during the latter half of the 20th century. In 2007, it was reported that 2.8% of the Iranian population consumed an opiate, compared to 0.58% in the United States in the same year. In 1956, Pakistan began licensing farmers in its Northwest Frontier Province to produce opium for its government-run monopoly. The raw opium was processed by the government and sold to registered addicts. Beginning in 1975, heroin laboratories began appearing in Pakistan. Illicit opium production escalated in Pakistan and peaked at 800 metric tons in 1979, when briefly Pakistan was the largest global producer of illicit opium. Pakistan continues to be a major transit country for illicit opium, heroin, and morphine base. However, the region of the Golden Crescent did not become a major player in the worldwide illicit drug market until after the 1979 invasion of Afghanistan by troops of the former Soviet Union. Local Afghan militants known as the *mujaheddin*, heavily subsidized by U.S. aid to help them resist the Soviet invasion, used profits from sales of opium, as well as hashish, to purchase arms and other supplies. By 1980, Afghanistan had become a major supplier of global opium. After the Soviet withdrawal, *mujaheddin* warlords became heavily dependent upon illicit drug trafficking to finance their hostile operations. By 1991, Afghanistan had become the leading global producer of opium. The Taliban regime rose to fill the political vacuum, capturing the capital of Kabul in 1996. By 1999, opium production in Afghanistan reached nearly 5,000 tons. Although initially tolerating opium cultivation, the Taliban banned it in 2000. Nevertheless, the Taliban exploited large reserve stockpiles of opium to gain control of drug trafficking in order to finance their terrorist activities both domestically within Afghanistan and around the globe.

Opium cultivation has never ceased in Afghanistan, and it resurged with the waning of the Taliban. By 2004, Afghanistan had risen to become the producer of three-quarters of the world's opium. By 2007, it is estimated that Afghanistan was supplying 90% of the world's opium. Heroin, as well as cannabis, from neighboring Afghanistan flow heavily into Pakistan, maintaining the dependencies of the estimated 6.7 million drug users and the 4.25 million addicts in the country. It is thought that around half of Afghanistan's illicit opiates are trafficked through its borders with Pakistan. Unfortunately, less than 1% of Pakistani drug abusers have access to intervention and treatment, most of which is provided by private nongovernmental organizations (NGOs). Further, about 70% of those receiving drug treatment in Pakistan relapse back into abuse. Even though drug traffickers caught in Pakistan face the possibility of the country's death penalty, they operate at unprecedented levels such that Pakistan is considered to be the most heroin-addicted country in the world. It is estimated that at least 44 tons of processed heroin is consumed in Pakistan each year, which is two to three times that of the United States and thought to generate about $2 billion annually. Other countries, notably Mexico and Columbia, have more recently come to serve as significant sources of opium for international drug traffickers. In fact, by 1999 about 65% of the U.S. heroin market was being supplied from Colombia. The flow has yet to be stopped, nor will it likely be while there remains high demand.

DEVELOPMENT OF MORPHINE

Before heroin, morphine addiction was recognized as a widespread problem in many countries. Prior to morphine, opium was the primary narcotic abused around the world. Morphine is the primary psychoactive component of opium and a highly addictive substance in its own right.

Morphine is essentially a derivative of the juice of the opium poppy. Morphine constitutes around 10%, by weight, of opium; although the amount varies considerably among different poppy varieties. As pure morphine is not very soluble in water, morphine is usually produced as morphine sulfate, an odorless white crystalline powder that is easier to administer and that tends to become darker when left exposed to light.

Morphine Use

Morphine is an opiate drug that acts specifically on the central nervous system to alleviate pain. In this regard, morphine essentially imitates our endogenous opioids. Morphine analgesia is produced by action at many sites within the central nervous system including both spinal and supraspinal sites, such as the periaqueductal gray matter, by means of the selective inhibition of various nociceptive reflexes; it also has gastrointestinal effects. Morphine analgesia is highly effective against both sensory and affective dimensions of pain. Morphine use also, unfortunately, results in drowsiness, alteration of mood, lessened gastrointestinal motility, diminished breathing, peripheral vasodilatation, and contraction of the pupils; these produce the array of negative side effects experienced by prescription or illicit users. Morphine use, on the other hand, may actually enhance the ability of some individuals to perform certain cognitive functions.

Morphine can be used in many different ways. It was sometimes spread on open wounds. Morphine can be administered orally, through injection, by inhalation, or by means of rectal suppositories, and it is also available as capsules and as extended-release tablets. The rate of onset and the intensity of morphine analgesia are related to the route of administration, being greatest with intravenous injection, although the duration of action is shorter by this method. A morphine-pump can even be implanted in some patients with chronic pain. Morphine is the only opiate that has been approved by the U.S. Food and Drug Administration (FDA) for intrathecal administration. Morphine is sometimes used for epidural injections. It is known that morphine crosses the placenta, and it has also been found in breast milk. Morphine is not indicated for use with patients with acute alcoholism, bronchial asthma, convulsive disorders, delirium tremens, head injury, acute pancreatitis, and renal failure.

Serturner's Isolation

Around 1805, Friedrich Wilhelm Serturner, a German pharmacist, became the first individual to successfully isolate and identify the organic alkaloid compound, morphine, from raw opium, which is basically the gum resin collected from opium poppies. Serturner created a process that used hot water to extract the opium, and then he applied ammonia to precipitate out the bitter crystalline form of morphine. This research paved the way for the subsequent identification of other potentially useful alkaloids, such as strychnine (1818), caffeine (1821), and nicotine (1828), as well as a succession of other opiates. Serturner named his new substance "morphium" after Morpheus, the Greek god of dreams. Ironically, Serturner experimented on himself with morphine and nearly died as a consequence.

Spread of Use

Morphine was available by the 1820s from Merck and from many other pharmaceutical companies scattered across Western Europe. Morphine pills were widely marketed in early-19th-century Europe and in the United States. In 1843, Alexander Wood, a Scottish physician at Edinburgh, discovered that administering morphine by means of hypodermic syringe injection produces a faster and more potent effect. The development in the 1850s of hypodermic syringes with hollow pointed needles, attributed by some to Charles Pravaz and Francis Rynd, permitted the widespread injection use of morphine. Morphine was first used as a remedy for addiction to opium as well as for its antitussive and analgesic effects. There was then little stigma directed against the occasional use of morphine. For instance, on the eve of the Civil War, a proper aristocratic southern lady, such as Mary Boykin Miller Chestnut, could casually note in her diary that she had a morphine bottle to travel with. Heroin, ironically, was first introduced some time later in order to treat addiction to morphine. However, heroin is, in fact, very rapidly metabolized by the body into morphine, essentially by removing the acetyl groups.

Soon after its introduction, as was the case with many other drugs, morphine was enthusiastically acclaimed to be a panacea. Regular use of morphine by soldiers during and after the American Civil War (1861–1865), as well as the subsequent Franco-Austrian (1866) and Franco-Prussian (1870–1871) Wars in Europe, led to the popular notion of morphine addiction being referred to as the "Soldier's disease." In fact, opium and morphine were both widely dispensed during the Civil War, which, particularly facilitated by syringe injection, resulted in dramatic increases subsequently in opiate addiction among veterans. Morphine, ether, and chloroform were the primary anesthetic agents available for military medicine until World War I, when nitrous oxide was added; during the war, morphine tended to be used along with other agents to produce a balanced anesthesia.

In the middle of the 19th century, reports appeared on the use of morphine to treat cases of insanity. Morphine was then being injected to treat myriad mental disorders, including mania and melancholia. However, by the late 19th century, cases of insanity were being attributed to the habitual use of morphine. Nevertheless, there is a considerable history to the use of opiates for treating various psychiatric disorders.

Physicians in the 19th century were, in fact, using morphine to treat an array of conditions. For example, in 1875, morphine was being administered hypodermically for treating puerperal eclampsia. The widespread use of morphine and other substances was among the issues that arose in the heated debates between practitioners of allopathic and other approaches to healing. An advocate of homeopathy, for example, could proclaim in 1885 that: "All cases of morphia disease may be referred to an allopathic initiative" (Ameke, 1885, p. 405). Further, after the middle of the 19th century, physicians were one of the most prominent demographic groups of morphine addicts as they had ready access. At any rate, awareness was also growing at the time of some of the personal and social problems associated with chronic morphine use. In fact, physicians and pharmacists were among the leaders in helping to shape public attitudes and policies toward narcotics. For example, in 1876, the Viennese psychiatrist, Maximilian Leidesdorf, published an influential report on morphine withdrawal.

Opium use was widespread across much of 19th-century America. For instance, in 1858, U.S. Customs Houses reported that about 300,000 lb. of opium were imported, of which it is estimated that around 90% was for recreational use. Opium was routinely administered as a soporific to infants and to soothe teething and other pains in infants. In this vein, the ubiquitous use of opium by all levels of society is indicated by the observance that individuals who conducted the Underground Railroad, like Harriet Tubman, used doses of it to quiet crying babies as they helped runaway slaves escape to the North.

During the 19th century, accordingly, morphine was regularly and freely used in remedies for treating a wide assortment of conditions, including colic, diarrhea, headaches, and menstrual pains. Morphine was also thought to be useful as a cure for treating alcoholics, even though by then it was known to be addictive itself. Morphine addiction was then often referred to as "morphinism" (Stanley, 1915). Physicians and other authorities, as well as society at large, then regarded alcoholism as a condition that was far worse to endure than morphine addiction. Consequently, morphine was commonly used as a component for a diverse array of patent medicines, and it could even be ordered through the mail, as could hypodermic syringes to administer it. Concern with this alarming situation aroused a loud public outcry that eventually led to the passage of the 1906 Pure Food and Drug Act during the second term of Theodore Roosevelt and then of the subsequent Harrison Narcotics Act in 1914 during the first term of Woodrow Wilson. Under the Harrison Narcotics Act, the original intent was mainly to regulate the marketing of morphine and other substances; however, enforcement agents interpreted its vague language to essentially effect a state of general prohibition. Unfortunately, legislative barriers led to the closing of the few drug treatment programs that were even in existence then. For decades after the passage of the Harrison Narcotics Act, there was considerable debate as to whether the narcotic addict should be regarded and dealt with as a criminal or as a medical patient. There was also considerable international pressure to deal with opiate abuse during the early 20th century. Under the International Opium Convention of 1912, for instance, nations agreed that governments should take measures to control morphine and other opium derivatives.

In 1925, the chemical structure of morphine was first elucidated by Robert Robinson at the University of Oxford, and the first synthetic form of morphine was made in 1952 by Marshall Gates at the University of Rochester. Further, hundreds of different compounds have been studied in the search for the as-yet-elusive morphine derivative that is an effective painkiller, but without the highly addictive potential. Morphine has a positive reinforcing effect on behavior both in humans and in laboratory animals. In fact, there is a long history of assessment for abuse potential of opiates and opioids in both humans and laboratory animals.

MODERN ERA

Opium, along with morphine and other opiates, helped in part to usher in the modern era. Some historians have suggested, for example, that the use of the term "hip" originated with early opium smokers who typically laid on one hip while smoking, which tended to produce bruising that helped users identify like-minded individuals. The related term "beat" was also acquired from the slang of addicts who used it to denote being in such a fallen, defeated state as to be beyond the possibility of rehabilitation.

Other Opiates

After Serturner successfully isolated morphine from opium in the early 19th century, efforts continued to isolate and identify other substances from opium and other sources. For instance, codeine, or methyl morphine, was first isolated in 1832 by the French chemist Pierre-Jean Robiquetin. Long-term codeine use has been strongly associated with the development of dependence as well as with depression and depressive symptoms. At any rate, several of the alkaloids contained in opium have been isolated, identified, and used for various purposes. In fact, 44 alkaloids have been isolated from opium. Various methods have been developed to determine the respective alkaloids contained in raw opium.

Morphine, of course, is among the major alkaloids contained in opium. The United States has the highest rate of morphine use in the world, as well as the highest global level of opioid use in general. The United States accounts for 56% of global morphine consumption, while Europe accounts for 28% and Canada for 6%. Elsewhere, the proportion of global morphine consumption is much lower; in Japan, for instance, the rate is 0.80%, while it is 0.02% in Africa. Although morphine is widely used around the world as a painkiller, the annual consumption of morphine is relatively low in many countries, including, as just noted, those in Africa; for example, Malawi is amongst the countries with the lowest morphine consumption rates, ranked 152nd in the world. The annual consumption of morphine is 0.6930782 mg/capita in Malawi. Nevertheless, the annual consumption of morphine per capita is even lower than that of Malawi in many other African nations; for instance, in Burkina Faso, the annual consumption of morphine is 0.000004627 mg/capita, the annual consumption of morphine is 0.011518 mg/capita in Burundi, 0.00277 mg/capita in Cote d'Ivoire, 0.0004226 mg/capita in Eritrea, 0.000285 mg/capita in Ethiopia, 0.071 mg/capita in Ghana, 0.575 mg/capita in Kenya, 0.003416 mg/capita in Lesotho, 0.1561 mg/capita in Madagascar, 0.011237 mg/capita in Mali, 0.004355 mg/capita in Mauritania, 0.440625 mg/capita in Mauritius, 0.24 mg/capita in Namibia, 0.011493 mg/capita in Niger, and 0.0118 mg/capita in Sierra Leone.

Codeine, thebaine, papaverine, and narcotine are among the major alkaloids contained in opium. The pharmacological properties and varied medical applications of these respective opium derivatives have been well examined. Narcotine is the second-most common opium derivative contained in raw opium after morphine. Narcotine, also known as noscapine, is used medically as a central cough suppressant. In addition to being an antitussive, it also has an antitumor agent that could potentially be useful in cancer treatment. Narcotine also has mild local anesthetic properties and does not cause constipation like codeine. Codeine is considered to have less potential than morphine for the development of tolerance and physical dependence. However, at equivalent doses, codeine is more toxic than morphine. In fact, codeine is metabolized into morphine by a cytochrome P-450 dependent process that is highly individualized due to metabolic issues; thus some individuals may metabolize codeine more quickly or slowly than others. Papaverine is a component of opium used medically as a vasodilator, such as for treating impotence by intracavernosal injection; it is also used as an antispasmodic for treating gastrointestinal disorders. Papaverine potentiates the analgesic, or painkiller, effects of morphine. Narceine is a minor component of opium that is occasionally used medically for treating a persistent cough. Narceine has no analgesic effect but has a depressant effect on blood pressure.

Many of these opiate drugs can also be synthesized. Codeine, for instance, although a natural opiate occurring in opium, can also be synthesized by methylation of the 3-hydroxy group of the morphine ring. These developments in the rapidly developing field of alkaloidal chemistry led to the subsequent work on semisynthetic and then synthetic opioids. Some concern has arisen more recently on the potential brewing of opiates with genetically modified yeasts. The microbial synthesis of substances like morphine and codeine and their related derivatives, it has been speculated, may in the near future come to serve as an alternative to traditional plant-based production. However, producing opiates by means of such processes will require highly controlled conditions and extremely specialized skills, for which at present no one has the technical capabilities. Nevertheless, the pharmaceutical industry, as well as illicit drug traffickers, are keenly interested in this potentiality.

Heroin and More

Interestingly, the study of the history of opiates clearly reveals that many substances initially used mainly for medical purposes were subsequently incorporated into decidedly nonmedical uses with commensurate personal and socioeconomic consequences. This was certainly the case with heroin, just as it had been earlier with morphine. In 1874, C. R. Alder Wright, a British chemist working at St. Mary's Hospital Medical School in London, boiled the anyydrous morphine alkaloid in acetic anhydride to acetylate it, and thereby invented the substance diacetylmorphine that was later called heroin. In August 1897, two weeks after he had successfully synthesized a pure and stable form of acetylsalicylic acid, or aspirin, Felix Hoffmann began work on diacetylmorphine, and he also successfully synthesized a stable version of it. The Bayer pharmaceutical company, which employed Hoffmann, coined the name "heroin" for marketing purposes after Heinrich Dreser recognized its commercial potential; the word is derived from the German for heroic, *heroisch*. It was initially thought by pharmaceutical and medical specialists that heroin was not addictive and that it would be useful for the safe treatment of morphine addiction. Heroin was first registered as a trademark in the United States in August 1899. In 1901, Bayer was selling 1-ounce packages of heroin hydrochloride in New York City for $4.85, less for larger quantities. In 1906, Squibb was selling a thousand 10-mg tablets of heroin for $1.20.

Heroin is a semisynthetic opioid, although it is chemically considered to be an opiate; it is produced by adding an acetyl group to morphine. Heroin is rapidly hydrolyzed by the human body into morphine and 6-monoacetylmorphine, or MAM. It is the presence of the acetyl groups that increases the lipid solubility of heroin, permitting more rapid passage across the blood-brain barrier. Fundamentally, the effects of morphine and heroin are similar, except that heroin is faster acting with greater potency. Accordingly, the major pharmacological effects of heroin are dependent upon the formation of morphine and MAM.

Part, at least, of the addictive potential of heroin is due to its pharmacokinetic properties. Specifically, as heroin is fat soluble, it passes through the blood-brain barrier about 100 times faster than morphine passes through. After crossing this lipid barrier, heroin is rapidly broken down and converted to morphine. It then spreads throughout the brain, binding to the respective opioid receptors. Interestingly, the rewarding properties of heroin appear to be dependent upon a dopaminergic neural substrate supporting the concept that both opiates and opioids, as well as other sources of reward, activate a similar process.

There had been concerted efforts by reformers, particularly Protestant missionaries, to prohibit opiate production and abuse. In 1868, for instance, the British Parliament passed the Pharmacy Act, which stipulated that opium could be sold only in pharmacists' shops. The Anglo-Oriental Society for the Suppression of the Opium Trade was formed in Britain in November 1874 for the primary purpose of opposing the opium trade. In 1878, Great Britain passed the Opium Act to regulate the sale and use of opium. In 1905, the U.S. Congress banned opium; in March 1905, the Congress passed a law that declared that as of March 1908, the importation of opium into the Philippines for other than medicinal purposes was banned, and that it was also illegal to sell nonmedical opiates to native Filipinos. In 1906, England and China signed a treaty agreeing to restrict the trading of opium. In 1906, the U.S. Congress passed the Pure Food and Drug Act, which made it illegal to sell medicines or food if the ingredients, particularly including opium, were not clearly stated on the label. In 1908, it became illegal to ship heroin and other drugs from one state to another. In 1909, the U.S. Congress passed the Opium Exclusion Act, which made the importation of opium for nonmedical purposes illegal.

In 1912, 12 nations plus the British Crown overseas territories signed the International Opium Convention, which was the first international drug control treaty. After World War I, the Convention was then incorporated into the Treaty of Versailles and registered with the League of Nations; it was thus effectively ratified by almost 60 nations. The Permanent Central Control Opium Board of the League of Nations supervised the legal international trading of opium, which was actually one of the most successful activities conducted by the League. In 1914, the U.S. Congress passed the Harrison Narcotics Act, which made possession of opiates and opioids without a doctor's prescription illegal, and it further required all doctors, dentists, and pharmacists who prescribed or handled narcotics to register and pay a special tax. In 1923, the Narcotics Division of the U.S. Treasury Department banned all legal sales of narcotics in the United States. These sorts of increased regulatory moves limiting the legal availability of opiates and opioids led to the growth of the black market. During the 1920s and 1930s, most of the illicit heroin smuggled into the United States came from China, usually after having been refined in either Shanghai or Tietsin. It appears to have first emerged in the Chinatown of New York City around 1925.

At any rate, the use of heroin and other similar drugs, even if mostly underground, continued over the next several decades. Prior to the 1950s, heroin was used by a relatively small number of jazz musicians and some Whites. During the 1950s, the use of heroin spread primarily to African American and Hispanic males in urban centers, notably in Harlem, New York City.

By the 1960s, there was a widespread perception of increased illicit drug use. In 1967, for example, it is estimated that there were 108,424 known opiate or opioid users in the United States; of this total, 30,885 reported their first use within that year. Most of the users of heroin and other similar drugs at that time were concentrated in metropolitan centers, unwilling or unable to maintain steady employment, and engaged in criminal activities. Many of them were of either African American, Mexican American, or Puerto Rican ethnic background. However, today's heroin users are somewhat different from those more typical during the 1960s through the early 1990s. For the decade from 2002 to 2012, the number of individuals in the United States who reported use of heroin within the past year rose from about 400,000 to about 665,000, or an increase of 265,000 individuals. Further, over the decade, there was a fourfold increase in the number of fatalities attributable to opiates or opioids, which amounts to almost 17,000 deaths each year from overdoses. Heroin-related overdose fatalities rose 39% between 2012 and 2013, reaching a total of 8,257 deaths; New York City alone had 420 fatal heroin overdoses in 2013. In addition, over 400,000 individuals in this country go to an emergency department each year due to opiate or opioid overdoses.

Today, heroin has reached into suburban communities where it is now often readily available, particularly to those with a cell phone and an automobile. Heroin users today tend to be younger, more affluent, better educated, and whiter than were their predecessors of earlier generations. In addition, the heroin available on the streets today is also often considerably more potent as well as relatively inexpensive compared to that sold on U.S. streets in earlier times. The current prolific availability with respect to heroin and other painkiller drugs in many communities, particularly with regard to the well-understood direct relationship between availability and abuse of respective substances, will in all reasonable likelihood result in even higher levels of painkiller abuse and addiction. A consistent, broadly supported and funded, multi-pronged societal approach to such an issue from education and prevention through to treatment, along with related legislation, regulation, and enforcement initiatives, is clearly called for to reverse these alarming trends.

Illicit Production of Heroin

There are several steps generally used by drug traffickers to produce illicit heroin. The first step is to collect the sap of opium poppies, *Papaver somniferum*. The collected sap is then boiled to produce a sticky gum substance. This gum substance is next soaked in water and then treated with various chemicals, such as a mixture of activated charcoal, ammonium chloride, hydrochloric acid, and lime; this chemical processing separates out morphine from the gum substance. This by-product is then dried and shaped into bricks, which then can be more readily transported or processed further on the spot. The bricks are mixed with an array of substances, typically a mixture of acetylic anhydride, more activated charcoal, and baking soda (i.e., sodium bicarbonate). The resulting mixture is dried and next treated with hydrochloric acid, which produces the pure white powder form of heroin. However, heroin sold on the streets varies considerably in purity; it is typically cut with assorted additives, such as baking soda, powdered cleanser, powdered milk, sugar, laundry detergent, lidocaine, procaine, starch, strychnine, and talc. Some of these adulterants can cause very dangerous side effects. Nevertheless, the purity of heroin sold on the streets today is generally much greater than that sold in previous decades. This fact alone can substantially increase the rate of fatal overdoses.

Other Painkillers

Numerous other opiates and opioids have been discovered or created. Apomorphine, for example, is a derivative of morphine and a potent emetic as well as an agonist for dopamine. Other pharmacological derivatives of morphine include dicodid, dilaudid, and dionin. Many other semisynthetic opioids, such as hydrocodone, hydromorphone, oxycodone, oxymorphone, dihydrodesoxymorphine, nicomorphine, and nalbuphine, were developed and then, in turn, myriad synthetic opioids have also been developed.

In addition to the various opiates or opioids, many other types of painkillers have been used. In the 5th century BC, Hippocrates prescribed the use of extracts of the white willow tree, *Salix alba*, to relieve pain. In 1763, Edward Stone of Oxford University's Wadham College identified salcyclic acid, the active ingredient in aspirin, in willow bark. In 1828, an extract of willow bark was purified by Johan Andreas Bucher; he called it salicin. The chemical structure of salicylic acid was derived in 1859 by Hermann Kolbe at Marburg University in Germany. As a student of Bucher's, Friedrich van Heyden, manufactured salicylic acid in Dresden; however, it irritated the stomachs of users, and many were not able to tolerate its harsh effects. However, other chemists had synthesized a somewhat less toxic formulation of acetylsalicylic acid that was more usable. Acetylsalicylic acid was first synthesized in 1853 by Charles F. Gerhardt, a French chemist, but his laboratory procedure did not produce a pure, stable form of the substance. A reliable process to successfully synthesize a chemically pure and stable form of acetylsalicylic acid was finally developed on August 10, 1897, by Felix Hoffmann; and then, after testing on human subjects, it was marketed as Aspirin by the Bayer pharmaceutical company of Germany beginning in 1899. Aspirin was initially produced as a white powder distributed in glass bottles. One of the first synthetic drugs, it was gentler on the stomach and less bitter than salicylic acid, of which aspirin is an analog. Salsalate, which is marketed under the trade name of Disalcid, is another salicylate painkiller.

Acetaminophen was first synthesized in 1909 by Joseph Freiher von Mering, a German physician; it is referred to as acetaminophen in the United States and Japan, while in most places elsewhere in the world, including the United Kingdom and Australia, it is called paracetamol. Widespread medicinal use of acetaminophen began only after 1949, when its specific mechanism of action was discovered with the realization that the body converts acetaminophen into phenacetin, which previously was a more popular but also more toxic drug.

Meperedine, also known as pethidine, was first synthesized in 1939 by Otto Eisleb, a German chemist, and its painkiller properties were first identified by Otto Schaumann of I. G. Farben, also in Germany. Although meperedine is widely used around the world as a painkiller, it is also often used by heroin addicts when the supply of heroin available on the streets is low. The annual consumption of meperedine is relatively low in many countries; for example, in Burkina Faso, the annual consumption of meperedine is 0.00167 mg/capita; in Burundi, it is 0.300966 mg/capita; in Chad, it is 0.00029 mg/capita; in Eritrea, it is 0.012208 mg/capita; in Ethiopia, it is 0.16131 mg/capita; in Kenya, it is 1.215 mg/capita; in Lesotho, it is 0.8692 mg/capita; in Madagascar, it is 0.0984 mg/capita; in Malawi, it is 2.6147052 mg/capita; in Mauritius, it is 4.132813 mg/capita; in Namibia, it is 2.20 mg/capita; in Niger, it is 0.031624 mg/capita; and in Sierra Leone, it is 0.0041 mg/capita.

Ketobemidone is another potent opioid painkiller drug that was first synthesized in 1942 by Otto Eisleb at I. G. Farbenindustrie at Hoechst, Germany, during World War II. A U.S. patent was issued for ketobemidone in 1949, and it is used mainly in Scandinavian countries, particularly in Denmark; it is listed under the Controlled Substances Act as a Schedule I drug in the United States. Dextromoramide, a potent synthetic opioid painkiller drug, was first discovered by Paul Janssen, a Belgian pharmacologist, in 1956, and it was first marketed in 1957 under the trade name of Palfium; and phenoperidine, another potent opioid painkiller drug, was first synthesized by Jansen in 1957. Dextromoramide and phenoperidine are both listed as Schedule I drugs in the United States.

Ibuprofen was discovered in 1958 by Stewart Adams, John Nicholoson, and Colin Burrows, British research chemists working for Boots Laboratories. A patent was filed for ibuprofen in 1961, and chemical trials were conducted in Edinburgh, Scotland, in 1966. It was first sold, by prescription, as ibuprofen in 1969 in the United Kingdom. In 1983, it was then made available without a prescription for use in the UK, marketed under the brand name of Nurofen; and, in 1984, ibuprofen became available in the United States as an NSAID medication that is marketed under the trade name of Advil. Indomethacin is another NSAID that was introduced in 1963 and that was marketed under various trade names such as Indocin, Indocin SR, Indo-Lemmon, and Indomethagan, all of which are available in the United States only by prescription; but with the introduction of safer alternatives, it has since fallen out of favor.

Research also continued into the development of new synthetic opioids. For instance, in 1960, Paul Janssen synthesized fentanyl for the first time; it was first marketed in 1963 under the trade name of Sublimaze. Janssen and his colleagues at Janssen Pharmaceutica also discovered several fentanyl-related synthetic opioid painkiller drugs, such as carfentanil and sufentanil in 1974 and alfentanil in 1976, the last of which is currently listed as a Schedule II drug in the United States under the Controlled Substances Act. Sufentanil was first marketed in 1979 under the trade name of Sufenta; carfentanil was marketed beginning around 1980 under the trade name of Wildnil; and alfentanil was first marketed in 1983 under the trade name of Rapifen.

Diclofenac is another NSAID medication that was initially developed in 1973 by Ciba-Geigy, which is now known as Novartis; it was first introduced in the UK in 1979 and is an NSAID available only by prescription. Marketed under trade names such as Cataflam and Voltaren, it is also produced in a combination formulation with misoprostol, which is marketed under the trade name of Arthrotec. Naproxen, another NSAID medication, was first released by the FDA in 1976 as a prescription-only painkiller, and it is marketed under various trade names such as Naprosyn, EC-Naproxyn, Naprelan, and Naprapac, the last of which is co-packaged with lansoprazole. In 1980, naproxen sodium, its salt form, was released by the FDA, and it was marketed under the trade name of Anaprox. The FDA subsequently granted approval in June 1994 for the over-the-counter sale of naproxen in low doses, and it is currently marketed under the trade name of Aleve, which is manufactured by Bayer HealthCare.

Numerous other NSAIDs have been developed, manufactured, and marketed. Fenoprofen calcium, for instance, is another NSAID medication that was approved for sale in the United States by the FDA on June 8, 1988, as a prescription-only painkiller, and it was manufactured by Mylan Pharms Inc. as a 600 mg oral tablet that has since been discontinued. It is currently marketed in the United States under the trade names of Nalfon and Nalfon 200 as an oral capsule, which is manufactured by Pedinol Pharmacal Inc.; it is marketed in the UK as Fenopron, which is manufactured by Typharm Limited. Ketorolac is an NSAID medication developed in 1989 by the Syntex Corporation, which is now a wholly owned subsidiary of Roche, and it was first marketed under the trade name of Toradol, which is available only by prescription.

Etodolac is another NSAID medication that is available in the United States only by prescription; the FDA first granted approval for its sale in the United States in January 1991, and it is marketed under trade names like Lodine and Lodine XL, which are manufactured by Almirall Limited, and Eccoxolac, which is manufactured by Meda Pharmaceuticals; it is also currently available in multiple strengths as generic formulations from many companies. Etodolac is sold under many other trade names in many other countries around the world; these include Flancox in Brazil; Etofree, Etova, and Proxym in India; Etopan in Israel; Haipen in Japan; Dualgan in Portugal; Etodin in South Korea; and Etoi in Turkey.

Tolmetin sodium is another NSAID medication that is only available by prescription; it was originally granted approval for sale in the United States on November 27, 1991, and manufactured by Teva as 400 mg oral capsules; a member of the arylakonic acid family of NSAIDs, it is marketed under various trade names such as Tolectin, Tolectin DS, and Tolectin 600. Diflunisal is another NSAID medication that is only available by prescription; it was originally granted approval for sale in the United States on July 31, 1992, and marketed under the trade name of Dolobid, which is manufactured by Teva as a 500 mg oral tablet; the FDA subsequently granted approval for diflunisal on March 8, 2012, for sale as a generic formulation manufactured by Emcure Pharms USA. Oxaprozin, also known as oxaprozinum, is another NSAID medication that was released by the FDA on January 31, 2001, as a prescription-only painkiller and it is marketed under various trade names such as Daypro, Dayrun, and Duraprox; it is manufactured as a 600 mg oral tablet.

Flurbiprofen, another NSAID medication available only by prescription, was first granted approval for sale in the United States by the FDA on June 20, 1994; it is marketed under trade names like Ansaid, which is manufactured by Pfizer, and as Froben, which is manufactured by Abbott. A flurbiprofen sodium formulation in a solution as eye drops was granted approval by the FDA for ophthalmic use.

Capsaicin and related capsaicinoids are, as mentioned previously, used in various topical formulations for the relief of minor pain and have actually been used for a considerable period of time, particularly in the pre-Columbian Americas, as chili peppers. Chili peppers were first domesticated over 6,000 years ago in Mexico. On Christopher Columbus's second voyage to the New World in 1493, a physician, Diego Alvarez Chanca, obtained chili peppers and was the first to bring them to Spain; in 1494, he wrote of their medicinal effects. In the 16th century, Portuguese traders brought the chili pepper to Asia, where it became widely used for culinary as well as medicinal purposes. In 1816, the compound capsaicin, in an impure crystalline form, was first extracted from chili peppers by Christian Friedrich Bucholz, who named it "capsicin." In 1876, John Clough Thresh isolated it in its pure form. In 1919, E. K. Nelson determined its chemical composition, and in 1930, it was first synthesized by Ernst Spath and Stephen F. Darling. Studies of capsaicin as a painkiller have yielded promising results for treatment of neuropathic pain, pain associated with fibromyalgia, post-therapeutic neuralgia, and pain associated with musculoskeletal disorders; it continues to be widely used today as a painkiller medication.

Piroxicam is yet another NSAID medication that was approved by the FDA on July 31, 1992, as a prescription-only painkiller of the oxicam family of NSAIDs and that was manufactured by Mylan and produced in 10 mg and 20 mg oral tablets; it is marketed under the trade name of Feldene, which is manufactured by Pfizer, but it is also marketed under many other trade names including Arantil, Feldan, Feldene, Flamoxin, Hawksone, Lubor, Remox,

Veral, and Vurdon. In Scandinavian countries piroxicam is marketed as Brexidol; in India, it is marketed under the trade name of Dolonex; in Thailand, it is marketed under the trade name of Fasden, in China, it is available as a patch that is marketed under the trade name of Trast. It is also marketed under the trade name of Roxam, which is manufactured by Bosnalijek and is available in Eastern Europe, including in Russia, and is also available in Africa and the Middle East.

There are far more numerous other substances that have been developed and identified as having painkiller properties than could be adequately covered in any one text. Nevertheless, further examination of some of those already mentioned and many additional other painkillers will be attempted in the remainder of this work. More thorough consideration of the external conditions under which respective painkillers were discovered or developed—that is, the factors that shaped their genesis and production—can be highly illuminating. In fact, the exegetical value of such studies seems indubitable, for they can only lead us to a deeper understanding and a fuller knowledge of these and related substances. Later chapters will take up these types of considerations, but first it would be highly advantageous to examine some of the science behind these painkiller drugs, including their effects and applications. As a general rule, these sorts of studies presuppose as complete an identification of the pharmacology of respective painkillers. Accordingly, we will next explore how respective painkiller drugs work.

DOCUMENT: "BAYER'S PHARMACEUTICAL SPECIALITIES"

An advertisement for "Bayer's Pharmaceutical Specialities" was published in the 19th century in the British Medical Journal. *Friedrich Bayer's pharmaceutical company, Farbenfabriken of Elberfeld, Germany, developed, manufactured, marketed, and sold heroin alongside its other products, including aspirin. Heroin was promoted and touted thus, as in this illustration: "Heroin has given excellent results in cases of bronchitis, pharyngitis, ..." Heroin, in fact, was introduced to the market as a powerful "heroic" panacea, as its name implies. It was, for a brief time at least, even thought to be nonaddictive and hailed as a remedy for myriad conditions. It was also mistakenly asserted that heroin "does not cause constipation," which, of course, is now recognized as a serious undesired side effect for users of heroin. Heroin, described in the advertisement as the "Di-acetic ester of morphia," was actively marketed, prescribed, and distributed for some time to many unsuspecting individuals until the reality of its highly addictive potential was more fully recognized.*

BAYER'S

Pharmaceutical Specialities.

Trional
(Diethylsulphon Methylethan).

THE most reliable of the hypnotics. Acts quickly and surely, and is not attended by any secondary effects. The sleep produced by Trional is as calm and refreshing as the natural one; it is deep and dreamless, and the patient awakes without showing the least sign of drowsiness. In small doses, Trional prevents the night sweats of Phthisis.

IN simple insomnia TRIONAL will produce sleep in from 15 to 30 minutes with absolute certainty.

DOSE.—15 to 30 grains, followed by a hot drink. A good method of administration is in the form of Palatinoids (Messrs. Oppenheimer, Son & Co., 179, Queen Victoria Street, E.C.), or in the form of Oxy-Carbonated Trional Water (manufactured by Messrs. Cooper & Co., 80, Gloucester Road, S.W.).

Lycetol
(Tartrate of Dimethyl Piperazine).

THE best product yet introduced in the treatment of the uric acid diathesis. Combines the acknowledged uric acid solvent properties of Piperazine with the diuretic properties of Tartaric Acid.

INCREASES considerably the alkalinity of the blood.

DOSE.—16 to 32 grains daily. Best administered either in effervescing form (Effervescing Lycetol, Messrs Bishop & Sons, Ltd., Spelman Street, E.), or in the form of Oxy-Carbonated Lycetol Water (Messrs. Cooper & Co., 80, Gloucester Road, S.W.).

Salophen
(Acetyl para Amidosalol).

INVALUABLE IN INFLUENZA.

A PERFECT substitute for salicylate of sodium, as it acts quite as promptly, but without producing any of the unpleasant after effects so frequently attending the use of this drug. Its action is sure and quick.

ABSOLUTELY non-toxic. Specially indicated in acute articular rheumatism, sciatica, chorea, migraine, and neuralgia.

DOSE.—16 grains, three or four times a day, in powder or in the form of lozenges.

Heroin
(Di-acetic ester of Morphia).

AN excellent substitute for Codeine. In doses of 5 milligrammes Heroin has given excellent results in cases of bronchitis, pharyngitis, catarrh of the lungs, and in asthma bronchiale. In the latter two cases the dose may be increased to 1 centigramme.

HEROIN does not cause constipation. Its dose is much smaller than that of morphine. Heroin can be administered to patients with a weak heart who cannot tolerate morphine. It is best given in the form of powder, mixed with sugar, or may be dissolved in brandy or water accidulated by the addition of a few drops of acetitic acid.

TANNIGEN, TANNOPINE, IODOTHYRINE, CREOSOTAL (Pure Carbonate of Creosote), DUOTAL (Pure Carbonate of Guaiacol), ARISTOL, EUROPHEN, PROTARGOL, PHENACETINE-BAYER, SULPHONAL-BAYER, PIPERAZINE-BAYER, ANALGEN, LOSOPHAN, TETRONAL, SOMATOSE, IRON SOMATOSE, MILK SOMATOSE, &c.

Samples and Literature may be had on application to—

THE BAYER CO., Ltd., 19, ST. DUNSTAN'S HILL, LONDON, E.C.
ALSO AT MANCHESTER, BRADFORD. AND GLASGOW.

Wellcome Images

Source: Wellcome Image Library: http://wellcomeimages.org/

DOCUMENT: "PERRY DAVIS' PAINKILLER"

An advertisement for "Perry Davis' Painkiller" was published in the 19th century in The Chemist and Druggist. *This advertisement claimed that this product was "The Oldest, Best, and most Widely Known Family Medicine in the world." However, no mention was made as to its contents, which was typical for the marketing of proprietary patent medicines. Another common ploy used was to make fantastic claims as to the efficacy of these products. This advertisement claimed that "Perry Davis' Painkiller" would cure "Weak Nerves . . . Painful Nerves . . . Shaky Nerves . . . Depressed Nerves . . . Debilitated Nerves . . . Sleeplessness . . . Tremulous Nerves. . . Painful Headache . . . Painful Neuralgia" and so forth; rather impressive, perhaps, but unsubstantiated claims. The production and use of patent medicines like "Perry Davis' Painkiller" facilitated the widespread administration of potent painkillers, particularly opium, morphine, and codeine, to uninformed consumers. However, most of these proprietary products like "Perry Davis' Painkiller" did not openly declare the nature of their contents. Accordingly, many individuals were giving these drugs to their loved ones, including children, often completely unaware of the dangers. Recognition of these pernicious phenomena led to widespread public outcries that stimulated reforms, such as that embodied in the Pure Food and Drug Act.*

Source: Wellcome Image Library: http://wellcomeimages.org/

Chapter 4

How Painkillers Work

Adequate control of pain is a laudable and very worthwhile goal around the world. Unfortunately, lack of appropriate pain management has created one of the most urgent health problems in the United States and globally as well. There are many different types of pain, both acute and chronic. Accordingly, there are varied methods available to assess an individual's pain. Pain, in a most fundamental sense, is an issue of neurotransmission. Different painkiller drugs address pain at the cellular level by means of respective mechanisms of action.

WHAT IS PAIN?

Pain serves as a warning system to alert the body to potentially dangerous injuries or situations. Pain, accordingly, is part of the body's way of protecting itself from injury and other damage. Biologically, pain serves to warn us of impending harm to the body that requires action to avoid. Pain is strictly defined as the unpleasant sensory and/or emotional experiences associated with actual or potential damage to bodily tissues. Pain, in fact, adversely affects more Americans than all cancers, heart disease, and diabetes combined.

Pain has a substantial emotional component. How we feel about a particular pain sensation is to some degree at least mediated by our personal and cultural repertoire of experiences and resources. The degree of disruption, if any, resulting from a particular painful situation experienced is highly variable among different individuals. Our own individualized emotional and psychological well-being can, of course, influence how well we are able to cope with any respective challenge. Suffering and misery are, after all is said and done, fundamentally cognitive constructs that are products of our minds.

There are also profound cultural dimensions to pain. What is perceived of as painful, for example, or how to appropriately deal with a painful situation, or even when and how to describe a pain sensation, are all culturally learned patterns of behavior. However, not everyone in any specific culture, of course, conforms to a rigid set of expected pain beliefs or behaviors.

There are different theories to explain pain. One of these, the pattern theory, suggests that pain results from a pattern of intense neuron activity encoding the pain sensation. The gate theory, on the other hand, which was originally proposed by Ronald Melzack and Patrick David Wall, suggests that the spinal cord receives messages not only from the pain receptors, but also from other sensory neurons, as well as getting descending signals going through centrifugal pathways outward from the brain. These competing messages might block the gate, it is speculated, so that an incoming pain message cannot get through; this theory has been used, for example, to explain how acupuncture works with the signals from the acupuncture needles blocking other pain messages from reaching the brain. These and other theories about pain are not mutually exclusive but are, in fact, compatible and can potentially help explain different aspects of pain.

Acute Pain

Pain varies along the dimension of the time of duration. Acute pain is the short-acting type and generally lasts for just a few seconds, minutes, hours, days, or, at most, weeks. Acute pain signals are transmitted along A-delta nerve fibers, which are insulated with myelin so that the messages can be transmitted rapidly. These fibers seem to signal the occurrence of an injury along with its location and extent. The fast pain signals are transmitted through the A-delta nerve fibers that end in the dorsal horn of the spinal cord, where they cross synapses to stimulate dendrites of neurons of the neospinothalmic tract. These neurons cross through the anterior white commissure and ascend contra-laterally; they transmit signals through the ventrobasal complex of the thalamus to the somatosensory cortex.

Acute pain is that type of pain that occurs suddenly and then dissipates after the underlying cause is eliminated. Acute pain, accordingly, serves as a mechanism for protection and survival, since the natural reaction of any healthy being is to try to avoid harmful circumstances that triggered the pain sensations. Perhaps the clearest example is that we will tend to automatically pull our hands away from a hot object, which often helps us to avoid serious burns.

Acute pain is generated rapidly and then is suddenly gone when the underlying trigger ceases. It thus serves a useful biological service of self-preservation, since the natural reaction is to avoid dangerous circumstances if possible. The most primitive pain response occurs as a reflex. Perhaps the clearest example is that we will automatically pull our foot away from a sharp object stepped on, which often helps us to avoid serious damage. The nociceptors in the sole of the foot send a pain message to the spinal cord, which sends a message back to the muscles that bend the foot and cause it to instantly withdraw from contact with the sharp object. This reflexive response happens very quickly, even before the pain signal reached the brain, and thus there is not even any cognitive awareness of the pain. There tends to be less of an emotional component associated with acute pain incidents. Acute pain thus tends to be tuned on and then, once the stimulus stops, turned off equally fast.

Chronic Pain

Chronic pain persists over time from months, years, or even over a lifetime. Chronic pain often worsens and intensifies over time. Chronic pain signals are carried over C nerve fibers, which transmit dull, chronic aches and burning sensations. C nerve fibers are unmyelinated, which allows them to transmit slower pain messages. Slow pain signals are transmitted through these C nerve fibers to the second and third laminae of the dorsal horns of the spinal cord, which is also referred to as the *substantia gelatinosa*. The signals then pass through the fifth lamina of the dorsal horn, crossing through the anterior white commissure ascending contra-laterally to the brain stem, some terminating in the thalamus and others to the medulla, the pons, and the periaqueductal gray of the midbrain tectum. Painkillers can mediate the intensity of these pain signals in several ways, such as by modifying them as they cross through the periaqueductal gray matter before they reach the thalamus, and are consciously perceived.

Evidence suggests that chronic pain is associated with a dysregulation of descending pain modulation. In this view, disruption of the balance of descending pain modulatory circuits is being implicated in the development and maintenance of chronic pain. It is thought that the higher cortical and subcortical centers of the brain that control emotional, motivational, and cognitive processes may communicate directly with the descending modulatory circuits, which would provide a more mechanistic explanation of how various exogenous factors can facilitate the development of chronic pain in susceptible individuals.

Chronic pain might have begun with an injury, like a sprained ankle, or from an ongoing condition, like arthritis or cancer. Some of the common types of chronic pain include chronic neck, back, and shoulder pain; chronic knee, hip, and joint pain; chronic muscle pain; central pain syndrome; and carpal tunnel syndrome. Unfortunately, in chronic pain, the individual's nervous system adapted to a situation that began with signals triggered by a certain condition or event, but that even after that initial condition or event was corrected, the pain signals are still being transmitted. It is estimated that about 116 million Americans currently suffer from chronic pain, but that only about 25% of them receive appropriate treatment.

There are several different ways by which the body creates chronic pain. Repetition of a specific painful experience can create a central sensitization, whereby the nervous system achieves a heightened sensitivity. With such a conditioned heightened sensitivity, even a normal stimuli can provoke an abnormal pain response. Damage to the nerves in our extremities can result in peripheral nerve pain, which heightens the sensitivity of the nociceptors, which are discussed immediately below. The sympathetic nervous system, which normally responds to emergencies with a flight-or-fight response, can become overstimulated, and the resulting hypersensitivity can produce chronic feelings of pain. Chronic pain can be debilitating and interfere with sleep, even leading to depression.

Chronic pain appears to enhance depressive symptoms and may also reduce motivation. It is speculated that a protein that normally aids in neuronal transmission, galanin, influences the brain's reward circuitry in the nucleus accumbens during episodes of chronic pain. The nucleus accumbens is situated in the ventral base of the forebrain and has been implicated in motivation, rewards, and addiction, particularly with respect to learning to predict pleasurable experiences. Experiencing greater levels of distress during an acute pain episode seems to result in higher levels of galanin produced, which increases the likelihood that it will evolve into chronic pain.

Management of chronic pain is typically intended not necessarily to eliminate the pain entirely, but rather to be able to have a good quality of life while managing the pain at a more tolerable level. Use of both over-the-counter and prescription painkillers, as well as of alternative and complementary medical techniques, are some of the common ways used by individuals to try to better manage these chronic pain feelings. For instance, Mindfulness Based Stress Response (MBSR) meditation techniques are sometimes recommended for those afflicted with chronic pain. Central pain results from a lesion in the central nervous system and typically involves the spinalthalamic cortical pathways, such as occurs in a thalamic infarct; the pain sensations are usually constant and are very resistant to painkiller treatment. Physicians and other health care providers in the medical community need to diligently monitor the dosages and effects of opiate or opioid use to assure that they are providing effective relief from chronic pain, but that they are not being abused. There is a general consensus that opiates and opioids prescribed and used in low and stable doses, at least for short-term purposes, can be safe and effective. In fact, some evidence even suggests that increasing the dose of opiates or opioids too much and too soon can have adverse effects not only of significantly increasing the likelihood of dependence, but also of reducing the pain relief and functioning.

Nociceptive Pain

Nociception is an instantaneous, intense perception of pain. The term "nociception" was coined in a 1906 medical text written by Charles Scott Sherrington and was created to distinguish between the physiological processes of nervous activity and the subjective experience of feeling pain. Nociception, as it is now understood, produces various autonomic responses in the body, and it may also create a subjective experience in the individual. Nociceptive pathways produce trails of action potentials when intensely stimulated. The frequency of the firing of the neurons will determine the intensity of the nociceptive pain.

Nociceptors are specialized types of neurons that change harmful stimuli into electrical energy. Nociceptors, more specifically, are specialized peripheral terminal branches of sensory nerve fibers that are sensitized to respond to noxious stimuli. The electrical energy of the signal is transmitted along the pain neural pathway, through the spinal cord, and then finally up to the brain. Nociceptive pain appears to activate the hippocampus, amygdala, basal ganglia, cerebellum, thalamus, somatosensory cortices, prefrontal cortex, frontal cortex, and anterior cingulate cortex.

Nociceptors are found in many different types of body tissues, like the skin, muscles, tendons, and subcutaneous tissue. However, the nociceptors are not evenly distributed throughout the human body. The skin, for example, contains far more nociceptors than internal structures; similarly, the eyes contain many more than the arms or legs. The different types of nociceptors include the cutaneous ones, which are situated in the skin; the somatic ones, which are located in the joints and in the bones; and the visceral ones, which are within some, but not all, of the internal body organs. More specifically, the nociceptors found in the epidermis of the skin are referred to as Meissner corpuscles, while those located in subcutaneous tissues are known as Pacinian corpuscles. Nociceptors are activated by tissue damage resulting from intense mechanical stimulation, such as occurs from pinching or crushing part of the body; from intense chemical stimulation, such as from exposure to an acidic substance; and from intense thermal stimulation, such as from heat or cold.

The signals from these nociceptors can stimulate the transmitting neurons to release the excitatory neurotransmitter glutamate.

It takes a fairly high stimulus threshold to elicit a nociceptive pain sensation. Consequently, nociceptive pain is fundamentally adaptive in that it helps prevent or at least lessen damage to bodily tissues. In this type of pain, the switch is rapidly turned on in reaction to the noxious or unpleasant stimulus, and then turned off again quickly as the stimulus is removed.

Inflammatory Pain

Inflammatory pain is produced when bodily tissues become damaged and swollen. This type of pain has a relatively low stimulus threshold; once swelling occurs, the inflammatory pain receptors generate a pain sensation signal. Unfortunately, inflammatory pain signals tend to hypersensitize the central nervous system, priming the nerves in the spinal cord and brain to be overactive, and this amplifies the transmission of other pain signals transmitted over these pathways. In this sense, inflammatory pain is nonadaptive as it can result in the perception of higher levels of pain than would otherwise be the case.

Inflammatory pain happens abruptly in response to an assault on the integrity of bodily tissues at the cellular level. The inflammatory response is part of the body's innate immune system response. The precipitating cause can be things like arthritis, autoimmune disorders, burns, extreme cold, fractures, infections, penetration wounds, and vasoconstriction. Some common types of inflammatory pain conditions include arachnoiditis, which is associated with inflamed tissues that surround the spinal cord; and inflammatory bowel disease, which is often associated with Crohn's disease and ulcerative colitis, and it principally affects the colon and small intestine.

The initial stage of inflammation is irritation, which triggers the actual inflammation in an attempt to protect the damaged area and to initiate the healing process. The inflammation is followed by the discharging of pus or suppuration, which, in turn, is followed by granulation to surround the damage and close any open wound. There is both acute inflammation and chronic inflammation.

Acute inflammation can be associated with conditions like appendicitis, bronchitis, meningitis, sinusitis, and tonsillitis. Acute inflammation begins within seconds of the triggering stimulus. The arterioles, which branch out from the arteries to the capillaries, dilate, which results in increased blood flow. As the capillaries become more permeable, fluids and blood proteins accumulate in the interstitial spaces between cells. The primary mediators of acute inflammation are the eicosanoids and the vasoactive amines. Neutrophils, a type of white blood cell that is a granulocyte, are released into the interstitial spaces where the damage occurred; they release enzymes from their vesicles to break down any microorganisms or other foreign matter. If parasites or worms are part of the cause, then eosinophils are sent to respond to their threat. Basophils aid in the inflammatory response as well. Edema, or swelling, follows as fluids build up in the interstitial spaces. This can result in immobility and some loss of function. Increased blood flow to the area produces redness and heat to promote the healing process. Acute inflammation is generally of short duration, typically only lasting a few days ending with resolution.

Chronic inflammation can result if an acute inflammation incident does not successfully end in resolution. This can be the result of various conditions, including infection with certain kinds of viruses, the persistent pressure of foreign bodies not removed in a timely manner, the presence of nondegradable pathogens creating continued inflammation, or an overactive immune system response. Chronic inflammation can lead to the development of atherosclerosis, asthma, cancers, hay fever, hepatitis, peptic ulcer, periodontis, rheumatoid arthritis, or tuberculosis. The major types of cells involved in chronic inflammation are the fibroblasts, lymphocytes, macrophages, and plasma cells. The primary mediators of chronic inflammation are the cytokines, the hydrolytic enzymes, growth factors, and reactive oxygen species. Chronic inflammation can last in duration from several months to years. The outcomes of chronic inflammation usually include thickening and scarring of connective tissue, known as fibrosis; the destruction of tissue; and the death of cells or tissue, referred to as necrosis.

COX enzymes activate prostaglandins and leukotrienes, which produce the swelling effects. Consequently, NSAIDs, such as aspirin, ibuprofen, and naproxen, are the preferred painkillers for treating inflammatory pain as they help reduce inflammation and swelling. Immune selective anti-inflammatory derivatives (ImSAIDs) are a group of peptides that also have anti-inflammatory properties and that may, in the future, be approved for human use; however, they are not, strictly speaking, painkillers. Some herbs, such as ginger, hyssop, and turmeric, also have anti-inflammatory properties, and their use, along with NSAIDs, may be helpful in reducing inflammation.

For treating pain associated with inflammatory arthritic conditions, such as ankylosing spondylitis, lupus, psoriatic arthritis, and rheumatoid arthritis, a combination of multiple drugs is typically recommended, usually including NSAIDs and other painkillers. Methotrexate is often recommended as a disease modifying antirheumatic drug; however, it may take several weeks before the inflammation is sufficiently reduced to lessen pain.

In an inflammatory pain situation, precursor substances are flooded to the affected area, but unfortunately, they are also carried by blood vessels to other areas of the body that can hypersensitize them. Thus inflammatory pain can become self-perpetuating and stimulate more widespread inflammation, which, in turn, results in its own associated inflammatory pain sensations.

Dysfunctional Pain

Dysfunctional pain is troubling as it is completely useless and serves no productive purpose. It is actually maladaptive and lacking in any redeeming values. There are selected health problems, such as irritable bowel syndrome, fibromyalgia, and certain types of headaches that manifest with dysfunctional pain sensations, but lack, as far as we can presently tell, any specific external pain stimulus.

Complex regional pain syndrome is a severe type of debilitating body pain that can occur after an injury to a limb or other body part. Large areas of the limb or other body part can become excruciatingly painful, even virtually untouchable, such that a small air draft can even be difficult to tolerate. In this syndrome, the brain appears to develop abnormal neuroplasticity where it retains the memories of the traumatic injury along with the associated pain sensations. Further, analysis of the blood of individuals suffering with complex regional pain syndrome revealed that it contained higher levels of autoantibodies, specific immune substances that seem to bind to peripheral tissues to cause pain sensations, perhaps by making sensory nerves in the impacted area misfire. These autoantibodies seem to be activated by trauma-induced inflammation.

Trigeminal neuralgia, also known as *tic douloureux*, is another debilitating condition that is characterized by intermittent, shooting pain in the face, usually on one side of the jaw or cheek. Antiseizure drugs such as carbamazepine, originally granted FDA approval in August 1986 and marketed as Tegretol, or gabapentin, originally granted FDA approval in September 2003 and marketed as Neurontin, are commonly used to treat trigeminal neuralgia. Other antiseizure medications, such as clonazepam, originally granted FDA approval in September 1996 and marketed as Klonopin; or divalproex sodium, originally granted FDA approval in July 2008 and marketed as Depakote, are sometimes coadministered with painkillers to enhance their effectiveness; as well as use of some antidepressants. Any of these strategies may help achieve pain relief for this condition.

Neuropathic Pain

Neuropathic pain, also known as deafferenation, is caused by injury to nerves or by nerves that are not functioning as they should, and as a consequence, it is one of the most difficult types of pain to understand and treat. Unlike somatic pain caused by injury to specific tissues, which tends to be highly localized; visceral pain caused by stimulation of pain fibers in some internal organs, usually in the abdomen or chest, such as that associated with gall bladder disease, pancreatitis, or peptic ulcers; and referred pain, which usually originates in a visceral organ but is felt elsewhere, individuals suffering from neuropathic pain often use terms like "burning," "electric-like," or "shooting" to describe their pain sensations. Referred pain, by the way, has been speculated to result from the spinal convergence of visceral and somatic afferent nerve fibers of spinothalamic neurons and can manifest as autonomic hyperactivity, hyperalgesia, or muscular contractions. Deafferentation occurs from the loss of afferent input to the central nervous system. It can arise either from the periphery, such as in peripheral nerve avulsion, or from within the central nervous system, such as happens in multiple sclerosis or from spinal cord lesions. The cause of neuropathic pain is not always completely understood, but it can often be traced to specific types of nerve damage or to a particular disease.

Neuropathic pain is commonly seen in individuals with cancers whose tumors have invaded nerve bundles, such as occurs in diabetic neuropathy or in shingles associated with *Herpes zoster*. There is also an HIV-related neuropathy as well as that related to exposure to toxins, including alcohol, arsenic, and thallium. Several other types of neuropathies are associated with respective disorders, such as Fabry's disease and Guillain-Barre syndrome, which can manifest via neuropathic pain. Damage from carpal tunnel syndrome, chronic alcoholism, kidney disorders, degenerative disk disease, and sciatica can also manifest as neuropathic pain.

Mechanisms of neuropathic pain include both noninflammatory states and inflammatory states. Peripheral neuropathic events can be complicated by either short-term or long-term central nervous system changes, such as central sensitization, and then also by reorganization of the pain pathways at the level of the dorsal horn. Sympathetic efferent activity can, at least in part, sustain neuropathic pain; this activity could be the result of expression of alpha-adrenergic receptors on damaged C nerve fibers, essentially messages sent from abnormal nociceptors.

Selected painkiller drugs are given specifically for managing neuropathic pain, such as that associated with complications of diabetes, fibromyalgia, rheumatoid arthritis, sciatica, and reflex sympathetic dystrophy. These specific neuropathic painkillers include amitriptyline, duloxetine, gabapentin, and pregabalin. Amitriptyline hydrochloride, which is marketed with trade names such as Elavil or Endep, is generally used as an antidepressant and was originally granted approval for such in September 1997; but at low doses, it can be used for neuropathic pain caused by arthritis or fibromyalgia. The starting dosage for amitriptyline is usually 5 to 10 mg, with doses gradually increased; the maximum recommended daily dosage is 50 to 75 mg. Some of the most common side effects associated with the use of amitriptyline include drowsiness and a dry mouth. Use of amitriptyline should be avoided in individuals with heart rhythm problems and those with certain forms of glaucoma. Duloxetine hydrochloride, another antidepressant that was originally granted FDA approval in 2004, is marketed by Eli Lilly and Company as Cymbalta, and is also available in several generic formulations, is sometimes used for treating diabetic neuropathy or fibromyalgia, for which use it was granted FDA approval in June 2008. The most common side effects associated with the use of duloxetine are dizziness, sleepiness, and weight gain. Gabapetin, marketed under various trade names such as Fanatrex, Gabarone, Gralise, Neurontin, Nepentin, and Neogab, was initially developed as an anticonvulsant drug synthesized to mimic the chemical structure of the endogenously produced neurotransmitter gamma-aminobutyric acid (GABA) to treat epilepsy; it is now also commonly used to manage neuropathic pain, such as that approved in 2004 by the FDA for treating postherpetic neuralgia associated with an outbreak of shingles. Pregabalin was designed by Richard Bruce Silverman of Northwestern University to be more potent than gabapentin, and as such, is another drug originally developed as an anticonvulsant medication, but that is subsequently now used for managing neuropathic pain; it is also sometimes used for treating generalized anxiety disorder. Pregabalin is considered to have a limited liability for dependence and thus a low potential for abuse; it is accordingly currently listed as a Schedule V drug by the FDA, and it is marketed by Pfizer as Lyrica, which was initially approved by the FDA in December 2004 for treating epilepsy but also for postherpetic neuralgia and diabetic neuropathic pain. It has been available on the U.S. market since the fall of 2005, and it was approved in June 2007 as a treatment for fibromyalgia.

Traditional painkillers, such as the opiates and opioids, are also used for managing neuropathic pain. However, higher opiate and opioid doses are often needed for neuropathic pain compared to nociceptive pain. Buprenorphine appears to have a distinct benefit in controlling symptoms of neuropathic pain due to differences in its specific pharmacological profile. Buprenorphine was first approved for use in the United States by the FDA on October 8, 2002, and is listed as a Schedule III narcotic, which means that it has an abuse potential but can still be legally prescribed as a medication; it has a rather wide margin of safety and a relatively long duration of action, serving as a partial agonist at the mu receptors and an antagonist at the kappa receptors. Buprenorphine has a high safety profile as it causes less respiratory depression and carries less risk of overdose than do full mu agonist painkiller drugs such as morphine, heroin, methadone, and oxycodone. Sustained release formulations, including transdermal preparations, appear to have even greater patient compliance. Further, slow dose titration seems to help reduce the incidence of some typical adverse events, like nausea and vomiting.

Pain Assessment

Pain assessment has always generated a myriad array of issues of concern. These issues include those related to the purpose of assessment and the way in which it is to be conducted. Psychometric issues of concern include those of reliability and validity, particularly with respect to the selection of pain assessment instruments.

Pain assessment involves the orderly collection of data that reflects the health status of the individual. Assessment is the initial phase in helping an individual with pain concerns to understand treatment options and to eventually realize their full potential. The client is understood to be the primary source of data and should be informed of his or her mutual roles and responsibilities in the assessment process. By definition, pain assessment is a comprehensive and interdisciplinary review of a person's behavioral, cognitive, emotional, and other abilities in relationship to the functional demands of the environments in which they are expected to participate. These collaborative assessments include social, educational, and vocational evaluations, among others, to develop a holistic but also individualized plan of pain treatment and rehabilitation. Understood as a comprehensive process within an ecological paradigm, pain assessment should focus on the individual's ability to function as an independent actor in the community, family, school, vocational, and other situations without undue suffering. A pain assessment, in this strictest sense, should endeavor to provide an overall picture of the individual, consisting of both abilities and deficits of that individual. Unfortunately, however, in practice we all too often focus on the dysfunctions and limitations of an individual.

An important aspect of pain assessment rests in the way that the health care professional approaches individuals and, hopefully, is able to form a therapeutic relationship based on a sense of mutual trust and rapport. This should minimally include being nonjudgmental, being willing to listen, and maintaining an openness toward other opinions. It may also be quite helpful to be flexible and, if needed, to be willing to meet at different places and at irregular times. Active listening and creating an atmosphere of professional confidence can be very useful in conducting a pain assessment. Getting the individual involved to actively engage in the pain assessment process is extremely crucial to being able to obtain meaningful results.

Any method of pain assessment involves selecting some method of observation that enables us to collect relevant information on the individual. We then analyze and interpret this data to produce some understanding of the individual and his or her condition. This gives us the opportunity to then make predictions about how that individual might function under particular circumstances, including participation in a specific pain treatment regimen. Pain assessment instruments are one of the most typical tools used to quantitatively measure an individual and his or her level and severity of pain, and then to thereby attempt to estimate the scale or size of the problem, if in fact there is any.

The purpose, intended target population, administrative options, and psychometric properties are some of the issues to consider in the selection of specific pain assessment instruments. The sensitivity and specificity of specific pain assessment instruments vary, and any can generate either false negative or false positive results. In addition, the purpose of a specific pain assessment instrument is unfortunately often ignored by health care practitioners in its application. A common misuse is to employ a screening instrument for the purposes of diagnosis. In a similar manner, diagnostic instruments have sometimes been used for clinical research studies. Clearly, the use of a pain assessment instrument should be consistent with its intended purpose. However, if used appropriately, such tools can reduce bias on the part of clinicians during pain assessment.

In selecting a pain assessment instrument, it is essential to consider its suitability for a given individual with respect to the intended target population. Many instruments developed for and on adult populations have been administered to adolescents and children. A related issue is whether there are norms available to compare the performance of a given person to that of a sufficiently relevant, large group of comparable individuals. The ethnic background and other demographic characteristics of an individual must also be considered in evaluating whether appropriate normative information is available, which could seriously affect the interpretation of a score on a particular pain assessment instrument, as well as perhaps influence the choice of pain treatment recommended. Further, no single specific pain assessment instrument has been shown to be appropriate for use with all possible populations.

Administrative options that may or may not be available with the use of a respective pain assessment instrument must also be examined. Alternative administration procedures include written self-reports, interviews, computer administered, and collateral inquiry formats, such as via a spouse or significant other; some of these approaches have demonstrated greater engagement of clients in the pain assessment process as well as heightening the accuracy of responses. Some assessment instruments require substantial training for proper administration as well as for interpretation of the results. Related issues of concern with the use of these types of pain assessment instruments are the availability of computerized scoring and the fee, if any, for use. There are also some simple-to-use Internet-based pain assessment tools, such as the Pain-QuiLT, previously known as the Iconic Pain Assessment Tool, for the visual self-reporting and tracking of pain.

Psychometric properties of respective instruments raise a significant set of issues with respect to pain assessment; principal areas of concern are those of reliability and validity. There are several different types of reliability and validity issues that should be considered. The importance placed upon these particular psychometric issues varies in accord with the nature of the instrument and its intended application.

Reliability refers to the likelihood that one would tend to get the same or at least similar results with repeated assessment administrations. Thus reliability is concerned with the generalizability of the pain assessment instrument across different evaluators, settings, times, and so forth. Any pain assessment technique that has low reliability would, of necessity, also have low validity. On the other hand, a pain assessment technique may have rather high reliability, being very consistent across administrations and administrators, but may or may not actually be a valid assessment.

Some of the most common types of reliability issues considered are those of test-retest, split-half, internal consistency, and parallel forms. The similarity of results for administration of the same pain assessment measure at two different points in time is known as test-retest reliability. For instance, an assessment instrument may be administered to a sample population and then again in six weeks. There should be sufficient time between assessment administrations so that the test subjects could not simply recall their earlier item responses. The correlation coefficient between the first and second administration of the instrument is generally used to indicate the degree of test-retest reliability. We would generally expect higher test-retest reliability scores on measures of relatively stable characteristics, such as those considered as traits as opposed to those considered as more transient states. Split-half reliability is measured by correlation coefficients calculated between half the items of a pain assessment instrument with those of the other half, such as the odd-numbered items compared to the even-numbered items. Internal consistency measures evaluate how well responses of individual items in an instrument correlate with those of the other items. For pain assessment instruments intended to assess a single phenomenon, we would expect high correlation coefficients for internal consistency. Split-half and internal consistency measures assess the agreement of content covered within the instrument itself. Parallel forms reliability refers to the degree of obtaining comparable results from two different sets of items designed to address the same pain-related issue; this necessitates creating equivalent forms of the same assessment instrument, an endeavor that is rarely ever engaged in.

Validity refers to the extent to which the pain assessment instrument actually measures what it purports to assess. Some of the most commonly considered types of validity usually considered are content validity, construct validity, criterion validity, concurrent validity, and discriminant validity. Content validity is concerned with the extent to which pain assessment items appear to appropriately and comprehensively sample the domain of interest; content validity is generally built into an instrument by means of careful construction and selection of pain assessment items. Construct validity is supported when a pain assessment instrument correlates highly with measures of other variables that would typically be expected to be associated in predictable ways with what the instrument purports to measure. Criterion validity is concerned with how well the pain assessment instrument scores relate to relevant and significant behaviors. Concurrent validity generally refers to the degree of agreement between the pain assessment instrument results and those of some other measure of the same variable that is obtained at approximately the same time, or concurrently. Some pain assessment instruments have subscales; discriminant validity refers to the ability of the instrument to discriminate between the respective subscales; inter-scale correlations can be used to indicate the degree of discriminant validity.

Pain assessment is fundamentally an exploratory exercise by its very nature. Although the specific content and respective methodologies employed for conducting a pain assessment are extremely variable, the process engaged in is always intended to gain a better understanding of the individual client before taking any action. From a clinical perspective, the primary benefit of pain assessment is to efficiently and accurately determine the treatment needs, if any, of a particular individual. Pain assessment should ideally be broad enough in scope to consider multiple variables that might potentially play a significant role in the functioning of an individual such that they could warrant targeted intervention in an individualized pain treatment plan. Pain assessment is essentially concerned with individualizing each case. It can provide useful individualized feedback that can enhance an individual's motivation for change. Pain treatment programs that incorporate formal assessment procedures have been found to have higher client retention and to be more successful. It is also a dynamic process that should be ongoing throughout the course of pain treatment delivery. Health care professionals should continuously collect data that are accurate, comprehensive, and systematic. Pain assessment should be regarded and utilized as an integral part of the treatment process, not separate and apart from it.

Optimal pain management clearly begins with appropriate pain assessment. Unfortunately, pain is highly subjective and very difficult to quantify. It has a substantial affective component that is learned as an individual grows and develops. Any definition of pain should certainly recognize that it is a very complex phenomenon that is composed of an array of experiences that include cognition, emotion, intensity, motivation, space, and time. At any rate, pain is fundamentally a highly subjective experience that cannot be completely identified or measured by an observer.

The emotional component of painful sensations are transmitted to areas of the hindbrain and reticular formation, as well as to the limbic regions of the cortex by way of the thalamus, which serves fundamentally as a relay station. The anterior cingulate cortex, which has a high concentration of dopaminergic receptors, functions as the attentional processing of the pain sensations, while the primary and secondary somatosensory cortices are where the pain is actually perceived. The amygdala, which is a limbic structure, seems to link sensory experiences to levels of emotional arousal as well as to negative emotional associations; accordingly, it helps us to link the intensity of positive or negative stimuli to motivationally relevant events, including the process of becoming drug dependent. Although pain has definitive physiological aspects and is influenced by genetic and other biological factors, it is significantly modulated by psychological and societal factors, particularly with respect to the degree of distress experienced. This can generate a considerably wide range of apparent differences in the capacity to tolerate pain. Further, belief in the efficacy of a painkiller can enhance its perceived effectiveness. When under the influence of certain painkillers, we can experience pain without feeling its emotional impact.

Although the pain perception threshold—that is, the point at which a stimulus is perceived of as being painful—has been found to be comparatively similar across groups of individuals, the point at which a stimulus is regarded as being tolerable, or the pain tolerance threshold, has been found to be extremely variable. Emotional states can substantially impact these two respective pain thresholds in human beings. Cultural expectations of what is considered to be a tolerable level of pain can significantly influence both thresholds of pain. Anxiety or depression, for just two general examples, can lower both thresholds of pain, while conditions like anger or high engagement on tasks at hand can lessen or somewhat blur pain sensations, at least temporarily.

Interestingly, intense pain experienced at one place in the body can increase the threshold of pain at other places. For example, intense pain felt in the arm of an individual can make it less likely that the same individual will experience chronic low back pain, or other types of pain for that matter, that is less intense. This is an instance of what is known of as perceptual dominance, under which an individual with pain at many places in the body tends to report only the most intense pain. A corollary of this is that as the dominant pain is reduced, then the individual is more likely to identify other painful sites.

Contrary to what might be assumed, pain tolerance is typically diminished as one experiences repeated exposures to painful stimuli. Pain tolerance tends to be diminished by factors such as anger, apprehension, boredom, fatigue, and sleep deprivation. On the other hand, one's pain tolerance tends to be raised by factors such as alcohol consumption, engaging in distracting activities, hypnotic suggestion, medication use, and warmth. An individual's pain tolerance can vary considerably over time, and it is also highly variable among different people.

Appropriate pain management is more likely to be provided when there is an independent objective clinical assessment of pain. The two major categories of pain assessment tools are the single-dimensional scales and the multidimensional scales. A simple assessment, such as that using a numeric scale with zero being "no pain" and 10 being "worst possible pain" can sometimes suffice. The American Chronic Pain Association (ACPA) developed a Quality of Life scale as a measure of function for people with pain. The scale is scored by a self-report of choosing a number from "0" for "Non-functioning" to "10" for "Normal Quality of Life." For example, a "0" might indicate that you are depressed, feel hopeless about your life, and stay in bed all day; while "7" might indicate that you can walk or volunteer for a few hours at a time each day; or a "10" would indicate that you can go to work each day and conduct a normal social life. The Present Pain Intensity (PPI) and the Numeric Pain Scale (NPS) are other examples of single-dimensional verbal pain scales. There are, in addition to numeric and verbal scales, also visual scales that have been created to help assess pain. As it can sometimes be difficult to explain how pain makes us feel, visual scales have been developed to help address this area of concern. For example, the Wong-Baker Faces Pain Rating Scale, which was developed for use with children age 3 years and older, uses six facial images to identify how their pain symptoms make them feel, from "No Hurt" to "Hurts Worst." The single-dimensional pain scales are self-reports that assess a single dimension of pain intensity. They are most useful for assessing acute pain situations.

The multidimensional pain scales measure various aspects of pain, such as the nature, intensity, and location of pain, and, in some cases, they also assess the impact of pain on an individual, such as its impact on their mood or on their level of activity and so forth. Multidimensional pain scales are useful in assessing individuals with conditions like chronic pain or those with complex pain disorders. Some tools have been developed that use a combination of behavioral and physiological measures to attempt to assess pain in infants. One of these instruments that was developed to assess neonatal postoperative pain is the CRIES; it is based upon five variables rated on a 0–2 scale; these variables, respectively, are *C*rying, *R*equires oxygen, *I*ncreased vital signs, *E*xpression, and *S*leeplessness. The Modified Behavioral Pain Scale (MBPS) is another assessment instrument that uses three variables—facial expression, crying, respectively—and movements to attempt to assess pain in children 2 to 6 months of age. The Functional Pain Scale (FPS), on the other hand, was developed incorporating both objective and subjective components to assess pain in the elderly.

Another approach used to assess pain is a Pain Diary, in which you log in what type of pain you are feeling, the intensity of the pain, what you did right before it appeared or worsened, and what if any treatments you used, particularly what, if any, painkillers were used. A diary can be very useful in providing a pain profile, and then that can be used to design individualized ways to help manage your pain.

One method currently used to evaluate the effectiveness of painkillers is the number needed to treat (NNT). This approach is based on a 50% or greater reduction in pain during clinical trials due to the painkiller alone. For example, two standard tablets or capsules (400 mg) of ibuprofen will produce 50% pain relief in 2 out of 5 cases of acute pain. Similarly, two tablets of acetaminophen (1,000 mg) will produce 50% pain relief in slightly over 1 out of 4 cases, while two aspirin tablets (600 mg) will produce 50% pain relief in slightly less than 1 out of 4 cases of acute pain.

Different technical devices are available to help diagnose the cause of pain using an array of techniques. A physician would invariably perform a physical examination and would often order blood tests and other measures as well, beginning with X-rays. Focus of the physical examination should be on the anatomic pattern of the pain as well as the localization of the abnormal neurologic deficits and of other abnormal sensory symptoms. Biopsies of the skin and nerves are sometimes necessary. Computed axial tomography (CAT) or computed tomography (CT) scans utilize X-rays and computer imaging capabilities to generate cross-sections of the body and/or its respective parts. Magnetic resonance imaging (MRI) does not use X-rays, but rather a large magnet and radio waves to produce images of the body and its parts. Myelograms utilize a contrast dye injected into the spinal canal to enhance the capability of X-rays to identify herniated vertebral discs or vertebral fractures that can cause nerve compression along the spinal cord. Discography utilizes a contrast dye injected directly into the spinal disc believed to be causing the pain to enhance the image of the damaged area. Ultrasound imaging or sonography utilizes ultrasound high frequency waves to produce visual images of the inside of the body. An electromyogram (EMG) utilizes very small needles inserted into muscles to measure the electrical response produced by signals to the muscles sent from the brain or spinal cord. Bone scans utilize a minute amount of radioactive material that is injected into the bloodstream and then settles in bones; this allows scanners to produce computer-generated images, making it easier to identify specific areas of abnormal blood flow or areas of irregular bone metabolism.

NEUROTRANSMISSION

Neuron: Structure and Function

In order to understand how painkillers work, it is necessary to understand a little about how the brain and nervous system work. The main nerve cells that make up the brain and nervous system are called neurons, which communicate with each other by means of chemical and electrical messages. The average adult human brain weighs about 1,400 grams, or about 3 pounds; has an average volume of 1,600 cm cubed; and is composed of approximately a billion neurons arranged in a complex array to transmit and receive these electrochemical signals. These messages are how the pain signal gets to the brain and how it is processed. The brain can send out messages to the rest of the body at a speed of 268 miles per hour to direct how to avoid or lessen the cause of pain, if there is, in fact, an actual physical cause.

Each neuron consists of several major areas. The dendrites are the beginning of the neuron; they protrude out from the cell body in branchlike extensions and contain receptor sites where chemical messages from neighboring neurons can be received. Small extensions spread out in all directions from the dendrites. A single dendrite can have as many as 30,000 small extensions spreading out to collect information from nearby receptors and neurons. Dendrites are constantly making new connections and severing old ones; this is how learning takes place dynamically. The cell body of the neuron is called the soma; it contains the cell nucleus and, accordingly, helps conduct activities related to metabolism and other main internal cellular functions. The area between the cell body and the axon is generally known as the axon hillock. The major lengthwise extent of the neuron is provided by the axon that serves as the path along which to transmit the electrical message of the action potential; it extends from the soma and ends at the synaptic terminals. Specialized neurons that have short axons or no axon at all are referred to as interneurons; they function by integrating neural activity within a particular brain structure, not by conducting messages from one structure to another. There are actually perhaps a thousand different types of neurons. Each neuron typically consists of one axon, which can vary from 0.05 inches to over 3 feet in length. Bundles of axons in the peripheral nervous system are referred to as nerves, while those in the brain and spinal cord of the central nervous system are called tracts. The synaptic terminals, also referred to as terminal boutons, buttons, or presynaptic endings, are specialized protuberances that hold the endogenously produced neurotransmitters in vesicles, which are signaled to be released by the action potential that converts the electrical signal into a chemical one. The synaptic vesicles are spherical membrane packages that hold neurotransmitter molecules waiting to be released near the synapses. The Golgi complex of the neuron is responsible for packing the neurotransmitters into the synaptic vesicles. An electrical signal traveling down a neuron opens up calcium ion channels in the synaptic terminal, which cause the vesicle to move and then fuse to the neural membrane; then the neurotransmitter can be released into the synapse, a process referred to as exocytosis. The surfaces of the receptive areas of most neurons can potentially be exposed to thousands of synapses. Synapses, also referred to as synaptic clefts, are the spaces between neighboring neurons. A synapse is generally about an 18 millionth of an inch wide, and it is estimated that a normal human brain contains over a hundred trillion synapses—an extremely large number of connections through which pain signals can be transmitted. Different painkillers affect the functioning of different parts of the neurons in different ways.

The release and uptake of neurotransmitters is how neurons communicate across a synapse. Neurotransmitters are continually produced, released, broken down, and recaptured as the communication between neurons occurs. Over 60 different types of neurotransmitters have thus far been identified, and more no doubt will; in fact, it has been speculated that there may be as many as 2,000 different neurotransmitters. There are two major types of neurotransmitters, excitatory and inhibitory ones. Excitatory neurotransmitters tend to stimulate adjacent neurons to fire and inhibitory neurotransmitters tend to prevent their firing. The vast majority of neurotransmitters at fast-acting, directed synapses are amino acids, like aspartate, glutamate, glycine, and gamma-aminobutyric acid (GABA); as compared to the neuropeptides, like substance P, dynorphins, and enkephalins such as leucine and merhionine, which tend to have slower, more diffuse effects. For example, GABA is an inhibitory neurotransmitter that mediates gate control in the dorsal horn by synapsing neurons containing substance P. In addition to neurotransmitters, there are other chemical messengers that influence the type, frequency, strength, and magnitude of neuron signaling; these include neuromediators, neuromodulators, and neuroregulators.

After crossing a synapse, each respective neurotransmitter must bind to a receptor in the postsynaptic membrane. Each receptor is a protein that contains sites to which only a particular neurotransmitter can bind. However, any particular type of neurotransmitter can generally bind to several different subtypes of receptors. Any neurotransmitter that does not successfully bond to a receptor must be eliminated from the synapse. Many neurotransmitters are removed by reuptake by means of which they are drawn back into the presynaptic neuron. Other neurotransmitters are broken down by enzymes, the products of which are then used in the synthesis of more new neurotransmitters. For example, the neurotransmitter acetylcholine is degraded by the enzyme acetylcholinesterase. Drugs can inhibit, or increase, at many different points, the synthesis, release, action, and deactivation of neurotransmitters.

Neurons constantly monitor the total amount of the two different types of neurotransmitters. When the level of the excitatory neurotransmitter exceeds that of the inhibitory neurotransmitters by a critical amount, then the neuron can succeed in firing its signal on to the next neuron along the pathway. Once the incoming pain signal reaches the brain, neurons in respective areas of the brain must be stimulated in order for the pain to be perceived. Although there is a close association between the firing of brain neurons and the perception of pain, there are many cognitive factors that will impact the meanings attributed to that particular sensation as well as help to formulate an appropriate response. By the way, contrary to the popular misconception, nearly all of the brain is being accessed all of the time by the firing of neurons.

Impulse Transmission

Neurons generate electrical signals that then are converted into chemical signals that can be transmitted across the synapse, the space between two neurons. Substance P, a neuropeptide first isolated in 1931, is the neurotransmitter that signals the intensity of the pain message. The message travels down the axon of the neuron as an electrical signal that stimulates vesicles, specialized sacks located at the synaptic terminal that contain various neurotransmitters, to release these substances. Pain messages travel down the axon at a speed of about 300 feet per second.

The electrical signal carried along the axon is also known as a nerve impulse or an action potential, as it may be able to convert the electrical transmission to a chemical one at the end of the dendritic branches known as the synaptic terminal. The action potential only lasts about 1 millisecond. The axon is sometimes coated with a myelin sheath that consists of a lipid bilayer embedded with proteins. There are two major classes of these membrane proteins; some are signal proteins that transfer signals to the inside of the neuron after specific molecules from outside the neuron bind to them; the others are known as channel proteins through which certain molecules can pass. Gaps between sections of the myelin sheath are known as nodes of Ranvier. The myelination of the axons of the peripheral nervous system is performed by Schwann cells. Neurons covered with a myelin sheath can transmit pain signals over 100 times faster than those without it.

Ions in solution cannot pass across the myelin on their own as its membrane acts as an insulator. The solution outside the neuron is called extracellular fluid, and that inside is called intracellular fluid. Both fluids have positive and negative ions dissolved in them. Positive ions include those of calcium (Ca), potassium (K), and sodium (Na), while chloride (Cl) is a negatively charged ion. The difference in electrical charge between the inside and the outside of a resting neuron, which is referred to as its resting potential, is almost 70 millivolts. At that point, the neuron is said to be polarized.

Ions, on their own, tend to naturally flow from areas of higher to those of lower concentrations, otherwise known as moving down their concentration gradients. Ions are salts that are distributed at different concentration levels throughout the body, including inside and outside of our neurons. These ions pass through the membranes of neurons by flowing through specialized pores known as ion channels. The exchange of ions is thus highly essential to the normal functioning of neurons. Since ions are charged either positively or negatively, their varying levels of concentrations generate variable electrical potentials.

Protein pumps help to maintain an ionic imbalance. An important example of such is the sodium-potassium pump, which pumps out the influx of sodium ions that flowed into neurons and pumps in potassium ions that tend to flow, or efflux, out of neurons. Some neurotransmitters have been found to open or close ion channels that allow rapid changes in electrical states of the neurons. Neurotransmitters with a positive charge can depolarize the membrane potential of the receptive neurons, while those with a negative charge can hyperpolarize or increase the membrane potential. This serves to recharge the electrical potential of the neuron. This rapid exchange of positive or negative charges is one way that an electrical signal is sent down the length of the axon.

As the sodium enters the upper part of the neuron, it becomes depolarized or excited; then, as the potassium is passed to the outside of the neuron, it becomes hyperpolarized or inhibited. This process continues along the length of the axon; when it gets to the terminal of the neuron, the vesicles are stimulated to release their neurotransmitter contents. Thus, the electrical signal is transferred into a chemical signal, which can, in turn, be transmitted across the synapse to the next neuron along the pain pathway. A postsynaptic depolarization is known as an excitatory postsynaptic potential, while postsynaptic hyperpolarization is known as an inhibitory postsynaptic potential; the former increase the likelihood that the receptive neuron will fire, and the latter decrease the likelihood.

The neurotransmitters float across the synaptic cleft and, hopefully, bind to receptor sites located on the next neuron along the pathway or circuit. The receptor sites consist of specialized proteins that may be activated by a specific neurotransmitter. The receptor sites can be carrier protein gated, enzyme gated, guanine coupled gated, or ion channel gated. In addition, there are also assorted intracellular hormone gates; any gate can contribute to a change in the firing rate of a neuron. Neurons in the central nervous system typically fire about every 4 milliseconds. The released ions crossing the synapse can begin to either stimulate or inhibit an excitation in the postsynaptic neuron. Neurons can combine or integrate many individual signals into one overall signal. They can accomplish this either through spatial summation or through temporal summation of signals. Each neuron must continuously integrate signals over both space and time as they are constantly bombarded with stimuli across thousands of synapses. When enough of the neurotransmitter binds to receptors, a new electrical signal is generated in the receiving neuron, and this travels down its axon to repeat the process all over again, and so on down the line. At high levels of continual stimulation, each neuron can fire up to a rate of about 1,000 times a second. Some neurons can release more than one type of neurotransmitter.

If the pain sensation is too intense, the body can try to lessen the intensity of the signals to protect itself. It can accomplish this by releasing large quantities of endorphins and enkephalins into the synapses of the brain and spinal cord. These naturally, or endogenously, produced substances, released by secondary terminals, can bind to the opioid mu, delta, and kappa receptor sites. On the neurons sending and receiving messages, these opioid receptors can slow down the firing rate and inhibit the release of substance P. Opiate and opioid drugs, like morphine or heroin, are effective painkillers as they function similar to the endorphins and enkephalins by binding to primary and secondary receptor sites and thereby inhibiting the release of substance P and also by blocking it from getting across the synapse to receiving neurons. However, small changes in the molecular structure of respective opiates and opioids can produce substantially different effects with respect to how readily they bind to receptors sites, how long they last, and, consequently, how effective they will be as a painkiller.

CELLULAR LEVEL OF PAIN

When something stresses part of your body enough, pain sensors known as nociceptors send neuro-electrical signals to your brain, which you interpret and experience as pain. The neurobiological manifestation of pain is the result of a complex cascade of neurochemical events that occur within and between numerous brain structures that function in tandem and create neurological pathways. Painkillers block or interfere with the transmission of these messages, either at the site of the injury itself, along the spinal cord, or in the brain. Nociceptors are specialized nerve cells that transmit a pain signal only if their firing threshold is reached. Nociceptors are free nerve endings located in your skin, muscles, spinal cord, teeth, membranes around bones, cornea of the eye, and some internal organs.

When cells in your body are damaged, arachidonic acid, an endogenously produced substrate, is one type of chemical released; it normally binds to COX-1 and COX-2 enzymes and thereby produces prostaglandins, as well as prostacyclins and thromboxanes, as part of the inflammatory response. Prostaglandins stimulate the release of fluids from the blood to surround and protect the injured tissues. The prostaglandins thereby produce swelling and inflammation around the injury site, which helps to insulate and protect the area from further damage. However, the swelling and inflammation can also cause some tissue damage as well as restrict mobility, particularly if joints are involved. The COX-1 enzyme controls production of prostaglandins and thromboxane that help regulate gastrointestinal, renal, vascular, and other physiological functions.

COX is a bifunctional heme containing protein that sequentially catalyzes two different reactions. The first one involves the cyclooxygenation of arachidonic acid to form some of the prostaglandins. The second one is a peroxidase reaction within the COX catalytic system. Several variables, such as substrate concentrations, incubation time, and hydro-peroxide concentration, influence the rate and extent of COX inhibition, which, in turn, determines the relative anti-inflammatory effectiveness of the respective drug. The chemical structure of COX-2 is similar to that of COX-1, except that a valine is substituted for an isoleucine that is on COX-1; thus, the COX-2 enzyme can accommodate larger chemical structures, up to those that, in fact, have about 25% greater volume. The COX-2 enzyme was discovered by Daniel Simmons of Brigham Young University in 1988. The COX-2 enzyme helps control production of prostaglandins involved in pain, inflammation, and fever.

Mechanisms of Painkiller Action

Different types of painkillers actually work quite differently. Some painkiller drugs, such as NSAIDs like aspirin and ibuprofen, block the production of prostaglandins in different ways by blocking the ability of arachidonic acid to bind to COX-1 and COX-2 enzymes; they essentially raise the nociceptor-firing threshold, but this can be done in several different ways. We now understand that aspirin, which was originally introduced to clinical medicine in 1899, deactivates the COX-1 and COX-2 enzymes permanently by covalent modification, while ibuprofen does so temporarily until it is broken down. Aspirin unlike other NSAIDs, orientates within the cyclooxygenase active site by means of a weak ionic bond. Aspirin thus exhibits rapid but reversible binding along with covalent modification of both COX-1 and COX-2 enzymes. Ibuprofen, which was originally granted approval by the FDA on September 24, 1985, binds quickly, but weakly, to the active binding site on the cyclooxygenase or COX enzymes, as the drug is broken down, the inhibitory effect on these enzymes is reversed. Thus, ibuprofen, as well as piroxicam and mefenamic acid for instance, all exhibit rapid competitive but easily reversible tight binding to COX-1 and COX-2 enzymes; they all dissociate rapidly from the COX active sites. Acetaminophen, which was originally granted approval by the FDA on April 22, 1980, also appears to inhibit COX-1 and COX-2 enzymes, as well as probably inhibiting COX-3 enzyme in the brain. Although acetaminophen inhibits COX enzymes effectively in the central nervous system—that is, the brain and spinal cord—it does not have any appreciable effects in the peripheral nervous system. Consequently, it can be effective in treating headaches and other minor pains, but it is ineffective against musculoskeletal pain; the recommended maximum daily dose of acetaminophen is 4 grams. Acetaminophen, along with fenoprofen calcium, which was originally granted approval for use in the United States by the FDA on June 8, 1988, and sulindac, which was originally granted approval by the FDA on March 3, 1988, also suppresses progesterone production in women and thus may potentially be useful for promoting clinical reproductive toxicity. Diclofenac as well as indomethacin and flurbiprofen are all NSAIDs that exhibit rapid but lower affinity reversible binding to both COX-1 and COX-2 enzymes, followed by time-dependent but higher affinity and slowly reversible binding. Flurbiprofen is actually one of the most potent inhibitors of both COX-1 and COX-2 enzymes.

All NSAIDs inhibit COX-1 and COX-2 enzymes, but they vary in the extent to which, and the rate at which, they can do so. The variation in this COX inhibition parallels the therapeutic efficacy of the respective medications as well as the potential adverse side effects that may be experienced by users.

Selective COX-2 inhibitors work primarily by altering the functioning of the COX-2 enzyme, but they also impact COX-1. Celecoxib has slow competitive binding to COX-2 and, at high concentrations, does so irreversibly. Nimesulide, on the other hand, is a weak competitive COX-1 inhibitor but is a potent but time-dependent inhibitor of the COX-2 enzyme. The selective COX-2 inhibitors all lack a carboxyl group, but are large methylsulfonyl-phenyl derivatives that block the COX-2 channel in a time-dependent manner; they are able to do this since they have access to a hydrophobic side pocket that simple NSAIDs do not.

The use of NSAIDs in individuals with kidney or liver diseases can result in kidney failure. Gastrointestinal toxicity results from the inhibition of COX-1, which creates a reduction in the synthesis of the mucosal protective prostaglandins. Adverse renal effects result from the role the prostaglandins play in regulation of vascular tone and electrolyte hemodynamics.

The opiates and opioids are different types of painkillers that work in two other main ways than those of the NSAIDs and other over-the-counter as well as prescription painkillers. First, opiates and opioids block or interfere with the transmission of pain signals throughout the nervous system, particularly including the spinal column and brain as well as in the gastrointestinal tract. Second, these drugs work in the brain itself to modulate the perception of pain. The periaqueductal gray and other areas of the brain contain receptors that opiates and opioids, as well as internally produced, or endogenous, endorphins bind to and thereby block the transmission of pain signals. At least four different types of endorphins have been identified; these include dynorphin, beta-endorphin, methionine (met) encephalin, and leucine (lek) encephalin. Encephalins have a short duration of action due to their rapid hydrolysis by peptidases. Encephalins are thought to be contained in short interneurons known as synaptosomes. Since opiate and opioid drugs have chemical structures that closely resemble those of the endogenously produced endorphins, they are able to bind to the same mu and kappa receptors to which these substances would bind. This binding not only effectively diminishes pain, but also triggers the release of dopamine in the brain and thereby creates the experience of the individual feeling euphoric.

Dopamine is the major neurotransmitter involved in the brain's reward system. Dopamine is a neuromodulator that is involved in, among other things, motivation and reward; it also plays a primary role in our experiencing emotion, cognition, and regulation of movement. Behaviors associated with natural rewards, like eating and sex, elicit a substantial release of dopamine, which enhances the reinforcing potential of these stimuli. Recreational drug use can also heighten dopaminergic activity and thereby activate the reward system of the brain. Abnormally high dopamine levels for an extended period of time can generate receptor site down-regulation along the neural pathways. Accordingly, the dopaminergic brain network plays a central role in the mechanics of opiate and opioid drug addiction. The down-regulation of dopamine receptors in the mesolimbic pathway can produce a diminished sensitivity to both natural reinforcers and to opiate or opioid drugs consumed. High sustained levels of dopamine in the synapses between neurons of the brain result in the intense euphoric feeling associated with recreational opiate or opioid use. After this intense euphoria, dynorphin and related proteins are produced; these substances block the further release of dopamine and also temporarily inhibit the brain's reward pathway. This suppression creates the need in the user to use progressively larger doses to reach the same effect, which is referred to as the development of tolerance, which, in turn, means that the user is likely to be dissatisfied and somewhat depressed. This downward state routinely triggers the user to be unable to experience feelings of pleasure from activities that were previously enjoyable; consequently, individuals in this situation tend to resort to administration of another dose of the drug. This drug seeking often progresses to dependence. Similarly, sustained naturally high levels of dopamine in the nucleus accumbens appears to increase the production of substance P, which, in turn, leads to increased dopamine synthesis in the ventral tegmental area of the brain. However, this natural positive reward feedback loop seems to be dampened by repeated drug use. The fact that opiate and opioid drugs can bind to these receptor sites not only in the brain, but also in the spinal column and in the gastrointestinal tract, helps to explain the ability of these substances to manage both pain sensations and the symptoms of withdrawal.

The dopamine reward pathway is one of the most well-studied neurological systems of opiate and opioid addiction. This pathway begins in the ventral tegmental area of the brain and projects into several other reward-related regions in the forebrain, particularly the nucleus accumbens and the medial prefrontal cortex. Nearly every neurochemical system has a functional role in the dopamine reward pathway for opiate and opioid addiction; these systems, in addition to dopamine, include but are not limited to the endogenous opioids, corticotropin-releasing factor, gamma-aminobutyric acid, glutamate, and serotonin. Nonetheless, when opiates or opioids are administered, dopamine neural activity within the ventral tegmental area is increased and dopamine released within the nucleus accumbens results in changes to neuronal activity projecting to other regions of the brain, including the medial prefrontal cortex. In fact, dopamine levels are increased in the nucleus accumbens in a dose-dependent manner; that is, the consumption of an opiate or an opioid, as well as the anticipation of its consumption, can result in an increase in dopamine. Other brain structures, such as the amygdala, hippocampus, thalamus, and ventral pallidum, are also thought to contribute to the euphoric end result state by means of the interconnectivity with the reward pathway. Accordingly, the underlying neurobiological basis of opiate and opioid addiction is by nature a complex, elaborate, and interrelated phenomenon that becomes further complicated when an individual is habitually consuming these substances.

There are many other types of drugs that have other primary purposes but that are also, from time to time, used as painkillers; these include certain anti-anxiety medications, antidepressants, anti-seizure drugs and muscle relaxants. Certain antianxiety medications, also referred to as anxiolytic drugs, can serve as effective painkillers since they can help lower anxiety, help relax muscles, and help individuals cope with the discomfort of pain. However, use of antianxiety medications, particularly those of the benzodiazepine group, can cause drowsiness; while abrupt cessation of their use can result in serious withdrawal symptoms, including seizures and possibly even death. Certain antidepressant medications, particularly the tricyclics, appear to help reduce pain transmissions through the spinal column. However, use of many antidepressants can cause drowsiness as well as suicidal thoughts; and some, particularly the tricyclics, have serious side effects when used in combination with many other drugs, possibly affecting the heart, and synergistic effects can even result in fatalities. On the other hand, antidepressants, as a group, are considered to be a relatively safe, highly effective, and nonaddictive class of medications with no abuse potential. The serotonin norepinephrine reuptake inhibitors (SNRIs) have several serious side effects including anorexia, constipation, dizziness, dry mouth, ejaculatory and other sexual function difficulties, headache, insomnia, nausea, nervousness, and sweating. Certain antiseizure, otherwise referred to as anticonvulsant, medications can help in relieving pain from assorted neuropathies, possibly by means of stabilizing impacted nerve fibers. However, individuals using antiseizure medications should be monitored for suicidal signs and symptoms; common side effects experienced with use of antiseizure medications include drowsiness, dizziness, and swelling of the lower extremities. Certain muscle relaxants are used to lessen pain in tense muscle groups, probably achieving this effect by means of the sedative effects of these drugs upon the central nervous system. However, use of muscle relaxants can cause drowsiness. In addition, chlorzoxazone, originally approved by the FDA for use in the United States on September 29, 1995, and marketed as Parafon Forte and DSC; and metaxalone, originally approved by the FDA on March 3, 1995, and marketed by King Pharmaceuticals as Skelaxin, should be used only with extreme caution in treating individuals with liver disease; and dantrolene sodium, approved by the FDA on March 1, 2005, and marketed under trade names such as Dantrium, Revonto, and Ryanodex, can be toxic to the liver; while chronic use of carisoprodol, originally approved by the FDA on January 24, 1996, and marketed as Soma, can result in the development of dependence as it is converted into a substance chemically similar to barbiturates. Methocarbamol, originally approved by the FDA on October 22, 1974, and marketed as Robaxin in the United States by Actient Pharmaceuticals and in Canada by Pfizer, can discolor urine to brown, green, or black; and use of cyclobenzaprine, originally approved by the FDA on February 29, 1988, and marketed under trade names such as Amrix, Fexmid, and Flexeril, can cause constipation, confusion, dry mouth, and loss of balance.

Pain has a decidedly negative emotional component. The emotional component of a pain stimulus is transmitted along specific pathways to the areas of the hindbrain and the reticular formation that function in pain arousal, as well as relayed through the thalamus to the limbic areas of the cortex. The raphe nuclei, which produce serotonin, are the source of descending pain inhibition. The emotional responses to pain are mainly learned responses. Cognitive factors are therefore highly involved in the overall emotional response to pain, even though it is fundamentally a cellular experience. There are several areas of research that support this view. For example, hypnotic suggestions of greater or lesser unpleasantness of pain stimuli produced associated changes in brain activity as observed with PET scans. For another example, individuals who have had undergone a prefrontal lobotomy, which damages the anterior cingulate cortex, typically have reduced emotional reactions to pain, but no changes to their threshold of pain.

Different pain neurons are activated by varying levels of stimulation. The different types of pain neurons use different types of neurotransmitters, endogenously produced chemical messengers that bind to different receptor sites. This fact has led to the development of various new types of painkillers to manage pain more effectively. Endorphins, for example, are neurotransmitters that can block the synapses of nerve fibers that would otherwise transmit pain signals. Serotonin is another neurotransmitter that is released by neurons that descend from the brain. Some drugs can inhibit the effects of these natural painkiller neurotransmitters, while others can enhance the effects.

There are, as already noted, many other different types of drugs that are sometimes used as painkillers. For example, some antidepressants—such as fluoxetine hydrochloride, originally granted FDA approval in August 2001 and marketed under various trade names such as Prozac and Sarafem; paroxetine hydrochloride, originally granted FDA approval in July 2003 and marketed as Paxil and Pexeva; and sertraline hydrochloride, originally granted FDA approval in June 2006 and marketed as Zoloft—can help lessen the arousal level of the nervous system and thereby make it less sensitive to pain. These particular medications are all selective serotonin reuptake inhibitors (SSRIs), which have several adverse side effects; these side effects include substantial sexual dysfunction, such as decreased arousal, lack of interest, and absent or delayed orgasm, as well as conditions like agitation, insomnia and restlessness common during the initial phase of treatment. Antiseizure medications—such as ethosuximide, once marketed under trade names such as Emeside or Zarontin and now been discontinued from production, leaving only generic formulations; phenobarbital, marketed as Luminal; and phenytoin, marketed as Dilantin—are central nervous system depressants, and use of some can lead to overdose fatalities, typically by means of decreased respiratory drive. This fatal overdose risk is more likely to occur when the antiseizure medications are used in combination with opiates, opioids, or alcohol. The benzodiazepines—such as alprazolam, which was first released by Upjohn and marketed as Xanax and is now available in generic formulations; chlordiazepoxide, marketed under trade names such as Angirex, Elenium, Librium, Mesural, and Tropium; diazepam, first marketed by Hoffman-La Roche as Valium and now sold under about 500 brand names worldwide available in oral, inhalation, injectable, and rectal formulations; and lorazepam, first introduced in 1977 by Wyeth Pharmaceuticals and marketed as Ativan and Temesta, but subsequently been marketed under more than 70 other brand names such as Almazine, Bonton, Control, and Donix—are the most commonly used antianxiety drugs; however, long-term use of benzodiazepines carries a high risk for physiological dependence. Nevertheless, the benzodiazepines are considered to be generally safe and well tolerated as there is a wide margin between the therapeutic dose and the dose likely to cause a harmful overdose. Benzodiazepines can also be prescribed for their muscle relaxation, or myorelaxant, effects, which can be helpful for some pain patients. Anesthetic medications or steroids can be injected directly into injured areas to provide localized pain relief. For example, epidural injection of corticosteroid is a commonly used intervention for managing spinal pain, with the strongest evidence of efficacy for providing short-term pain relief for a period or six weeks or less. Corticosteroids have profound anti-inflammatory effects. Although generally injected at the site of an injury, corticosteroids can also be administered orally for use as painkillers, such as for treating arthritis.

DOCUMENT: NOCICEPTIVE VERSUS NEUROPATHIC PAIN

Neuropathic pain, as opposed to nociceptive pain, is that caused by either damage to body structures or by dysfunction of nerve cells in either the peripheral or the central nervous system; it tends to be persistent pain even in the absence of stimuli. Nociceptive pain, on the other hand, tends not to be associated with sensory dysfunction; depending on the nociceptors activated, it can be subdivided into either somatic or visceral pain. The table "Differentiating Features of Nociceptive and Neuropathic Pain" from the World Health Organization, 2012 WHO Guidelines on the Pharmacological Treatment of Persisting Pain in Children with Medical Illness, *provides an overview of how a clinical distinction is made between nociceptive and neuropathic pain, whether it is localized or diffuse, and whether it is characterized as burning, dull, or sharp pain.*

Differentiating features of nociceptive and neuropathic pain

Type of pain	Origin of stimulus	Localization	Character	Referral and radiation of pain/ sensory dysfunction	Examples
Nociceptive pain Superficial somatic pain	Arises from nociceptors in skin, mucosa of mouth, nose, urethra, anus, etc. Nociceptive stimulus is evident.	Well localized	Usually sharp and may have a burning or pricking quality.	None	• abscesses • postsurgical pain from a surgical incision • superficial trauma • superficial burn
Nociceptive pain Deep somatic pain	Arises from nociceptors in bone, joint, muscle and connective tissue. Nociceptive stimulus is evident.	Usually well localized with tenderness to palpation.	Usually dull or aching or throbbing in quality.	In some instances, pain is referred to the overlying skin. No associated sensory dysfunction.	• bone pain due to metastasis • fractures • muscle cramps • sickle cell vasoocclusive episodes
Nociceptive pain Visceral pain	Arises from nociceptors in internal organs such as the liver, pancreas, pleura and peritoneum.	Poorly localized, diffused. Palpation over the site may elicit an accompanying somatic pain.	Usually vague, dull, aching, cramping or tightness, deep pressure, spasms, or squeezing or colicky in nature. Nausea, diaphoresis and emesis are frequently present.	In some instances, pain referred to skin supplied by same sensory roots that supply the diseased organ. There may be radiation of the visceral pain, but it will not be in a direct nerve distribution. No associated sensory dysfunction.	• pain from acid indigestion or constipation • pain due to stretching from liver metastasis, pleura stretching due to pleuritis, as in pneumonia or tuberculosis

(continued)

Differentiating features of nociceptive and neuropathic pain

Type of pain	Origin of stimulus	Localization	Character	Referral and radiation of pain/sensory dysfunction	Examples
Neuropathic pain	Is generated at various sites, and is not always stimulus dependent	Poorly localized, diffuse pain in an area of sensory dysfunction in the area of anatomical distribution of nerve supply.	Difficult to describe and different words may be used in different populations: • burning, pricking or needle like pain; • sharp or shooting. The pain may be persisting or recurrent.	Neuropathic pain is perceived within the innervation territory of the damaged nerve. There may be abnormal radiation. The pain is associated with sensory dysfunction (dysesthesia, hypoesthesia, hyperesthesia and allodynia).	• central neuropathic pain due to spinal cord injury from trauma or tumor • painful peripheral neuropathies, due to HIV/AIDS, cancer or anticancer treatment pain (e.g. chemotherapy with vincristine) • phantom limb pain

Source: Table 1.2, Differentiating features of nociceptive and neuropathic pain. *WHO guidelines on the pharmacological treatment of persisting pain in children with medical illnesses*, © World Health Organization 2012. Online at http://apps.who.int/iris/bitstream/10665/44540/1/9789241548120_Guidelines.pdf. Used by permission of the World Health Organization.

Chapter 5

Effects and Applications

There are many varied ways that painkiller drugs are presently administered, and there have been other approaches used in the past. The different routes of administration of painkillers impact the dosage levels needed to bring about the desired therapeutic effects. About 100 million American adults now are living with chronic pain. It is estimated that 9.4 million Americans are currently taking opiate or opioid painkiller drugs for long-term pain; of these, it is thought that about 2.1 million are dependent and at risk for use of the illicit drug market. This has become a worldwide problem as well.

WAYS TO USE PAINKILLERS

Administration

Many different ways have been found to use opium, morphine, heroin, and other opiate and opioid drugs, as well as the many other painkillers. In this regard, it should be noted that narcotic addicts in many settings have been observed to engage in elaborate rituals in order to obtain and to administer their substances of choice. Different methods of administering respective substances, such as the eating of opium or the smoking or intravenous injection of heroin, have come into and subsequently gone out of fashion in different places over time. Eighteenth-century physicians also engaged in external, topical applications of opium. In 1843, Dr. Alexander Wood, a Scottish physician, discovered that injecting opiates substantially increased their effectiveness. In this regard, the hypodermic syringe was first used for the injection of drugs, principally by physicians for administering opiates, in the middle of the 19th century, becoming more widespread probably after 1856 when they were first brought to the United States. For example, by 1902, one could, through the Sears Roebuck catalog, order various hypodermic syringes with two needles, vials, and extra wire, which came in a basic version for $1 each, a "more complete" version for $1.50, and the "best grade" for $2 each and $0.08 postage for whichever model was selected. At any rate, it is estimated that about 200,000 Americans had become addicted to opiates by the end of the 19th century.

The injection of drugs and other methods of their administration have certainly followed different courses of historical development in numerous places around the world. The indiscriminate use of injection morphine and opium administration during the U.S. Civil War (1861–1865) created an estimated 400,000 painkiller-addicted veterans. Soon thereafter, the Franco-Austrian War (1866) and then the Franco-Prussian War in Europe (1870–1871) similarly created populations of painkiller addicts. World War I witnessed a similar situation and the common practice of morphine injection of wounded military personnel persisted, with, not surprisingly, similar personal and societal results. For example, in 1918, the health commissioner for New York City, Dr. Royal S. Copeland, estimated that there were between 150,000 and 200,000 addicts in the city, most of whom were heroin dependent and many of whom were recently discharged veterans.

On August 21, 1897, Felix Hoffmann was the first to synthesize the substance that would later be called heroin; he had synthesized aspirin just 2 weeks before. In 1888, David Dort and Ralph Stockman reported from Edinburgh, Scotland, that heroin was stronger than morphine. Heroin injection by physicians rapidly increased in popularity, and it was not too long before its illicit use displaced that of both opium and morphine. For instance, by 1915, heroin had surpassed morphine as the primary cause of addiction admissions at Bellevue Hospital in New York City.

In 1934, the Hisamitsu Pharmaceutical Company of Japan introduced a pain-relieving patch with a combination of active ingredients of 1.2% camphor, 5.2% menthol, and 6.3% methyl salicylate; it is still produced and marketed under the trade name of Salonpas. This product initiated the use of transdermal patch administration of painkiller drugs.

In the 1990s, heroin imported from Mexico and Colombia became cheaper and of higher potency than earlier supplies of heroin in the United States had generally been. It is estimated that in 1997, around 600,000 Americans were using heroin as their drug of choice. Emergency room visits related to the use of heroin doubled between 1990 and 1995. Morphine is 10 times more potent a painkiller than opium, while heroin is 25 times more potent a painkiller than morphine. It takes about 10 units of opium to produce 1 unit of heroin; this mass differential has been well exploited by drug smugglers. This greater potency of the drug allowed individuals, including adolescents, to initiate heroin use by means of nasal administration rather than by injection, which had a much greater stigma associated with it. Whatever the route of administration selected, frequent use of opiates or opioids tends to lead rapidly to the development of tolerance and intense craving in some individuals. However, it must be recognized that if opiates or opioids are taken, even for long periods of time, at moderate doses and in pure forms—which is not generally the situation with illicit use such as, for example, with heroin sold on the streets—there may be no severe medical problems resulting from it other than, of course, addiction. On the other hand, injection drug use of opiates, opioids, or similar drugs as typically done can readily cause serious health complications to users, such as abscesses, gangrene, necrosis, and severe vein damage. Furthermore, injection drug users are at substantially higher risk for various diseases, such as human immunodeficiency virus (HIV), hepatitis C, and other blood-borne infections.

Many other methods have been developed for the varied routes of administration of painkiller drugs. Transdermal patches, intranasal sprays, sublingual tabs, suppositories, topical applications, and many more other approaches have been utilized to administer respective painkillers. There are also other approaches under development, such as a subdermal implant that can deliver 6 months of buprenorphine that is currently pending FDA approval. However, there are both positive and negative points associated with each respective method of administering painkiller drugs. For instance, transdermal patches slowly administer a dose of the painkiller through the skin. Painkiller patches, such as fentanyl transdermal patches, are usually used for long-term relief of pain, and some can be effective for a few days (72 hours) at a time. However, use of heating pads, hot baths, and even the heat of the sun can accelerate the rate of the release of fentanyl and similar painkiller medications from transdermal patches. Many painkillers are also formulated in a suppository form. Opioid suppositories, for example, are most often used for treating cancer pain. With the use of a suppository, there is a slow release of the painkiller drug over a period of time, which can be for up to 12 hours. Unfortunately, painkiller patches and suppositories do not have a rapid onset of action and therefore are not recommended for situations where such is needed.

Combinations

Opiates and opioids are often mixed with other substances for their combined effects. For example, heroin and cocaine are often abused together in an illicit form commonly referred to as "speedballing." Of great concern in this regard of mixing drugs is that heroin-related deaths are highly associated with the use of alcohol or other drugs. Historically, opium and morphine were also often used in combination with alcohol and other substances. Laudanum, a mixture of alcohol and opium, along with selected herbs, for example, was introduced in the 16th century by Paracelsus, a Swiss physician, and it was even used to ease suffering from the plague. He is credited with the repopularization of opium in Europe as it had fallen out of use due to its toxicity. Paracelsus is reputed to have always carried some laudanum and referred to it as the "immortality stone." Laudanum became particularly popular in the later Victorian era, both in the United States and in Europe. Thomas Sydenham, the famous 17th-century English physician, for instance, promoted the use of laudanum. Sydenham, in fact, was such an enthusiastic supporter of opium that he was sometimes referred to as "Opiophilos" (that is "lover of opium").

Many other combinations of opiates were and are made and used. For example, morphine and cannabis were combined in a product known as chlorodyne, which in the early 20th century was prescribed as a cough suppressant. The painkilling effectiveness of a drug can often be enhanced by using it in combination with other painkillers, as well as with other non-painkiller drugs. Many pharmaceutical products have been developed and marketed by combining different painkillers and other substances. For example, Percodan is oxycodone hydrochloride combined with aspirin, which was originally granted approval for use in the United States by the FDA on April 12, 1950; and Endo Pharms manufactured it as 4.835-mg and 325-mg tablets marketed under the trade name of Endodan. Percocet is oxycodone combined with acetaminophen, which was originally granted approval for use by the FDA on August 31, 1976, and Vintage Pharms manufactured it as 5-mg and 325-mg tablets; and Talacen is pentazocine hydrochloride combined with acetaminophen, which was originally granted approval for use by the FDA on September 23, 1982, and Sanofi Aventis US manufactured it as 650-mg tablets.

Painkillers can be combined in formulations with other painkillers, which often increases their effectiveness. Excedrin and Excedrin Migraine, as examples of legally produced and sold multiple combination products, both contain acetaminophen, aspirin, and caffeine; Excedrin Migraine was originally granted approval by the FDA for use in the United States on January 14, 1998, and it was manufactured by Novartis as 65-mg and 250-mg tablets. Vanquish is another similar product that is used for the acute management of headache, and it consists of 227 mg of aspirin, 194 mg of acetaminophen, and 33 mg of caffeine.

Painkillers are often combined with other non-painkiller drugs as well, for both illicit and licit use. For instance, a study of recent illicit injection drug users in Ukraine found that the most common drug used was *hanka*, which is a homemade product using poppy straw and which is often mixed with diazepines, hypnotics, and other substances. In 1928, Merck & Co. introduced a combination product consisting of scopolamine, oxycodone, and ephedrine, which it initially marketed as SEE and then later renamed it Scophedal; the ephedrine was added to reduce its adverse respiratory and circulatory effects. Midol is an over-the-counter product manufactured by Bayer for the relief of menstrual pains; it contains acetaminophen, caffeine, and pyrilamine maleate, an antihistamine, which reduces the effects of histamine, a naturally produced chemical substance in the body. Pamprin is a similar over-the-counter combined product that contains acetaminophen, pyrilamine, and pamabrom, a diuretic. NyQuil contains acetaminophen and dextromethorphan, a cough suppressant, and NyQuil Cold and Flu capsules also contain doxylamine succinate, an antihistamine.

Some NSAIDs are included in various over-the-counter as well as prescription products in formulations combined with other substances. For instance, many over-the-counter combination products contain aspirin; these include Alka-Seltzer, Kaopectate, Maalox, Pepto-Bismol, and YSP. Many prescription combination products also contain aspirin along with other substances; these include Aggrenox, Equagesic, Gelprin, Halfprin, Helidac, Magan, Magsal, Myogesic, Norgesic, Robaxsial, Roxiprin, Salflex, and Trilistate.

Some barbiturates, such as butalbital, are also combined in formulations with painkiller drugs; these combination products are generally prescribed for treating pain and headache. Butalbital and acetaminophen are combined in products that are marketed under trade names such as Axocet, Bucet, Bupap, Cephadyn, Dolgic, Phrenilin, Pherenilin Forte, and Sedapap. Butalbital, acetaminophen, and caffeine are combined in products marketed under trade names such as Esgic and Fioricet. Butalbital and aspirin are marketed in a combination product sold under the trade name of Axotal. Butalbital, aspirin, and caffeine are combined in products marketed under trade names such as Fiornal, Fiormor, Fiortal, Fortabs, and Laniroif. A combined butalbital, acetaminophen, caffeine, and codeine phosphate product is marketed under the trade name of Fioricet #3 with Codeine; and a butalbital, aspirin, caffeine, and codeine phosphate combined product is marketed under the trade name of Fiorinal #3 with Codeine. These are but a few examples of the numerous pharmaceutical products that contain combinations of painkillers and other drugs and that, consequently can be used to relieve various types of pain sensations.

Smoking

Opium smoking became popular in the Orient during the 18th century, inspired at least in part by the smoking of tobacco. An influx of opium-smoking Chinese laborers brought the practice to the United States. Opium smoking spread rapidly in America beginning in the latter half of the 19th century, commonly associated with the various Chinatowns established in urban centers across the country. In this regard, it has been estimated by the U.S. Public Health Service that about 7,000 tons of crude opium and 800 tons of smoking opium were imported into the United States between 1859 and 1899. Opium became popularly demonized, and Chinese immigrants were further vilified, as a result of their popular association with opium smoking; this led to the popular conception of the yellow peril, also sometimes referred to as the yellow terror or the yellow specter. Consequently, 11 states passed anti-opium laws between 1877 and 1900 hoping, in large part, to discourage Chinese immigration. By the 1920s, opium dens, where opium was typically smoked, were in operation in most U.S. cities that had a local Chinatown. Alarmingly, at least to many Americans at the time, opium smoking tended to induce sleep and dreams and was considered characteristically un-American. Of great concern was the paranoid fear that White women might be lured into these dens by lecherous Chinese men, and if a biracial child should result, it was felt that it would result in the demise of the American race. Opium smoking subsequently decreased substantially in popularity in this country. However, Indochinese refugees reintroduced opium smoking to the United States in the early 1980s.

The smoking of heroin, as another example, appears to have originated in the 1920s in Shanghai and to have begun with the use of bamboo tubes and porcelain bowls, while the "chasing the dragon" method was developed in the 1950s in or near Hong Kong and refers to inhaling the vapors produced by heating heroin, typically on tin foil above a small flame. Unfortunately, inhaling heroin smoke may lead to the development of toxic leukoencephalopathy and other complications. Smoking drugs can also damage the lungs and bronchi, and it significantly increases the risks of having several respiratory diseases such as bronchitis and pneumonia. Heroin, like opium, has gone through various cycles of popularity with a range of populations, such as that observed among inner-city African Americans in the 1960s. The smoking of heroin results in lower traces of use in the blood than results from injection use. Many heroin addicts do not prefer smoking as this method of administration results in a waste of much of the drug and sole use is very difficult. However, the drug is delivered faster to the brain by smoking than it is by an injection route of administration; this more rapid onset of action is generally associated with greater risks of developing dependence.

Strategic Resource

Opium and other related narcotics continued to be an area of strategic concern during World War II. In fact, the Japanese desire to retain the opium-producing area of Mengjiang was a significant factor that led to the opening of the Pacific front, with the extension of hostilities at Pearl Harbor in December 1941 that led directly to U.S. entry into the war.

Opium has been regarded by many countries as a key strategic resource for several centuries. During World War I, for instance, there was nearly a total cessation of shipments of medicinal supplies from Germany and its allies to the United States and its allies; Germany was a major producer of pharmaceutical products at the time. The entry of Turkey into World War I further threatened the availability of opium and morphine in Great Britain, the United States, and their allies, which was at least partially remedied by the development of Indian opium production. The supply problems resulted in increases in the price as well as in dramatic shortages of opium and its associated derivative medications, particularly morphine and codeine. For example, in 1916, the pharmaceutical company Merck reported that the cost of opium had by then escalated about 10%, that supplies were running low, and consequently, that higher prices were expected. Accordingly, in April 1916, Merck was selling opium for $16.50 per pound, morphine sulphate for $7.40 per oz., codeine sulphate for $9.00 per oz., narcotine sulphate for $7.50 per oz., and heroin for $10.80 per oz. However, by January 1917, Merck was selling opium for $18.75 per pound, morphine sulphate for $9.30 per oz., codeine sulphate for $10.45 per oz., narcotine sulphate for $8.25 per oz., and heroin for $12.50 per oz. Further, by April 1917, Merck no longer had supplies of opium to sell, and it was selling morphine sulphate for $13.50 per oz., codeine sulphate for $44.25 per oz., narcotine sulphate for $8.25 per oz., and heroin for $20.50 per oz. There were, therefore, dramatic price increases within just one year for opium and its derivative medications.

Opium and its derivatives, particularly morphine, continued to be a strategic resource during World War II. Field Marshall Hermann Goering was one of the Nazi leaders well known to be addicted to morphine. The Nazis certainly invested heavily in trafficking opium from Turkey, which they relied on as their primary source, while the Allies relied primarily on opium from India. In this regard, it is estimated that an average acreage of *Papaver somniferum* in India yields between 25 kg and 30 kg of opium.

Heroin use hit record lows in the United States during World War II. However, the postwar era of the late 1940s and 1950s witnessed a sharp rise in the numbers of young Black and Latino heroin users. Heroin addiction, mainly by means of injection, became a steady facet of the drug problem in the United States and around the world during the 20th century. In this vein, the Office of National Drug Control Policy has stated that since 1981, the median bulk price of heroin has dropped by about 93%. On the other hand, there was a cessation in the use of heroin for medical purposes in most, but by no means all, countries.

The International Narcotics Control Board is a United Nations agency that is currently responsible for regulating the global opium supply. This helps to insure that there is sufficient availability of this strategic resource. It does this by means of enforcing the rules of the 1961 Single Convention on Narcotic Drugs. This Single Convention stipulates that a country can purchase opium poppies only in an amount corresponding to its use of opium-derived drugs, such as codeine and morphine. It also empowers two UN policy bodies, the World Health Organization (WHO) and the Commission on Narcotic Drugs, respectively, to maintain and update schedules of controlled substances so that newly created drugs, such as novel synthetic opioids, can rapidly be addressed.

The strategic importance of opium is underscored by the fact that a reserve supply of raw opium and of processed morphine has been stored for decades in the U.S. Bullion Depository at Fort Knox, Kentucky. These strategic reserves were established in 1955 to meet the painkiller needs of the entire United States for a year if foreign supplies were cut off. In 1993, the opium reserves were refined into morphine sulphate and are still stored at the depository.

Patent Medicines

Opium, morphine, codeine, and heroin were all readily available up through the early part of the 20th century, either by prescription or through nonprescription means such as the array of patent medicine preparations, many of which were even available through mail order. Not surprisingly, a growing awareness of many problems surfaced with these practices. For example, Mrs. Winslow's Soothing Syrup was reported to contain so much morphine that it was alleged to be an "infant murderer" that "killed outright . . . [with] murderous efficiency . . . used, in a vast majority of cases, because they are supposed to be harmless" (Winterburn, 1884, p. 46). Bateman's Pectoral Drops, for another example, contained opium, along with camphor gum, powdered catechu, red saunders, anise oil, and 76% alcohol. In 1888, a review of 10,000 prescriptions filled at pharmacies around the city of Boston found that 15% contained opiates (Eaton, 1888). One investigation, also conducted in 1888, found that alarming quantities of opium and alcohol were contained in many children's proprietary medications, including products like Ayer's Cherry Pectoral, Dr. Bull's Cough Syrup, Hooker's Cough and Croup Syrup, and Mother Bailey's Quieting Syrup. This reality even led to numerous cases of unintended fatal overdoses of children, which, not surprisingly, were dramatically reported on in the media of the day. Many of these patent medicines also claimed to cure an extremely broad array of "female" complaints and problems. Some proprietary medications containing opium and alcohol were sold to the public as cures for various disabilities, such as epilepsy, hysteria, neuralgia, and paralysis.

These panaceas were essentially unregulated, and as they were considered proprietary products, their ingredients would typically not be revealed but were maintained as protected trade secrets. Many of these 19th- and early 20th-century cure-alls were, in fact, very effective painkillers as they often contained opium, morphine, or heroin along with whatever else one wished to add in—unfortunately, often including toxins like lead or mercury as well as extracts from many poisonous plants. Further, the problem of narcotic addiction was, of course, largely unrecognized at that time. Consequently, the major demographic group addicted to narcotics at this time were middle- and upper-class females, due in large part to their use of these proprietary products.

The Pure Food and Drug Act of 1906 required proper labeling of the specific contents and dosage of respective drugs. After labeling of ingredients was mandated, it is estimated that the sale of patent medicines that contained opiates decreased by about 33%. In the early 20th century, increased regulation of narcotics in particular and laws requiring disclosure of ingredients became the norm in many countries around the world. The manufacturing and distribution of products containing opiates became increasingly restricted, such as was stipulated in the Harrison Narcotics Act of 1914 in the United States, the *Loi des stupefiants* of 1916 in France, and the Dangerous Drugs Act of 1920 in Great Britain. These types of measures contributed to the eventual disappearance of patent medicines.

THERAPEUTIC LEVELS AND EFFECTS

There are considerable differences between respective painkiller drugs in terms of what dosages are necessary to attain therapeutic results as well as to what effects, both desired and undesired, might commonly be experienced by users. Opiate and opioid drugs vary substantially in potency, as do respective over-the-counter and other related painkiller drugs.

Opiates and Opioids

Human beings have used opium and its derivatives as effective painkillers for a considerably long period of time with, however, somewhat mixed results, including misuse, abuse, and dependence as well as, of course, therapeutic pain relief. Drugs typically enter the brain from the circulatory system transported by the blood. However, the brain is protected by the blood-brain barrier, a protective layer around blood vessels in the brain. Painkillers, like opiates and opioids, must pass through the blood-brain barrier prior to altering the functioning of cerebral neurons and thereby affecting the pain-signaling processes in the brain.

These opiate and opioid substances have their most profound pharmacological effects by bonding to opioid receptor sites located principally in the brain and nervous system, but also in the gastrointestinal tract. In fact, multiple opioid receptors were first speculated about and were then later identified in the human brain and gastrointestinal tract. Opiate receptors include delta, kappa, lambda, and mu subtypes, each of which has diverse respective functions. Further, neuro-pathological changes in the brains of opiate addicts have been well documented by researchers. There is even some evidence suggesting that at least certain opiates, such as morphine and codeine, may be synthesized in mammalian tissue, including human cells. The half-life of opiates and opioids varies considerably depending upon the chemical structure of the respective painkiller substance. For instance, the half-life of morphine is about 2 hours, and the half-life of oxycodone is between 2 and 4 hours, while the half-life of methadone is about 27 hours. The pharmacological effects of these respective painkiller substances is somewhat variable as well. At any rate, addiction to these substances is well known, and opioid intoxication and opioid withdrawal were specifically defined in the DSM-IV-TR. The DSM-V does not, however, separate abuse from dependence, but rather provides a set of criteria for a range of opioid use disorders from mild to severe, depending on the number of symptoms experienced by the person. The detection time in urine for the use of relatively low doses of these substances, such as 3 to 12 mg of heroin, is between 1 and 1.5 days when using the customary cutoff level of 300 mg/ml for total morphine.

The binding of opiates and opioids to receptor sites in the brain stimulates the production of dopamine, a neurotransmitter associated with feelings of pleasure experienced in the brain's limbic system. The neurons, or brain cells, involved in the dopamine reward system are located mainly in the mesolimbic pathway of the ventral tegmental area of the human brain. This pathway extends into other brain regions, including the nucleus accumbens, which is part of the emotional control center, and into the frontal cortex, where decision making takes place.

Opiates and opioids vary somewhat in their painkilling abilities. Codeine is about only 1/12 as effective a painkiller as morphine, but it is a much better cough suppressant. Globally, codeine is currently the most widely used opiate medication. It is available in various formulations, such as extended-release tablets, syrups, and injectable forms, and in some countries it is also sold as a suppository. Codeine is most effective as a painkiller when used in combination with other substances, such as aspirin or acetaminophen; for example, Nurofen Plus is a combination product of codeine and ibuprofen. Codeine is also available in combination formulations with acetaminophen, such as those marketed under trade names such as Capital and Codeine Suspension, Tylenol with Codeine #3, and Tylenol with Codeine #4. Meperidine, also known in many countries as pethidine, which was first synthesized in 1939 by Otto Eislib and then Otto Schaumann of IG Farber, both working on pharmaceutical products in Germany, were the first to recognize its painkiller properties; it is now marketed under the trade name of Demerol, and it is approximately one-ninth as effective a painkiller as morphine. Methadone and oxycodone are roughly as potent painkillers as morphine. Although heroin is no longer used medically in the United States, it has a long history of medicinal use and continues to be used in some countries, including the UK. For example, from 1900 to about 1925, terpin hydrate with heroin, known as Elixir No. 2, was the most common cough medicine in the United States. When given parenterally for treating acute pain, heroin is about 2 to 4 times more potent a painkiller than morphine, with a faster onset of action. However, when administered orally, heroin is only about 1.5 times more potent than morphine in managing chronic pain in cancer patients. In fact, when the potency difference is taken into account, the pharmacological effects of heroin do not differ from those of morphine to any appreciable degree.

There are many other opioid painkillers that have been developed and marketed. Hydromorphone, also known as dihydromorphinone, was first synthesized in Germany in 1924 and was released onto the market by Knoll in 1926; it is marketed under various trade names such as Dilaudid, Hydol, Hydromorphan, Opidol, and Palladone, is estimated to be about eight times more potent a painkiller than morphine. It has a high dependence potential and a half-life of 2 to 3 hours with a bioavailability of 30% to 35% when taken orally and 52% to 58% when taken intra-nasally; it exhibits only 20% protein binding. After an FDA advisory in July 2005 that warned of the high overdose potential when used along with alcohol, an extended-release formulation of hydromorphone, which was marketed as Palladone, was voluntarily withdrawn from the market. In March 2010, the FDA approved once-daily extended-release formulations of hydromorphone that are marketed under the trade name of Exalgo and is manufactured in 8 mg, 12 mg, 16 mg, and 32 mg tablets. Dihydrocodeine is a semisynthetic opioid used as a painkiller and as an antitussive; it was developed in Germany in 1908 and first marketed in 1911. Dihydrocodeine is usually taken orally either as tablets, as elixirs, or in other solutions and also as a suppository; while it can be administered subcutaneously and intramuscularly, it should not be administered intravenously as it has a high risk of resulting in anaphylaxis and pulmonary edema. Dihydrocodeine has a half-life of about 4 hours and a bioavailability of around 20%. Several other semisynthetic opioids are chemically closely related to dihydrocodeine; these include acetyldihydrocodeine, dihydrocodeine enol acetate, dihydroisocodeine, nicocodeine, and nicodicodeine. Acetyldihydrocodeine is an opiate derivative that was discovered in 1914 in Germany; since it has higher lipophilicity than codeine and is converted not into morphine by the body but into dihydromorphine, it is more potent and longer lasting, and has a higher bioavailability, than codeine. Nicocodeine was first synthesized around the same time as acetyldihydrocodeine, and it was first introduced to the market in 1957 by Lannacher Heilmittel in Austria; it is metabolized into morphine and is about as potent a painkiller as hydrocodone and has a faster onset of action. However, neither acetyldihydrocodeine nor nicocodeine has ever been used clinically for medical purposes in the United States, and both are listed as Schedule I drugs under the Controlled Substances Act, with DEA numbers respectively of 9051 and 9309. Nicodicodeine, first synthesized in 1904, is similar to nicocodeine but is metabolized into dihydromorphine; thus it is more potent and longer lasting than nicocodeine, and so it can be used as a cough suppressant and painkiller. Diphenoxylate was discovered in 1956 at Janssen Pharmaceutica; it is an opioid agonist that is used for treating diarrhea as it, like many other opiates and opioids, slows down intestinal contractions and peristalsis; it has a half-life of 12 to 14 hours and exhibits between 74% and 95% protein binding. Dextropropoxyphene is a mu opioid receptor agonist that was patented in 1955 by Eli Lilly and Company, which marketed it under the trade name of Darvon; dextropropoxyphene is a painkiller structurally similar to methadone but considered to be a much less effective painkiller; its onset of action is between 20 and 30 minutes and has been used as a painkiller, as an antitussive, for its local anesthetic effects, and to ease withdrawal symptoms in those addicted to opiate or opioid drugs; it has a half-life of 6 to 12 hours and a bioavailability of around 40%. However, dextropropoxyphene was withdrawn from the U.S. and European markets due to concerns with heart arrhythmias and fatal overdoses. Pentazocine, unlike the majority of opiate and opioid drugs, acts partially through the kappa receptors, and it must therefore be used with caution when taken along with other opiates or opioids as it can create withdrawal symptoms in those who are dependent. Pentazocine is a synthetic mixed agonist-antagonist opioid painkiller that has a half-life of 2 to 3 hours and a bioavailability of about 20% when taken orally.

There are several other mixed agonist-antagonist opioid painkillers similar to pentazocine; these include cyclazocine, dezocine, and phenazocine. Phenazocine is a more potent painkiller than pentazocone and has fewer side effects; it is about 4 times more potent a painkiller than morphine. However, due to adverse side effects, the use of cyclazocine, dezocine, and phenazocine has been discontinued in the United States. Morphine is pretty much the standard medicinal painkiller against which other similar substances are evaluated.

Morphine

Morphine is a very effective opiate painkiller drug. This narcotic medication is thus prescribed regularly for the relief of severe pain, like that associated with certain forms of cancer or as a painkiller administered after many types of surgery. The widespread popularity of the medical use of morphine is underscored by the fact that it is currently marketed under more than 100 different trade names.

The typical side effects of morphine use can include blurred vision, constriction of the pupils, constipation, lethargy, nausea, respiratory suppression, and vomiting. The subjective effects of morphine become even more pronounced as the dosage is increased; drowsiness leads to sleep, and nausea, vomiting, respiratory depression, and painkilling efficacy all increase. Extremely high doses of morphine and related painkillers can produce an onset of convulsions and seizures. Morphine metabolites are excreted primarily through the kidneys after being glucuronated, and depending on an individual's renal function, various metabolites can accumulate. The pharmacological effects of morphine are generally potentiated by alkaline substances and antagonized by acidic substances; its analgesic effects are potentiated, for instance, by the presence of other substances such as chlorpromazine, melatonin, and methocarbamol.

Although morphine has repeatedly been shown to be a highly effective painkiller for pain that is caused by a pathology that is generally associated with anxiety, such as a cancer, controlled laboratory studies have shown it to be not very effective in reducing pain not accompanied by anxiety. Similar evidence comes from observations that soldiers wounded on the battlefield request painkillers much less than civilians about to undergo a comparable major surgical procedure. The analgesic effectiveness of morphine and similar painkillers is heavily influenced by the mental state of the individual.

Morphine is a very addictive narcotic substance, with rapid development of tolerance and dependence often experienced. The early analgesic effect of morphine seems to abate over the course of repeated use. Continued use of morphine appears to produce a compensatory learned hyperanalgesic response that soon leads to the consequent development of tolerance, which has both physiological and psychological components. This tolerance reaction appears to be an amalgamation of the conditioned response to the rituals associated with use, as well as to the systemic effects of the substance itself. It has been recognized, at least since 1948, that the problem of relapse among addicts is associated with conditioning to the effects of morphine use. Similar morphine-conditioned responses have been observed in other animals, such as dogs and rats. It has been recognized that some apparent withdrawal symptoms are actually responses conditioned to either environmental or pharmacological factors associated with morphine use.

The duration of action of morphine after subcutaneous administration is about 4 to 5 hours; this is approximately equivalent to the duration of action of other opioids, such as hydromorphone, oxymorphone, metophan, dihydrocodeine, oxycodone, pholcodine, levorphanol, dextromoramide, and dipipanone, while that for other opiates and opioids is quiet variable. The duration of action of alphaprodine after subcutaneous administration is about 1 to 2 hours and that for phenadoxone is about 1 to 3 hours. The duration of action of both anileridine and meperidine after subcutaneous administration is about 2 to 4 hours. The duration of action of methadone after subcutaneous administration is about 3 to 5 hours, while that for heroin is about 3 to 4 hours. The duration of action of hydrocodone after subcutaneous administration is about 4 to 8 hours. The more lipid soluble substances have a more rapid onset of action after subcutaneous administration due primarily to differences in the rates of absorption.

The half-life of morphine is typically between 1.5 and 4.5 hours, with a bioavailability of around 30% to 40% when administered orally; it exhibits 35% plasma protein binding, has an onset of action of between 30 and 45 minutes, and a typical duration of action of 3 to 4 hours, while those variables for other opiates and opioids are quiet variable. For example, the half-life of LAAM is 48 hours, while the half-life of its active metabolites is up to 96 hours, while that for codeine is about 3 hours, with a bioavailability of about 70% to 90%, and its use is detectable for about 24 hours in blood and up to 3 days in urine. Heroin, which is 4 to 5 times more potent a painkiller than morphine, has 100% bioavailability for intravenous or intramuscular use, but has a half-life of just six-tenths of an hour. Buprenorphine is about 40 times more potent a painkiller than morphine with between 35% and 40% bioavailability when taken orally, exhibits 96% plasma protein binding, and has an onset of action of about 60 minutes, an average half-life of 36 hours, and a typical duration of action of 4 to 12 hours. Oxymorphone is about 7 times more potent a painkiller than morphine with only about 10 % bioavailability, exhibits 10% to 12% plasma protein binding, and has an onset of action of between 20 and 40 minutes, a typical duration of action of 3 to 4 hours, and an average half-life of 1.3 hours. Hydromorphone is about 5 times more potent a painkiller than morphine with between 20% and 35% bioavailability and an average bioavailability of 24% when administered orally, exhibits 8% to 19% plasma protein binding, and has an onset of action of about 30 minutes, a half-life between 2 to 3 hours with an average half-life of 2.6 hours, and a typical duration of action of 2 to 3 hours. Oxycodone is about 1.5 times more potent a painkiller than morphine with a range of about 87% bioavailability and between 60% and 80% bioavailability when administered orally, and a half-life of between 3 and 4.5 hours. Hydrocodone has about the same potency as morphine, with a bioavailability of greater than 80% and a half-life between 3.8 and 6 hours. Propoxyphene, a synthetic opioid marketed as Darvon, has a half-life of 4 to 6 hours and a duration of action of 6 to 12 hours; levorphanol has a longer half-life, an average of 11 to 16 hours, exhibits about 40% plasma protein binding, and is eight times more potent a painkiller than morphine, with about 50% to 70% bioavailability when administered orally, an onset of action between 20 to 40 minutes, and with a duration of action of 4 to 8 hours.

Methadone is somewhat different from most other opioids with respect to its potency as this varies depending on how long it has been used; when taken acutely from 1 to 3 days, methadone has a potency about 4 times more potent a painkiller than morphine, while when taken chronically for more than 7 days, it has a potency about 7 to 8 times more potent than morphine, with a bioavailability of between 40% and 90% and an average bioavailability of 80% when administered orally, exhibits 80% to 90% plasma protein binding, an onset of action between 60 to 90 minutes, a typical duration of action from 6 to 12 hours, and a half-life from 15 to 60 hours, with an average half-life of 22 hours. Methadone was first granted approval for use in the United States by the FDA in 1947.

The half-life of many opioids is quite variable depending on the method of administration. Fentanyl, for instance, has a half-life of 6.5 minutes for intranasal use, 10 to 20 minutes for intravenous use, 2 to 4 hours by tablet, and 20 to 27 hours for transdermal patch, with, of course, different respective levels of bioavailability. Morphine is eliminated primarily by means of renal excretion, with about 90% of morphine excreted in the urine within 24 hours of use.

There, of course, is a constellation of side effects that typically accompany the taking of morphine or other opiates or opioids. Constipation is a particularly common side effect of such use. In fact, among individuals taking opioids, up to 90% have constipation and other gastrointestinal side effects that not only affect their quality of life, but also adversely impact medication adherence. Unfortunately, opioid-induced constipation is not dose dependent, nor does it typically resolve over time. Further, there are some indications that higher doses of opiates and opioids are also associated with increased immunosuppressive effects.

Morphine use, as well as that of related painkiller drugs such as heroin, codeine, and other opiates and opioids, over a period of hours causes a glucose crash after transient hyperglycemia. This reaction is responsible for the commonly observed sugar cravings experienced by addicts.

Respiratory depression, or the reduced ability to breathe, is a very serious and potentially fatal side effect associated with the use of opiates and opioids; accordingly, individuals should inform their physicians or other health care providers if they have long-term breathing problems such as asthma or chronic obstructive pulmonary disease (COPD). As drowsiness and dizziness are classic side effects associated with opiate and opioid use and abuse, which are increased even more when combined with the use of alcoholic beverages, individuals must be particularly careful when driving or using electrical equipment and heavy machinery.

Continued use of morphine and other opiate and opioid drugs often leads to the development of tolerance. Tolerance is the phenomenon where one adapts, both physiologically and psychologically, to the effects of a drug, particularly the opiates and opioids, such that higher doses become necessary to achieve similar results that were previously produced by smaller amounts of the drug. Further, morphine and many of the opiate and opioid drugs exhibit cross-tolerance, whereby use of one can lead to the development of tolerance to other similar drugs, even if they never actually used those other drugs.

Tolerance is the cornerstone of developing a dependence upon a particular drug. The frequency of administration of the respective drug and its dosage taken are directly related to the development of tolerance. When opiate or opioid drugs are administered repeatedly, tolerance can develop rapidly, but it does not develop if there are prolonged periods of abstinence in between. Habitual users of opiate and opioid drugs can develop tolerance to the euphoric, as well as to the sedative and painkiller effects of the respective drugs.

Tolerance can also be developed to the respiratory effects such that a dose that would likely kill a naïve user may be tolerated by a habitual user without incident. Cross-tolerance, as noted, naturally occurs to most other opiate and opioid drugs. However, there is no cross-tolerance to other central nervous system depressants, including alcohol; accordingly, combined use of opiate or opioid drugs with alcohol or other depressant drugs can result in respiratory depression and possibly even death.

Physical dependence resulting from the use of morphine, as well as other opiate and opioid drugs, typically produces moderate to severe withdrawal symptoms when someone attempts to suddenly cease the use of that particular painkiller drug. Whenever chronic use of an opiate or opioid drug is discontinued or is dramatically reduced, then withdrawal symptoms can occur.

Continued use of the substance after dependence is developed is in some part at least due to the addict's perceived need to relieve the acute or protracted withdrawal symptoms, which is understood as a form of negative reinforcement. It must also be recognized that the drug user is not merely a passive subject in the development of an addiction, but is also actively involved in shaping its course.

Withdrawal signs associated with the cessation of morphine use can include a drippy nose, gooseflesh, restlessness, agitation, sleep disturbance, sweating, teary eyes, and yawning during the first 24 hours, with more symptoms, including dilated pupils, abdominal, leg and back pains, anxiety, diarrhea, extreme irritability, hot and cold flashes, insomnia, nausea, spasms and twitching of muscles, and vomiting, becoming more severe over the next 72 hours. The onset of symptoms varies with the respective painkiller used and its pharmacological characteristics, such as its half-life and duration of action. Withdrawal symptoms can typically start within 12 hours of the last heroin administration or within 30 hours of the last methadone administration. Withdrawal reactions from opiate and opioid painkiller drugs can be extremely uncomfortable and even painful, but they are not, in and of themselves, generally life-threatening. However, it is very crucial to maintain appropriate electrolyte and fluid balances during the course of the abstinence syndrome as diarrhea and vomiting can cause dangerous dehydration and electrolyte imbalances. Withdrawal treatment for these substances is largely supportive in nature and concerned primarily with the relief of symptoms, for which other drugs can be administered. Clonidine, for instance, is frequently given during opiate or opioid withdrawal as it helps reduce the symptoms of anxiety, agitation, runny nose, muscle aches, and cramping. Benzodiazepines, such as diazepam and oxazepam, are sometimes also used to help treat feelings of anxiety as well as for helping with issues like sleep and for muscle relaxation. Ibuprofen and related NSAIDs are sometimes also used for their anti-inflammatory and painkilling effects. Buprenorphine, which is marketed under trade names such as Suboxone and Subutex, can also be administered as it can help to shorten the length of detoxification.

There are, of course, a range of both individual and group differences with respect to the pharmacokinetics and pharmacodynamics of morphine and other opiate and opioid drugs. For example, individuals from East Africa, particularly Ethiopia and Eritrea, are known to metabolize codeine into morphine faster than those from other parts of the world. These sorts of population differences, mainly attributed to genetic variance, significantly influence the effects that respective dosages of morphine and other opiate and opioid painkiller drugs will have on different individuals.

Over-the-Counter and Other Painkillers

Many over-the-counter products can be highly effective painkillers. Aspirin and acetaminophen, for instance, can be used as appropriate painkillers for relief of musculoskeletal pains. However, much of the rather widespread use of over-the-counter painkillers is relatively ineffective, and they are also frequently used unnecessarily. Unfortunately, many individuals are unaware of the varied adverse side effects of such practices, some of which are not even very well understood.

The most common side effects associated with aspirin use include headache, heartburn, nausea, and an upset stomach, all of which are typically very mild and do not warrant discontinued use. However, there are more serious side effects that are sometimes experienced by use of NSAIDs, including aspirin; these are largely gastrointestinal in nature and consist of bloody or dark stools, severe stomach pains and ulcers, and severe diarrhea, as well as ringing in the ears and severe allergic reactions manifest by rashes, hives, facial swelling, and breathing difficulties.

Many Americans take daily low-dose aspirin in the hope of preventing a heart attack or stroke. In fact, one study reported on nearly 69,000 adults in the United States who are prescribed aspirin long term; many more Americans, of course, take daily aspirin without a physician's recommendation. The research evidence is clear that individuals who have already suffered a heart attack or stroke can substantially reduce the risk of having another by daily taking a low dose of aspirin. A daily low dose of 81 mg of aspirin is recommended when appropriate as larger doses may be associated with relatively excessive bleeding. However, the evidence does not necessarily support the practice for preventing a first-time heart attack or stroke. The risks associated with long-term aspirin use, particularly severe gastrointestinal bleeding and hemorrhagic stroke, or bleeding in the brain, do not outweigh the possible benefits of aspirin therapy. These risks increase as we age, and further if aspirin is used along with other NSAIDs, such as ibuprofen or naproxen. Actually, about 12% of U.S. adults prescribed long-term aspirin use in the study probably should not have been. Individuals with a history of stomach ulcer, for example, have up to 3 times the risk of suffering gastrointestinal bleeding compared to those without such a history. Nevertheless, most men aged 45 to 79 years old and women aged 55 to 79 years old are advised to talk to their doctor or other health care provider about prophylactically taking aspirin. In general, taking daily low-dose aspirin reduces the chances of having a first heart attack by about 32% in men. Although aspirin has not been shown to be very useful for preventing heart attacks in women, it has demonstrated utility for preventing strokes. Older individuals are more likely to have a heart attack or stroke, but they are also much more likely to have a serious stomach bleeding problem if they take aspirin long term. In addition, low-dose aspirin also appears to increase overall survival rate of individuals with various gastrointestinal tract cancers, such as cancer of the colon, rectum, or esophagus.

Aspirin is useful for relief of pain, fever, and inflammation from myriad conditions such as the common cold, influenza, neck and/or lower back pain, headache, toothache, dysmenorrhea, myositis, strains and sprains, arthritis, bursitis, synovitis, injuries, burns, and after surgical and/or dental procedures. Further, due to its ability to inhibit platelet aggregation, aspirin is also useful in lowering the risks for those with unstable angina and even those who have had a prior myocardial infarction, as well as reducing the risks for stroke and transient ischemic attacks (TIAs). Aspirin is, in fact, the only NSAID that inhibits blood clotting for an extended period, from 4 to 7 days, and thus it serves as an effective preventer of heart attacks and strokes. Aspirin is about 170 times more potent at inhibiting the COX-1 enzyme than the COX-2 enzyme. The relative strength of aspirin as a painkiller is only about one-360th that of morphine. Concomitant use of other NSAIDs is not recommended; particularly for those at high risk for cardiovascular events, other types of painkillers that do not interfere with its antiplatelet properties, such as acetaminophen, opiates, or opioids, should be considered.

NSAIDs all have a similar mechanism of action, but they differ considerably in their potency and duration of action. Some individuals who do not get an effective painkiller response from one NSAID may get so from others.

The half-life of many NSAIDs is somewhat variable depending on assorted characteristics of the users, such as the healthy functioning of their kidneys, whether they are pregnant, and so forth. Aspirin is rapidly absorbed from the stomach and small intestines with 100% bioavailability; the optimal pH range for aspirin absorption is from 2.15 to 4.10. The half-life of aspirin in a normal healthy individual, is about 3.5 to 4.5 hours for its effectiveness to be cut in half. However, the half-life of aspirin in circulation is between 13 and 19 minutes, as the level in the blood drops rapidly after absorption is completed. It can take up to 48 hours for complete elimination of urinary aspirin metabolites, essentially salicylate; generally, alkaline urine promotes excretion and acidic urine facilitates reabsorption by renal tubules. Diflunisal is a salicylic acid derivative that was developed in 1971 by Merck Sharp and Dohme, was first marketed under the trade name of Dolobid, and is currently available by prescription only in the United States; it is only about one-160th as potent a painkiller as morphine, with a bioavailability of 80% to 90% and a half-life of between 8 and 12 hours. Salsalate, also known as disalicylic acid, is another salicylate derivative drug that is currently available by prescription only in the United States; it is marketed under various trade names such as Disalcid, Nobacid, Salflex, Salina, and Sasapirin; and it has a half-life of 3.5 hours to 16 or more hours. Salsalate has weak inhibitory effects on COX-1 and COX-2 enzymes, but it inhibits the production of several other inflammatory substances, such as C-reactive protein, interlukin-6, and TNF-alpha; unlike aspirin, salsalate does not inhibit platelet aggregation. Salicylates are excreted primarily through the kidneys by means of glomerular filtration and tubular excretion. They are chiefly broken down into free salicyclic acid and salicyluric acid as well as phenolic and acyl glucuronides.

Ibuprofen is rapidly absorbed after oral administration and reaches its peak concentration after 15 to 30 minutes. It inhibits thromboxane synthesis and platelet aggregation. Ibuprofen also appears to decrease bacterial cell viability, while increasing leukocyte degranulation. Further, it inhibits the development of edema. Ibuprofen is recommended as the initial drug of choice for treating acute pain associated with musculoskeletal trauma in children. Findings from a randomized trial suggested that ibuprofen is at least as effective as orally administered morphine given every 6 hours for outpatient pain among children with uncomplicated fractures. Similarly, intravenous ibuprofen, which was granted approval by the FDA for use in the United States in 2009, appears to be more effective at reducing fevers in pediatric patients than acetaminophen taken orally or by suppository. It is well known that ibuprofen is associated with fewer adverse side effects than morphine when administered to children. Interestingly, prior ibuprofen oral administration has been shown to result in a doubling of beta-endorphin plasma levels, which mediate its painkilling ability. However, unlike aspirin, ibuprofen does not have long-lasting antiplatelet effects, nor does it produce comparable gastrointestinal irritation. Ibuprofen exhibits 98% plasma protein binding, has 87% to 100% bioavailability when administered orally and 87% bioavailability when administered rectally, has an onset of action of 30 minutes, and has an average half-life of approximately 1.3 hours to 3 hours. Over 90% of ibuprofen is excreted in the urine as metabolites or their conjugates.

Other profens, or propionic acid NSAIDs, chemically related to ibuprofen include carprofen, dexibuprofen, dexketoprofen, fenbufen, fenoprofen, indoprofen, loxoprofen, oxaprozin, pirprofen, and suprofen. Carprofen is used by veterinarians mainly for treating dogs; it has a half-life of about 8 hours, ranging from 4.5 hours to 9.8 hours in dogs; it exhibits 99% plasma protein binding, and it has around 90% bioavailability. Dexiprofen is the active dextrorotatory enantiomer of ibuprofen. Dexketoprofen trometamol is manufactured by Menarini and it is marketed in the UK under the trade name of Keral, under the trade name of Dolmen in Estonia and Lithuania, as Stadium in Mexico, as Ketesgel in Spain, as Menadex in Slovenia, and in Latin America under the trade name of Enantyum; it has greater painkiller efficacy and greater anti-inflammatory effects than ibuprofen. Fenbufen is an NSAID usually used to treat pain and inflammation associated with conditions such as ankylosing spondylitis, osteoarthritis, tendinitis, and other musculoskeletal disorders; it is marketed under several trade names, such as Cepal, Cinopal, Ctbufen, Lederfen, and Reugast, as well as under several generic formulations; it reaches its peak plasma concentration after 1.19 hours, and its plasma half-life is sufficiently long to permit twice-daily administration, in fact, it has a plasma half-life of 10.26 hours. Fenoprofen calcium is an NSAID used for relief of symptoms of rheumatoid arthritis, osteoarthritis, and other types of mild to moderate pain; it is marketed in the United States under trade names such as Nalfon; it has an average half-life of 3 hours. Indoprofen has a half-life of 2.3 hours and is metabolized by glucuronidation, but it was removed from the market in the 1980s due to reports of gastrointestinal bleeding. Loxoprofen exhibits 97% bioavailability, reaches peak plasma concentration in 30 to 50 minutes, has a half-life of about 75 minutes, and is metabolized by hepatic glucuronidation; it is marketed by Sankyo under the trade names of Loxonin in Brazil, Japan, and Mexico; as Loxomac in India; and as Oxeno in Argentina. Oxaprozin, also known as oxaprozinum, is an NSAID used for relief of inflammation, swelling and joint pain associated with rheumatoid arthritis and osteoarthritis. It was originally granted approval by the FDA in October 1992; it is manufactured as 600 mg tablets, available by prescription, and is marketed under various trade names, such as Daypro, Dayrun, and Duraprox. It exhibits 99% plasma protein binding, primarily to albumin; has about 95% bioavailability after being administered orally; has a rather long average half-life of 54.9 hours; and about 95% of oxaprozin is metabolized by the liver. Pirprofen is another propionic acid NSAID that was introduced to the market in 1982 as Rengasil manufactured by Ciba-Geigy, who voluntarily withdrew it in 1990 due to concerns over fatal liver toxicity.

Acetaminophen works as a painkiller primarily by seeming to raise the pain threshold; it accomplishes this apparently by inhibiting the nitric oxide pathway mediated by selected neurotransmitters like substance P and N-methyl-D-aspartate. Acetaminophen also works as an effective antipyretic by inhibiting arachidonic acid metabolism, thereby blocking the effects of internally produced pyrogens that elevate prostaglandin E levels and act on the preoptic area of the anterior hypothalamus to both stimulate heat gain and reduce heat loss. After swallowing an oral dose, acetaminophen is rapidly and nearly completely absorbed in the small intestine of the gastrointestinal tract. This results in ranges from 85% to 98% relative bioavailability; only a relatively small—10% to 25%—amount of acetaminophen is bound to plasma proteins. Acetaminophen is primarily metabolized in the liver, principally by conjugation with glucuronide and with sulfate, and by oxidation by means of cytochrome as well as by hydroxylation to form 3-hydroxy-acetaminophen and by methoxylation to form 3-methoxy-acetaminophen; it is eliminated primarily by formation of glucuronide and sulfate conjugates. The half-life of acetaminophen in normal healthy adults is about 2 to 3 hours; less than 9% of acetaminophen is excreted in urine. The elimination half-life is about 3 hours for the extended-release formulations of acetaminophen.

Ketoprofen is an NSAID that is currently available only by prescription and used for inflammatory pains associated with arthritis or severe toothache caused by gum inflammation. It is a nonselective COX inhibitor that has anti-inflammatory, antipyretic, and painkiller effects achieved by inhibiting the production of prostaglandins and leukotriene; it also appears to have lysosomal membrane-stabilizing action and antibradykinin activity. Ketoprofen was originally approved for use by the FDA on December 22, 1992. The bioavailability of ketoprofen taken by oral administration is approximately 90%, with peak plasma levels reached in around 3.9 minutes. The half-life of ketoprofen is about 2.1 hours. Within 24 hours, about 80% of ketoprofen is excreted in urine, mostly as a glucuronide metabolite.

Ketorolac is an NSAID used for short-term management of moderate to severe pain from an array of causes. It is a nonselective COX inhibitor that has anti-inflammatory, antipyretic, and painkiller effects achieved by inhibiting the production of prostaglandins. Ketorolac tromethamine was originally approved for use in the United States by the FDA on May 16, 1997; approval was granted to Cycle Pharms Ltd., Mylan, and Teva to manufacture 10 mg oral tablets. Subsequently, approval was granted by the FDA on June 5, 1997, to Hospira to manufacture injectable formulations of ketorolac tromethamine in multiple strengths, and several other manufactures were later also granted approval by the FDA. The half-life of ketorolac is between 3.5 and 9.2 hours in young adults and between 4.7 and 8.6 hours in the elderly. An average of 91.4%, ketorolac is excreted by the kidneys, and an average of 6.1% is metabolized by the liver.

Flurbiprofen is another NSAID that is used to treat the pain and/or inflammation of arthritis and related conditions. It is another nonselective COX inhibitor that inhibits the production of prostaglandins. Flurbiprofen was approved for use in the United States by the FDA in two different formulations; a flurbiprofen formulation that was initially granted approval by the FDA on June 20, 1994; and a flurbiprofen sodium formulation that was granted FDA approval on January 4, 1995. The half-life of flurbiprofen is between 4.7 and 5.7 hours. It is more than 99% protein bound and is metabolized by the liver and excreted through the kidneys.

Diclofenac, another NSAID, is of the acetic, also known as arylalkonic, acid family; it is used to treat pain and inflammation, such as that associated with arthritis or ankylosing spondylitis. It is also often used for treating mild to moderate postoperative or post-traumatic pain and for acute migraine headaches, menstrual pain, and endometriosis. The FDA approved Diclofenac for use in two different formulations; a diclofenac sodium formulation was granted approval on June 9, 1995, and a diclofenac potassium formulation was granted approval on August 6, 1998. Diclofenac should be used only to treat a migraine attack; it is not effective against a headache that has already begun and should not be used for cluster headaches. It is yet another nonselective COX inhibitor that inhibits the production of prostaglandins. The half-life of diclofenac is between 1.2 and 2 hours. It is more than 99% protein bound and is partly (ca. 40%) metabolized by the liver, with the remainder (ca. 60%) excreted through the kidneys in urine. Another arylalkonic acid NSAID closely related to diclofenac is aceclofenac, which is an analog of diclofenac, actually its glycolic acid ester.

Indomethacin, also known as indometacin, is another arylalkonic acid NSAID that is commonly prescribed for reducing fever, stiffness, swelling, and pain; it was discovered in 1963 and was originally granted approval by the FDA for sale in the United States in 1965. It is available in several different prescription-only formulations; for example, on April 20, 1984, Mylan received approval from the FDA to manufacture 25 mg and 50 mg oral capsules; on August 31, 1992, G and W Labs was granted approval by the FDA to manufacture a rectal suppository formulation; on March 17, 2010, Fresenius Kabi USA was granted approval by the FDA to manufacture an injectable formulation; and, on December 1, 2010, Amneal Pharms was granted approval by the FDA to manufacture a 75 mg extended release capsule. Indomethacin has a half-life of 2.6 to 11.2 hours in adults and of 12 to 28 hours in infants; it has about 100% bioavailability when taken orally and between 80% and 90% bioavailability when administered rectally. Acemetacin is an analog of indomethacin—actually, it is its glycolic acid ester that is a prodrug of indomethacin into which it is rapidly broken down; however, it causes less gastric damage than indomethacin. Acemetacin is manufactured by Merck and is marketed under various trade names in respective countries, such as: Emflex in the UK; Gamespir in Greece; Ost-map in Egypt; Rantudil in Germany, Mexico, and Portugal; Reudol in Spain; Rheutrop in Austria; and Tilur in Switzerland.

Other acetic acid NSAIDs include bromfenac, etodolac, nabumetone, sulindac, tolmetin, and zomepirac. Bromfenac is an acetic acid NSAID usually prescribed for treating ocular inflammation and pain after surgery for cataracts. It was first introduced to the U.S. market in July 1997, manufactured by Wyeth-Ayerst, and marketed as Duract, an oral formulation for short-term pain relief, but it was voluntarily withdrawn on June 22, 1998, after reports of hepatotoxicity; it was subsequently granted FDA approval in 2005 as a twice-daily formulation and marketed as Xibrom and in October 2010 as a once-daily formulation marketed as Bromday, and again in 2013 as Prolensa. Etodolac is another acetic acid NSAID available in the United States only by prescription; it is manufactured in 200 mg and 300 mg capsules, 400 mg and 500 mg tablets, and 400 mg, 500 mg, and 600 mg extended-release formulations. It exhibits 99% plasma protein binding, primarily to albumin; has 80% to 100% bioavailability when administered orally; has an average half-life of 7.3 hours, with a range of 3.3 hours to 11.3 hours; and it has a duration of action of between 4 hours and 6 hours. Nabumetone was developed by Beecham as an acetic acid NSAID that is prescribed to treat the pain and inflammation associated with rheumatoid arthritis, osteoarthritis, and related disorders like gout; it received FDA approval for use in the United States in December 1991 and is marketed under various trade names, such as Gambaran, Relaflen, and Relifex; it exhibits 99% plasma protein binding and has an average half-life of 23 hours.

Sulindac is an acetic acid NSAID available by prescription only to treat acute or chronic inflammatory conditions; it was first granted approval for use in the United States by the FDA in September 1978. It is marketed in the United States and the United Kingdom by Merck under the trade name of Clinoril, which comes in 150 mg and 200 mg tablets; it exhibits about 90% bioavailability when administered orally and has an average half-life of 7.8 hours. Tolmetin sodium is another acetic acid NSAID available only by prescription; it comes in both capsule and tablet formulations of variable strengths; it has an average half-life of 1 hour to 2 hours. Zomepirac sodium is structurally similar to tolmetin sodium; it was developed by McNeil Pharmaceutical, approved for use in the United States by the FDA in 1980, and marketed under the trade name of Zomax for treating all forms of mild to moderately severe pain; however, it was withdrawn from the market in March 1983 due to its tendency to cause dangerous anaphylaxis.

Naproxen is used to relieve pain such as that associated with dental issues, headaches, menstrual cramps, muscle aches, and tendonitis. It also reduces pain as well as swelling and joint stiffness, such as that associated with conditions like arthritis, bursitis, and gout. Naproxen was originally approved for use in the United States by the FDA and marketed under the trade name of Naprosyn on March 11, 1976. It was manufactured by Roche Palo and produced as 250 mg, 375 mg, and 500 mg tablets. Naproxen is now also marketed under various other trade names, such as Aleve, Anaprox, and Naprelan. The average half-life of naproxen is about 25 hours; it is O-desmethylated and conjugated into acyl glucuronides. Currently, naproxen is thought to carry the lowest risks among the NSAIDs for causing heart disease and stroke. Other propionic acid NSAIDs, or profens, closely related chemically to naproxen include benoxaprofen and flunoxaprofen. Benoxaprofen was marketed by Eli Lilly and Company as Oraflex in the United States and as Opren in Europe, but it was voluntarily removed from the market in 1982 after reports of adverse side effects including deaths. Flunoxaprofen is closely related to naproxen, but it has limited water solubility and must be formulated as a salt that has effective anti-inflammatory properties.

Flufenamic acid, meclofenamic acid, and mefenamic acid are some fenamic acid derivatives that function as NSAIDs. Flufenamic acid works by inhibiting the activity of prostaglandin F synthase and by activating TRPC6; it thus decreases both swelling and uterine contractions. Flufenamic acid has a half-life of about 3 hours and exhibits extensive protein binding. Meclofenamic acid, also known as meclofenamate sodium, is an NSAID used for relief of pain, tenderness, swelling, and stiffness associated with osteoarthritis, rheumatoid arthritis, and dysmenorrhea; it was initially approved for use in the United States by the FDA in June 1980 and was marketed under trade names such as Meclomen and Meclodium, but these are no longer available in the United States. However, meclofenamic acid is also sold under the trade name of Arquel for use in veterinary medicine, such as for treating dogs and horses.

Meclofenamic acid is rapidly absorbed in humans following oral administration with peak plasma concentrations reached from 0.5 hours to 2 hours; it exhibits nearly 99% plasma protein binding and has an elimination half-life from 0.8 hours to 5.3 hours. Mefenamic acid is a closely related NSAID that is used to treat pain, particularly menstrual pain; it has a half-life of around 2 hours and it has about 90% bioavailability and 90% protein binding. Mefenamic acid has been approved by the FDA in several 250-mg oral capsule formulations; this includes approval to Micro Labs Ltd. on November 19, 2010; Lupin Ltd. on July 22, 2011; Breckenridge Pharm on February 5, 2013; and Vintage Pharms LLC on June 2, 2014. Mefenamic acid is marketed under various trade names in respective countries, such as Ponstel in the United States and Ponstan in the UK and in Canada.

Several oxicam NSAIDs have been developed to treat painful inflammatory conditions such as arthritis. The oxicam family of drugs includes several chemically related painkillers such as piroxicam, isoxicam, droxicam, lornoxicam, meloxicam, and tenoxicam. Piroxicam is an NSAID of the oxicam family that was approved for use in the United States by the FDA in 1982. It is available by prescription only, is used for treating chronic arthritis, comes in 10 mg and 20 mg capsules in generic formulations, and is also marketed under various trade names such as Feldene, Novo-Pirocam, and Nu-Pirox; it has a 50-hour half-life and exhibits 99% protein binding. Isoxicam is a benzothiazine derivative of piroxicam, and it has anti-inflammatory and antipyretic properties; chemically it closely resembles piroxicam. Droxicam is an NSAID that is a prodrug of piroxicam. Lornoxicam, also known as chlortenoxicam, has a half-life of 3 to 4 hours and has between 90% and 100% bioavailability. Meloxicam is an NSAID that has painkiller and antipyretic properties; it was approved for use in the United States by the FDA in April 2000, is available by prescription only in 7.5 mg and 15 mg tablets in generic formulations, and is marketed under the trade name of Mobic, which is manufactured by Boehringer Ingelheim. It exhibits 99.4% plasma protein binding, has about 89% bioavailability after oral administration, has an onset of action of between 0.5 hours and 1 hour, and has an average half-life of 20 hours; it is also used in veterinary medicine. Tenoxicam has a half-life of between 30 and 40 hours and exhibits high protein binding. Droxicam and tenoxicam are currently available in other countries but not available for use in the United States.

Several NSAIDs of the pyrazolidine family of derivatives have been developed as painkillers. These include azapropazone, feprazone, phenylbutazone, oxyphenbutazone, and sulfinpyrazone. Azapropazone is a pyrazolidine derivative NSAID that was formerly available by prescription in the UK. It was manufactured by Goldshield and marketed under the trade name of Rheumox, but it has since been discontinued from the British National Formulary; it has an average half-life of about 20 hours. Feprazone is a pyrazolidine NSAID used for treating joint and muscular pain; it is available in a few countries and marketed under various trade names, such as Vapesin in Venezula and Xitong in China. Phenylbutazone, beginning in 1949, was initially used for treating gout and rheumatoid arthritis in humans, but it is no longer approved for human use in the United States and in the UK. However, it is still used for the short-term relief of pain and fever in animals; in horses the plasma elimination half-life is 4 hours to 8 hours, but the inflammatory exudate half-life is 24 hours, so it can be used for once-daily dosing. Oxyphenbutazone is a metabolic derivative of phenylbutazone; it exhibits 98% plasma protein binding; has an onset of action of 1 hour to 2 hours, and has a duration of action of 2 days. The FDA granted approval to Watson Labs to manufacture a 100-mg formulation of oxyphenbutazone; however, its use has been discontinued. Similarly, the FDA granted approval to Barr to manufacture sulfinpyrazone as 100 mg and 200 mg oral tablets on September 17, 1982; FDA approval was also granted to Ivax Pharms, Par Pharm, Vanguard, and Watson Labs for several other formulations of sulfinpyrazone; however, all have been discontinued due to adverse side effects.

Celecoxib is a selective COX-2 inhibitor and, as such, is a special type of NSAID. Celecoxib was first approved for use in the United States by the FDA on December 31, 1998, was manufactured in 50 mg, 100 mg, 200 mg, and 400 mg capsules, and sold under the trade name of Celebrex. Generic formulations were approved by the FDA on May 30, 2014, for sale in multiple strengths by Mylan Pharms, Teva, and Watson Labs; on October 29, 2014, Lupin Ltd. was also granted approval for sale of a generic formulation of celecoxib. The gastrointestinal toxicity of celecoxib appears to be similar to that of acetaminophen, but it also seems to be better than that of most NSAIDs. Celecoxib does not appear to increase small intestinal permeability or lower intestinal bleeding. Further, celecoxib has lower cardiovascular toxicity compared to NSAIDs as well as to other selective COX-2 inhibitors. Consequently, if an anti-inflammatory drug is needed, celecoxib should be the medication of choice when the overall risk of cardiovascular complications is relatively low. The use of celecoxib has also demonstrated effectiveness in reducing depressive symptoms, which is clearly beneficial for better pain management. Studies are currently being conducted to examine the use of celecoxib for treating various cancers and mental illnesses.

Several other selective COX-2 inhibitors, such as etodolac, etoricoxib, lumiracoxib, meloxicam, parecoxib, rofecoxib, and valdecoxib, have been developed. Selective COX-2 inhibitors reduce the risk of gastrointestinal complications but increase the risk of thrombo-embolic events. At therapeutically equivalent doses, both NSAIDs and selective COX-2 inhibitors provide equivalent painkiller and anti-inflammatory efficacy. Etodolac is another selective COX-2 inhibitor that was approved in 400 mg and 500 mg formulations by the FDA for Prosam Labs on February 28, 1997, for Teva on November 26, 1997, and for Taro on March 11, 1998. Extended-release formulations of etodolac were granted approval for sale in the United States by Actavis Elizabeth on July 31, 2000, by Teva on July 31, 2000, by Sandoz on July 26, 2002, by Taro on March 13, 2003, and by Zydus Pharms USA Inc. on January 23, 2014. Meloxicam is another selective COX-2 inhibitor that was approved by the FDA in April 2000 and is marketed under the trade name Mobic. Rofecoxib was voluntarily taken off the market in September 2004 by Merck, which marketed it as Vioxx due to concerns that its use was associated with a significant increase in heart attacks and strokes. By December 2011, similar concerns with other selective COX-2 inhibitors resulted in only celecoxib being available for purchase in the United States. Nevertheless, the selective COX-2 inhibitors do not substantially harm the gastrointestinal tract but are still able to exert desired painkiller and anti-inflammatory effects.

Many painkillers are combined in various formulations with other painkillers or with other substances to produce novel products. Vicodin, for an example of two painkillers combined in a product, is a combination of hydrocodone and acetaminophen. Several other hydrocodone-and-acetaminophen combination formulations are also available and marketed under various trade names, such as Hycet, Lorcety, Lortab, Maxidone, and Norco. Anacin, for an example of a painkiller combined with another nonpainkiller drug, was invented around 1916 by William Milton Knight and is a combination of aspirin and caffeine.

Several other types of compound painkillers consisting of two or more different types of painkillers have been formulated. These include co-codamol, which is a combination of 8 mg of codeine phosphate and 500 mg of acetaminophen that was originally granted approval by the FDA on April 26, 1996; co-codaprin, which is a combination of 8 mg of codeine phosphate and 400 mg of aspirin; and, co-dydramol, which is a combination of 10 mg of dihydrocodeine and 500 mg of acetaminophen. Many other combination formulations with painkillers have been approved for use by the FDA. For instance, an acetaminophen and hydrocodone combination was originally granted approval for use by the FDA on March 27, 1985; an acetaminophen, aspirin, and codeine phosphate combination was originally granted approval by the FDA on October 26, 1990; an acetaminophen, aspirin, and caffeine combination was originally granted approval by the FDA on November 26, 2001; and an acetaminophen and pentazocine hydrochloride combination was originally granted approval by the FDA on March 24, 2000. A combination of hydrocodone and ibuprofen is used for short-term management of acute pain, usually less than 10 days; this combination, which is marketed under various trade names such as Ibudone, Reprexain, and Vicoprofen, avoids some of the concerns with liver toxicity associated with the use of hydrocodone-and-acetaminophen combination products like Vicodin. Similarly, a combination product consisting of oxycodone hydrochloride and ibuprofen, such as that marketed under the trade name Combunox, is used for short-term relief of moderate to severe pain.

Likewise, there have been many other formulations of a painkiller and another drug. For instance, an ibuprofen-and-pseudoephedrine hydrochloride combination formulation was granted approval for use in the United States by the FDA on April 8, 2002; an ibuprofen–and– diphenhydramine citrate combination was originally granted approval by the FDA on December 22, 2008; an ibuprofen–and–diphenhydramine hydrochloride combination was originally granted approval by the FDA on November 22, 2010; and an ibuprofen–and–phenylephrine hydrochloride combination was originally granted approval by the FDA on July 3, 2014. Likewise, a naproxen–and–esomeprazole magnesium (a proton pump inhibitor that reduces stomach acid secretions) combination oral delayed-release tablet formulation manufactured by Dr. Reddys Labs Ltd., was granted approval for use by the FDA on September 27, 2013; and a naproxen sodium–and–pseudoephedrine hydrochloride (a decongestant) combination oral extended-release tablet formulation manufactured by Dr. Reddys Labs Inc. was granted approval by the FDA on September 27, 2006; while a diclofenac sodium–and misoprostol (a synthetic prostaglandin analog) combination oral delayed release tablet formulation manufactured by Actavis Labs FL Inc. was granted approval by the FDA on July 9, 2012. Lomotil is the trade name of a prescription-only combination product that consists of 25 mg of the painkiller diphenoxylate hydrochloride and 0.025 mg of atropine sulfate, an anticholinergic medication; it is designed such that nausea and severe weakness will result if the standard dose is exceeded. This combination formulation, manufactured by Mylan, was granted approval for use in the United States by the FDA on November 17, 1977, on February 21, 1978, FDA approval was also granted to Lannett and to Par Pharm on May 2, 2000.

There are also several formulations of combinations of two or more painkillers along with other drugs, such as Fioricet #3 with Codeine, which, as mentioned earlier in this chapter, is the trade name of a product that contains a mixture of acetaminophen, butalbital (a barbiturate), caffeine, and codeine. A combination of morphine and sequestered naltrexone was developed by King Pharmaceuticals as capsules that contained morphine pellets and an inner core with naltrexone, which was marketed under the trade name of

Embeda and used for managing pain severe enough to require long-term, daily, around-the-clock administration for which alternative treatment options were inadequate; however, Embeda was voluntarily withdrawn from the market in 2011 after complaints by the FDA that information was omitted as to the potentially fatal consequence of crushing and swallowing the capsules. These and many other compound painkiller combination formulations are used for treating mild to moderate pain, such as that caused by injuries and osteoarthritis. Of course, the various opiate and opioid painkillers and the numerous assorted combination products are generally used for treating more severe pain cases.

DOCUMENT: BIOAVAILABILITY AND POTENCY OF DIFFERENT OPIOIDS

The primary documents for this end-of-chapter consideration are two tables that come from an article by Rom Stevens and Salim Ghazi titled "Routes of Opioid Analgesic Therapy in the Management of Cancer Pain." These tables, collectively, provide useful information on the pharmacokinetic differences, particularly for the bioavailability of selected opiates and opioids by varied routes of administration and for the relative potencies of selected painkillers compared relative to the standard of morphine. Understanding the varied systems for the administration routes, such as oral, intravenous, subcutaneous, transdermal, rectal, and transmucosal, of these respective painkillers is essential in order for health care providers to choose the most efficacious as well as the most cost-effective approach to pain management with individual patients.

Bioavailability of Opioids by Route of Administration

Mode	Bioavailability
Oral	33% (morphine)
	60%-87% (oxycodone)
Intravenous	100% (all opioids)
Subcutaneous	80% (hydromorphone)
Transdermal	90% (fentanyl)
Transmucosal	30%-60% (morphine, fentanyl)
Rectal	30%-40% (morphine)

Relative Potencies of Opioid Analgesics Compared to Morphine*

Drug	Parenteral Relative Potency	Oral Relative Potency
Morphine	1	1
Hydromorphone	5	5
Meperidine	0.2	0.2
Methadone	1	2
Codeine	0.16	0.16
Oxycodone	1	2
Fentanyl	100	200

*The oral relative potency is the product of the parenteral potency compared with morphine multiplied by the oral bioavailability of the drug compared with morphine. For parenteral administration, the bioavailability of all drugs = 1.0. The oral bioavailability of morphine = 0.3. Thus, oral oxycodone is approximately twice as potent as oral morphine because its bioavailability is twice that of oral morphine.

Source: Tables from R. A. Stevens and S. M. Ghazi. (2000). Routes of opioid analgesic therapy in the management of cancer pain. *Cancer Control, 7*(2), 132–141. Used by permission.

Chapter 6

Risks, Misuse, and Overdose

Painkillers are not without their respective risks; they can actually cause a tremendous amount of pain and suffering as well as death. Opiates and opioids are powerful painkillers, but they also have a highly addictive potential. Opiate and opioid dependence affects almost 5 million people in the United States and results in around 17,000 deaths each year. Each day on average, 46 Americans die as a consequence of a prescription opioid overdose. A middle-aged American today is more likely to die from a prescription opioid overdose than from either an automobile accident or from a violent crime. Further, heroin and related painkiller drugs kill over 100,000 individuals around the world each year. Serious side effects of NSAIDs, such as gastrointestinal bleeding, result in more than 100,000 hospitalizations and thousands of deaths in the United States each year. It is estimated that at least 16,500 NSAIDs-related deaths occur annually among arthritis patients alone in the United States. Of the 100+ million Americans who suffer from chronic pain, many are undertreated and may therefore be more likely to resort to illicit painkiller misuse.

ADVERSE EFFECTS, DEPENDENCE, AND MISUSE

The legal or illicit use of painkiller drugs puts individuals at increased risk for a host of related problems, including psychological and physical dependence. There is, in fact, a vast array of adverse effects that individuals commonly experience as a result of the misuse or abuse of respective painkiller drugs. Unfortunately, the use, misuse, and abuse of the myriad semisynthetic opioid and synthetic opioid painkiller drugs has recently become more of a problematic concern. Levels of the use and abuse of these painkillers are continuing to increase globally, with North America among the regions with the most problematic rates. These and related substances have been around for some time, but the increased levels of use by more and more users have resulted in dramatically increased reports of adverse effects.

Risk Potential and Semisynthetic Opioids

The assemblage of effects associated, in general, with these semisynthetic opioids principally include the relief of pain; however, other common effects of their use include change of mood, typically resulting in euphoria as well as in lowered anxiety; decreased gastrointestinal motility, typically resulting in constipation; nausea; vomiting; pinpoint pupils; cough suppression; suppression of adrenocorticotropin hormone and corticotrophin-releasing factor; and respiratory depression, sometimes resulting in an overdose fatality. If semisynthetic as well as synthetic opioids are used chronically, then tolerance to the drug and to related drugs, along with physical and psychological dependence, typically occurs.

Several prescription semisynthetic opioids have been widely abused, particularly as alternatives to heroin abuse. Oxycodone is one of the most prolifically abused of these drugs; its salts in use include the hydrochloride, bitarate, camphosulphate, pectinate, phenylpriopionate, phosphate, sulphate, tartrate, and terephthalate. The first and last of these salts of oxycodone are used together in Percodan, while the hydrochloride version is the most common in formulations used in the United States. Oxycodone exhibits about 45% plasma protein binding, with an onset of action of 45 to 60 minutes, has an average bioavailability when administered orally of 60% to 80%, has an average half-life of 3.5 hours, and has a typical duration of action of 4 to 6 hours. In addition to oxycodone, these abused semisynthetic substances include hydrocodone, which has been marketed under trade names such as Vicodin, and hydromorphone, which has been marketed under trade names such as Dilaudid. Hydrocodone, also referred to as dihydrocodeinone, is a semisynthetic opioid, centrally acting antitussive drug that can be derived from either codeine or thebaine and was first synthesized in 1920 in Germany. It has an average oral bioavailability of 60% to 80%, with an onset of action of 45 to 60 minutes, an average half-life of 3.5 hours, and a typical duration of action of 4 to 6 hours. Hydrocodone is marketed in the United States only in combination with other substances, such as that consisting of hydrocodone bitartrate and homatropine methylbromide, an opioid antagonist, and sold under various trade names such as Hycodan and Tussigon. Hydrocodone may be a more effective analgesic than codeine for the relief of acute musculoskeletal pain. However, the administration of hydrocodone to individuals who have other drug dependencies has significant risk of leading to the development of dependence on prescription medications. Some of the hydrocodone administered is metabolized into hydromorphone, which can result in positive urine drug tests. Hydromorphone (also known as dihydromorphinone) is a semisynthetic opioid derived from morphine that was first synthesized in 1924 in Germany and then introduced to the United States in 1932. Hydromorphone exhibits only 8% to 19% plasma protein binding and has an average bioavailability of 24% when administered orally, an onset of action of about 30 minutes, an average half-life of 2.6 hours, and has a typical duration of action of between 2 and 3 hours.

Negative consequences—including, ultimately, death—have been reported from the abuse of these opioids. Further, certain populations appear to be at greater risk for the nonmedical use of these semisynthetic opioid drugs than others. Approaches are therefore necessary to help identify those who may be going down this slippery slope. Accordingly, various techniques, including analysis of hair and oral fluid by means of solid-phase extraction and gas chromatography–mass spectrometry, have been developed to differentiate the use of respective substances; additional analytical techniques are, of course, also available for testing urine. Interventions directed at discouraging drug diversion activities and other strategies employed by painkiller abusers are also helpful in curtailing abuse.

Dihydrodesoxymorphine, also known as desomorphine, was first patented in 1934, and declared an illegal narcotic painkiller in 1998 in Russia, where it is referred to as *krokodil* on the streets. *Krokodil* use first appeared in Siberia just before the turn of the millennium, but its use has subsequently spread to other areas of Russia and beyond. *Krokodil* is an illicit derivative of medications containing codeine. It is estimated that at least 100,000 individuals in Russia reportedly used *krokodil* in 2011 alone. In fact, *krokodil* use has already severely impacted over 50 cities in the former Soviet Union, including those in Armenia, Georgia, and the Ukraine. For instance, there are currently an estimated 20,000 users of *krokodil* in the Ukraine. The use and abuse of *krokodil* has become a serious health problem in many of these countries; adverse consequences associated with this include flesh-eating infections, necrosis, limb amputation, and death. A *krokodil* addict's life expectancy in the countries of the former Soviet Union is less than 2 years.

Tramadol hydrochloride, which has been marketed under trade names such as Ultram, is another opioid painkiller drug that has been diverted for abuse purposes. Tramadol is also another substance in the long history of opiates and opioids that was introduced with later-to-be-determined false claims of low abuse potential. It exhibits about 20% plasma protein binding, with a 60- to 90-minute onset of action, has a bioavailability around 68% to 72% when administered orally and an average half-life of between 5.5 and 7 hours. It was hoped that tramadol would be effective in treating pain but would tend not to be abused. It is only about one-tenth as potent as morphine, with a 100 mg tablet of tramadol hydrochloride needed to equal the painkiller effect of 10 mg of morphine. Nevertheless, increasing numbers of cases of abuse, dependence, and withdrawal were observed among users in various countries and, consequently, treatment approaches had to be developed, including those with the use of methadone. There are several potential complications associated with the use of tramadol; for one thing, it has an affinity for the mu opioid receptors, and it prevents the reuptake of serotonin and norepinephrine within the brain; it also appears to be particularly associated with a higher rate of hypoglycemia among individuals without diabetes. Unlike other painkiller drugs such as morphine, tramadol is dependent upon a cytochrome P450 enzyme for activation to its active metabolite; however, expression of this particular enzyme varies highly among individuals, which makes for substantial fluctuations of opioid receptor activation from individual to individual who use a given dosage of tramadol. At any rate, it presently appears that there is less abuse and dependence of tramadol than there is for hydrocodone. However, the U.S. Food and Drug Administration recently added a warning of suicide risk to the labels of tramadol. As its painkiller effects are, at best, moderate, its toxic effects merit consideration as do its negative side effects, which include seizures, hypoglycemia, and harmful drug interactions.

Fortunately, tapentadol is now available, and it can serve as a desirable alternative to tramadol hydrochloride. Tapentadol is similar to tramadol hydrochloride with a dual mechanism of action. Thus, tapentadol is a centrally acting painkiller that is both a mu opioid receptor agonist and a norepinephrine reuptake inhibitor. However, unlike tramadol hydrochloride, tapentadol has only weak effects on serotonin reuptake and no known active metabolites. It has been demonstrated that tapentadol provides comparable pain relief to oxycodone. Tapentadol exhibits about 20% plasma protein binding, with an average of 32 minutes for its onset of action, and has a bioavailability around 25% to 39% when administered orally, with a duration of action between 4 and 6 hours and an average half-life of about 4 hours. Developed by Grunenthal in collaboration with Johnson and Johnson Pharmaceutical Research and Development, it is marketed as both immediate-relief and extended-release tablets under the trade names of Nucynta and Nucynta ER, respectively. The FDA approved tapentadol for use in the United States on

August 26, 2011. It has an improved tolerability profile, particularly with respect to gastrointestinal tolerability; it also has relatively low rates of discontinuation as well as of adverse event-related discontinuations compared to oxycodone hydrochloride.

Over-the-Counter and Related Painkiller Concerns

There are some side effects that are common to most NSAIDs. Some of these common side effects include nausea, vomiting, constipation, diarrhea, headache, dizziness, rashes, and drowsiness. More serious side effects may be life-threatening and include ulcers, gastrointestinal bleeding, anemia, shortness of breath, and gastrointestinal perforation. Persistent headaches are a less common side effect that occur in about 10% of daily users of NSAIDs. Prolonged use of NSAIDs may also lead to swelling of the arms and legs since their renal effects cause retention of fluids. NSAIDs, specifically the nonselective COX inhibitors, differ substantially in their tendency to cause ulcers and gastrointestinal bleeding. NSAIDs, other than aspirin, may increase the risks of heart attack, stroke, and similar conditions that can result in fatality. Chronic use of NSAIDs is likely to cause impaired renal function due to sodium and water retention, suppression of bone marrow, and bronchial asthma.

Individuals with certain medical conditions should avoid use of NSAIDs. For instance, individuals with cirrhosis, congestive heart failure, or renal insufficiency should avoid use of NSAIDs as these drugs inhibit the synthesis of prostaglandins that are needed to maintain renal perfusion; this can result in unopposed vasoconstriction. NSAIDs also should never be used right before or after coronary artery bypass surgery.

Specific NSAIDs, of course, have their own respective set of side effects as well as the more general ones. Ketorolac, for instance, tends to cause ulcers more than other NSAIDs and therefore should not be used for more than 5 days in a row. Ketoprofen can have both minor and more serious side effects. Minor side effects include trouble falling and staying asleep, ringing in the ears, anxiety, headache, dizziness, diarrhea, and constipation. Some of the more serious side effects include difficult or painful urination, abnormal weight gain, excessive exhaustion, vision changes, itching, rashes, blisters, irregular heartbeat, jaundice, abnormal bleeding, and having trouble swallowing. Diclofenac is among the better-tolerated NSAIDs, and only about 2% of patients on long-term treatment discontinue use of the drug due to side effects, which are principally gastrointestinal in nature.

The more commonly used NSAIDs are not without their own sets of serious adverse side effects. Some studies have suggested that use of aspirin may be ineffective as a primary cardiovascular prevention strategy among older adults at elevated risks for cardiovascular disease. Aspirin use does not appear to improve overall mortality outcomes, but does seem to help prevent nonfatal myocardial infarcts and transient ischemic attacks, although also promoting a higher risk of serious extracranial bleedings. Adverse effects associated with use of acetaminophen include rash, disorientation, dizziness, gastrointestinal hemorrhage, kidney damage, and liver failure. About 33,000 hospitalizations are due to acetaminophen poisoning each year in the United States, and the FDA has linked around 980 deaths annually due to drugs containing acetaminophen. Since acetaminophen use may cause oxidative stress on the airway, calls have been made for further research to examine the effects of acetaminophen use on pulmonary function. Some of the more common adverse side effects associated with the use of naproxen include gastrointestinal toxicity, jaundice, heptatoxicity, and nephrotoxicity.

Reye's syndrome is an extremely rare but potentially fatal condition that damages many organs, particularly the brain and the liver, and it also lowers blood sugar. It has been associated with aspirin use by infants, toddlers, and other children who have a viral illness; however, no age group is immune. Epidemiological research has indicated a link for the development of Reye's syndrome when using aspirin to treat influenza-like illnesses, such as colds and chicken pox, in children. Symptoms of Reye's syndrome usually occur in the order of restlessness, listlessness, drowsiness, personality change (like irritability, slurred speech, or sensitivity to touch), disorientation, combativeness, and even sometimes resulting in delirium, convulsions, or loss of consciousness. The condition causes the development of a fatty liver with slight inflammation, alterations to the kidneys and swelling of the brain, known as cerebral edema; it can result in severe brain damage, especially in infants, and even, possibly, in death. More than 30% of the cases reported in the United States resulted in fatality. Consequently, it is recommended that aspirin and combination products that contain aspirin not be given to children under 19 years of age when they are experiencing fever or viral illnesses.

Reye's syndrome was first identified as a distinct entity in the early 1960s. By the 1980s, over 500 cases were being diagnosed each year in the United States alone. In 1980, the CDC cautioned about the possible dangers of aspirin administration to children. In 1982, the U.S. Surgeon General issued an advisory about the dangers of giving aspirin to children. Since 1986, the FDA has required a Reye's syndrome warning to be included in the labels for all medications containing aspirin. More recently, as a result of these types of initiatives, there are now usually fewer than 5 cases identified per year in the United States.

Due to concerns with Reye's syndrome as well as with other issues, attention should be directed to considerations of breast feeding. Aspirin in particular passes into breast milk and consequently should be avoided if nursing, as should combination formulations containing aspirin. Similarly, ibuprofen passes into breast milk and thus use should be avoided while nursing, as should ibuprofen in formulations with hydrocodone bitartrate and similar drugs. Naproxen also passes into breast milk, and thus it should be avoided or discontinued while nursing, as should any combination formulations. Although there do not appear to be any problems associated with use of acetaminophen by nursing mothers, use of acetaminophen combination formulations, such as acetaminophen with codeine phosphate or with aspirin and caffeine, should be avoided as these other drugs may pass into breast milk. Use of most other NSAIDs should be avoided while nursing as many, like diclofenac, diflunisal, indomethacin, ketoprofen, ketorolac, salsalate, sulindac, tolmetin sodium, and tramadol hydrochloride, are known to pass into breast milk. Likewise, use of opiates and opioids should also be avoided or discontinued by nursing mothers as most, such as codeine, fentanyl, oxaprozin, oxycodone hydrochloride, propoxyphene, and methadone hydrochloride, are also known to pass into breast milk.

The selective COX-2 inhibitors, also known as coxcibs, significantly reduce the incidence of serious gastrointestinal complications, such as gastric bleeding, perforations, and ulcers, associated with the more typical NSAIDs. Nevertheless, the selective COX-2 inhibitors are still associated with some chronic inflammation of the intestines. Furthermore, the selective COX-2 inhibitors are associated with an increased incidence of thrombotic events and hypertension due to the inhibition of the COX-2 dependent vascular prostacyclin.

MISUSE

Various painkiller drugs are sometimes misused. Whether to self-medicate for real or imagined pain or to get "high," if not used as advised or prescribed, such use is misuse. Individuals misuse painkillers by taking their own prescription or over-the-counter products improperly, stealing or getting medications intended for others, seeking out multiple health care providers to get an extra supply, or by purchasing them from drug dealers and other unauthorized individuals.

Long-term or acute use of NSAIDs not only can lead to adverse effects to the gastrointestinal system, but it can also result in peptic ulcers and other complications, like bleeding or perforations, particularly in the upper gastrointestinal tract. Adverse effects to the cardiovascular system from misuse of NSAIDs can result in cardiac, cerebral, and peripheral thrombotic events. Such serious adverse effects are highly unlikely if NSAIDs are used as indicated and approved.

Individuals who are actively consuming alcoholic beverages should avoid using most painkillers. Acetaminophen, as well as the opiate and opioid drugs, are not recommended for individuals who are drinking alcohol.

Misuse of opiate or opioid drugs can have serious adverse effects, including death. The first-time misuser of heroin, fentanyl, or similar potent painkiller drugs could possibly overdose. Further, drugs obtained through the illicit market are often impure and frequently may contain hazardous ingredients. Continued misuse of these types of painkillers may lead to the development of tolerance and then dependence.

ABUSE AND ADDICTION

The levels of the potential for abuse and addiction to respective painkiller drugs has become an alarming concern both in the United States and elsewhere around the world. The opiate and opioid painkillers, in particular, are associated with a much higher risk of dependence than many other drugs. This is due both to their unique pharmacological properties, but also to societal factors.

Risk of Dependence

There is no sure way to predict which user of a painkiller—opiates and opioids are of particular concern here—will become dependent upon the particular drug. If they ever become dependent and how rapidly they might progress to an addiction to a particular painkiller, as well as subsequent likelihood of treatment success, depends on many factors; these include their age, gender, genetic background, and environmental factors. While some individuals who use a particular substance for a few or even many times may experience no ill effects, another individual might overdose on their first use or become dependent after only a few administrations of a particular drug. Nevertheless, we do know several powerful risk factors to establishing such a vulnerability, such as having a family history of drug addiction, having a preexisting psychiatric condition, and so forth.

The genetic predisposition to drug addiction appears to account for about half of the overall susceptibility. In support of this view, several studies have indicated that if one identical twin becomes drug addicted, there is then about a 50% probability that the other twin will also become addicted. The other 50% or so of the susceptibility to developing an addiction appears to be related to various environmental factors, such as socioeconomic status, family background, peer groups, smoking or other drug use, and stressful events experienced during childhood. The young brain is still developing up through adolescence and even beyond, and it is highly susceptible to traumatic experiences, such as the early loss of one or both parents, witnessing a very violent event, and incidents of physical or sexual abuse. These types of experiences seem to create neurochemical changes in the developing brain, which places the individual at a much greater risk for developing drug addiction at some point later in his or her life. The euphoric pleasure experienced from the misuse of an opiate or opioid painkiller drug, in particular, seems to actually rewire the dopamine reward pathway of the brain, which in turn can lead to the compulsive drug-seeking behaviors, cravings, and continued use despite an awareness of the negative consequences of such actions.

If someone snorts, smokes, or injects the crushed painkiller drugs, then they can get a stronger, more intense reaction than if they swallowed the tablets or capsules as they are generally intended to be used. The abuse of opiate or opioid painkiller drugs can cause serious health complications, particularly the cessation of breathing and then even death. Other problems that are also commonly associated with the abuse of these painkiller drugs include nausea, vomiting, and constipation. The rampant use, misuse, and abuse of these highly powerful painkiller drugs has led to dramatic increases in the numbers of those who are dependent or addicted to them. This, in turn, has led to the need to develop more therapeutic alternatives to these substances that can be integrated into comprehensive treatment strategies.

ADDICTION TREATMENTS

There are several evidence-based approaches available for treating opiate and opioid addiction. Effective treatments can include behavioral therapies, such as cognitive behavioral therapy (CBT) or contingency management (which will be discussed in a later chapter); medications; and combined approaches of both behavioral therapy and medication.

These treatment medications can help painkiller-dependent individuals restore normal brain functioning, reduce cravings, and also help prevent relapse. The FDA has approved several medications for treatment of opiate and opioid dependence, respectively—oral naltrexone, injectable extended-release naltrexone, buprenorphine, buprenorphine-naloxone combination formulations, and methadone. Several studies have found that injectable opioid treatments are more cost effective and have greater effectiveness, as well as higher levels of pre- and post-treatment satisfaction, than oral methadone approaches for treating chronic refractory heroin addicts.

The success, or lack thereof, of specific medication-assisted treatments, like those based on opioid agonists, for those who became dependent is probably influenced by a range of individual characteristics including variable gene profiles. Genetic studies have examined the response to methadone maintenance treatment and similar approaches; these types of studies often focus on opioid receptor genes, like OPRM1, and methadone metabolism genes, like ABCB1 and CYP450. However, additional research is needed in this area, particularly that with larger samples and more diverse populations. In addition, multiple genes must be evaluated simultaneously to examine polygenic effects on the likelihood of experiencing low treatment response. Nevertheless, we can be optimistically hopeful that these future developments will help us better individualize treatment for enhanced success.

Methadone

Methadone (4, 4-diphenyl-6-dimethylamino-3-heptanone) was developed around 1939 by Max Bockmuhl and Gustav Ehrgart working for I. G. Farbenindustric at Hoechst-am-Main, Germany, and was first called Hoechst 10820 and then polamidon; after World War II, Eli Lilly, an American pharmaceutical company, began marketing it as Dolophine. It was first approved for use in the United States by the FDA in 1947. Methadone functions as a full opioid agonist that competes with other opioids by suppressing cravings and managing withdrawal symptoms. From very early on it was recognized that methadone has a high addiction potential. Methadone was initially used for analgesic purposes as a substitute for morphine, and it is still widely used for this purpose.

Methadone metabolization is significantly impacted by co-ingestion of various foods, herbs, and other drugs, which can raise important metabolic issues. Nevertheless, methadone has a very high fat solubility as well as a slow metabolism; thus, it tends to last longer than many other opiate or opioid drugs. Methadone exhibits between 41% and 99% bioavailability when administered orally. The usual elimination half-life of methadone is between 15 and 60 hours, with an average elimination half-life of around 22 hours.

Use of methadone can affect the heart and, accordingly, individuals being considered for methadone therapies should first get an electrocardiogram (ECG or EKG) to test for heart abnormalities. Methadone hydrochloride when administered chronically leads to tolerance, sedation, lethargy, and edema; however, the onset of the acute abstinence syndrome is slower than that produced by morphine or heroin. Methadone use also impairs learning and immediate recall. Nevertheless, methadone is a commonly used medication to manage narcotic addiction. It is also less expensive than its closest therapeutic alternative, buprenorphine.

Fentanyl

Fentanyl is another synthetic opioid that is much more potent than morphine or heroin. Fentanyl was first synthesized in 1959 by Paul Janssen at a pharmaceutical company he started in Belgium. Sandoz manufactures a generic formulation of fentanyl, which it markets as Duragesic. Sufentanil citrate, initially synthesized at Janssen Pharmaceutica in 1974 and approved by the FDA on December 15, 1995, and marketed under trade names such as Sufenta and Sufentil, and alfentanil hydrochloride, initially synthesized at Janssen Pharmaceutica in 1976 and approved by the FDA on October 28, 1999, and marketed under trade names such as Alfenta and Rapifen, are two other opioid analgesics closely related to fentanyl and that are used for similar purposes; they are both listed as Schedule II drugs in the United States under the Controlled Substances Act. Sufentanil can be synthesized from N-benzyl-4-piperidine. In its intravenous formulation, fentanyl is considered to be between 70 and 100 times more potent a painkiller than morphine. Sufentanil is even more potent than fentanyl; about 5 to 10 times more potent a painkiller than fentanyl and 500 times more potent than morphine. Alfentanil, as an analogue of fentanyl, is estimated to be about one-quarter to one-tenth as potent as fentanyl, with about one-third the duration of action; but it has about 4 times as fast an onset of action. Fentanyl and its several synthetic analogues have been abused; however, none of these substances are detected by urine drug-screening tests focused on morphine-like substances as fentanyl and its analogues are not structurally related to morphine and the other opiates or opioids.

Etorphine and Dihydroetorphine

Etorphine is a semisynthetic opioid that was first prepared in 1960 as a derivative of oripavine, which is found in poppy straw and in *Papaver orientale* and *Papaver bracteatum*, but not in *Papaver somniferum*; it was first synthesized by Kenneth W. Bentley and Denis G. Hardy of MacFarlan Smith in 1963 in Edinburgh, Scotland, and it is mainly used as a sedative in veterinary medicine; it can also be synthesized from thebaine. It is used mainly for sedating wild and exotic animals; a 4 mg dose of etorphine can immobilize a 5,000 kg elephant, while a 1 mg dose can sedate a 2,000 kg rhinoceros. It has a very rapid onset of action and short duration of action with a high abuse potential. Etorphine is listed as a Schedule I drug under the Controlled Substances Act with DEA number 9056; although its hydrochloride salt form—whose chemical name is 6, 14-endoetheno–7a (1-(R)-hydroxyl–1 methylbutyl)–tetrahydro-nororipavine hydrochloride—is listed under Schedule II, and its DEA number is 9059. Etorphine hydrochloride is marketed under the trade name of M99, which is manufactured by American Cyanamid. It is estimated to be up to 12,000 times more potent a painkiller than morphine. Etorphine must be handled with extreme caution as even a very small amount can cause respiratory paralysis.

Dihydroetorphine is a potent semisynthetic opioid which is a derivative of etorphine. It was developed in the late 1960s by Kenneth W. Bentley for MacFarlan Smith. It is many times a more potent painkiller than morphine; estimates range from 1,000 to 12,000 times more potent depending on the method used for comparison. It is used primarily in China as a painkiller where it is available in a sublingual formulation and also as a transdermal patch. In the United States, it is listed as a Schedule II drug under the Controlled Substances Act. Dihydroetorphine is occasionally used in China as a mainte-nance drug for treating opiate or opioid addicts in a manner similar to the sub-stitution use of methadone or buprenorphine in the United States. Dihydroetorphine is considered by some experts to have a lower risk for addic-tion than many other opioids.

LAAM

LAAM, or levo-alpha-acetylmethadol, is a synthetic opioid drug that was developed in the 1940s and that has a slow onset of action and a long duration of action that made it unsuitable for purposes of pain management, but that seemed to be appropriate for treating those chronically dependent on opiates or opioids. Thus, LAAM was being administered to some individuals who were on methadone maintenance. In fact, LAAM can block the effects of opiate and opioid drugs for up to 72 hours. However, the availability of buprenorphine in 2003, which does not cause heart problems, led to the discontinuation of the use of LAAM.

Buprenorphine

Buprenorphine was first synthesized in 1969 by Rickett and Colman in the UK, now Rickett Benckiser, and human clinical trial testing was begun there in 1971. Buprenorphine is a semisynthetic derivative of thebaine that was approved by the FDA for treating opioid addiction in the United States in October 2002. However, buprenorphine can also be prescribed as a painkiller as well as for treating nausea in individuals who are antiemetic intolerant. Buprenorphine has also been used for treating neonatal abstinence syndrome, which sometimes occurs in newborn babies who were exposed to opiates or opioids during pregnancy and exhibit withdrawal symptoms. Buprenorphine is regarded as a partial agonist as it produces less respiratory depression than opiates such as morphine. Buprenorphine is estimated to be 25 to 50 times more potent a painkiller by weight than morphine. Buprenorphine has a relatively long duration of action, which makes it well suited to be used as an opiate or opioid substitute in drug treatment programs. A single dose of buprenorphine can block many of the pharmacological effects of morphine for up to 30 hours. In fact, buprenorphine has a half-life ranging from 20 to 70 hours, with an average half-life of 37 hours; it exhibits 96% protein binding and has a bioavailability of 55% when administered sublingually and of 48% when administered intra-nasally. Prolonged occupation of opioid receptors by buprenorphine means that antagonists like naloxone have limited effectiveness if administered after the buprenorphine; while if administered prior to buprenorphine, then the naloxone can readily block its effects.

U.S. physicians can complete specialized training as authorized by the Drug Addiction Treatment Act of 2000 to be able to prescribe buprenorphine products. Buprenorphine is used elsewhere as well, such as in France for maintenance treatment of opiate addicts. Buprenorphine is being used along with methadone for the treatment of opioid dependence; the effectiveness of addiction treatment based on either buprenorphine or methadone is roughly equivalent. Drug interactions must, of course, be an area of concern. Cocaine, for instance, has effects on the pharmacokinetics of both buprenorphine and methadone. There are also clinically important drug interactions between methadone and buprenorphine, and substantial interactions between buprenorphine and various antivirals. Buprenorphine is usually administered as a sublingual tablet, such as that marketed under the trade name of Temgesic, which is recommended for the relief of moderate to severe pain. However, a buprenorphine transdermal patch is being considered as an alternative way to conduct opioid detoxification; there are also buprenorphine suppository formulations. Buprenorphine transdermal preparations include those marketed under trade names such as Butrans and Norspan; these transdermal patches are not indicated for treating short-term acute pain or for postoperative pain. There are also solution formulations of buprenorphine that are available for injection administration and commonly used for relief of acute pain in primary care settings, such as that marketed under the trade name of Buprenex.

The generic formulations of buprenorphine have been available in the United States since 2009.

Since the use of buprenorphine alone has the potential for abuse, it is produced in a formulation combined with naloxone that is marketed under trade names such as Suboxone, Bunavail, or Zubsolv, which is hoped to reduce the likelihood of abuse. Suboxone and Zubsolv each consist of a ratio of 4 parts of buprenorphine to 1 part of naloxone; Zubsolv, which consists of a formulation with high bioavailability oral tablets, with a rapid dissolve time and a menthol flavor that was granted approval for sale in the United States by the FDA in July 2013. Bunavail was approved for sale in the United States by the FDA in June 2014, and it consists of a ratio of 6 to 7 parts of buprenorphine to 1 part of naloxone, manufactured in a buccal film form that causes less constipation than either Suboxone or Zubsolv. When taken orally, as is prescribed, the naloxone has little appreciable effect; but if the tablets are crushed, mixed in a solution and injected, the naloxone can induce withdrawal symptoms. The generic formulation of the combined buprenorphine and naloxone medication became available as a generic drug in 2013. This combined formulation of a partial mu opioid agonist and a kappa opioid agonist was first approved by the FDA for use in the United States in 2002 and marketed as Suboxone. It competes at receptor sites with other opioids and effectively suppresses cravings and withdrawal symptoms. Suboxone, however, is estimated to be about 20 times more powerful than morphine. There are now generic versions of a combined buprenorphine-naloxone formulation that were first made available in the United States in 2013. The combined buprenorphine-naloxone formulation has a low abuse potential by means of injection use.

Opioid Antagonists

Antagonist medications block or inhibit the communication between neurons by changing the actions of opiates or opioids, as well as of similarly structured neurotransmitters, at the postsynaptic receptor. An antagonist drug is a substance that binds to a receptor site, but that does not activate its intrinsic activity. Thus, the antagonist drug binds to the receptor and blocks the ability of other substances to bond with it and to potentially activate it. It essentially functions as an inhibitor, blocking the effects of various drugs and other substances.

Some antagonists work by directly blocking the effects of a painkiller drug by binding to postsynaptic receptors, while others work indirectly by decreasing the activity at receptors by acting remotely. Antagonist medications, accordingly, work in several different ways. Some antagonists decrease the amount of neurotransmitters synthesized in presynaptic neurons; others inhibit the storage of neurotransmitters in vesicles. Still others inhibit the release of neurotransmitters; or enhance the reuptake process, thereby reducing the amount of neurotransmitters present in the synaptic cleft; or function by enhancing enzymatic degradation of neurotransmitters.

An array of opioid antagonists, like nalorphine and cyclazocine, has been synthesized. Opioid antagonists bond to the opioid receptors and thereby block the effects of opiate and opioid painkillers. Nalorphine was one of the first narcotic antagonists developed and examined beginning in 1915, when it was observed that nalorphine abolished the respiratory depression induced by either morphine or heroin. In the 1950s, it was found that nalorphine could serve as an antidote for morphine poisoning and that it could help initiate abstinence in treating those dependent on morphine; it also has a low abuse potential. Clonidine has also been used as an effective agent for minimizing symptoms in individuals undergoing heroin detoxification. Good treatment, ideally, should be multimodal and recognize that detoxification may not be the objective for all individuals.

Naltrexone is an opioid antagonist that seems to help reduce the cravings and thus, as a consequence, may help reduce the consumption of opiates and opioids. Naltrexone, a longer-acting nonselective, competitive opioid receptor antagonist, can be given to prevent relapse. It essentially blocks those opioid receptors that are associated with the euphoric effects of opiates and opioids. The formulation of naltrexone that can be taken orally was first approved for use in the United States by the FDA in 1984, and an extended-release formulation that can be injected was first approved by the FDA in 2010. Naltrexone, which is marketed under trade names such as Depade or Revia, does not cause sedation, nor does it result in physical dependence. Unfortunately, opioid-using patients treated with naltrexone have been reported to have a higher mortality rate than those treated with methadone due primarily to lower post-treatment cessation rates. Naltrexone is effective in blocking the effects of heroin while being used, but it has rather low rates of compliance and retention. Further, there is a high risk of overdose on heroin upon relapse following naltrexone cessation. Naltrexone has been most successful in addiction treatment when used with highly motivated individuals involved in structured treatment programs based on an abstinence goal. There is a long-acting injectable formulation of naltrexone that is marketed as Vivitrol, which is administered once a month and will hopefully result in greater rates of patient compliance.

Oral naltrexone, which is used for the treatment of opiate or opioid dependence, is on the Preferred Drug Lists (PDLs) for all 51 Medicaid programs.

Oral naltrexone was initially granted approval by the FDA in 1994 and is marketed under trade names such as Depade and Revia. However, as of 2013, only 13 state Medicaid programs covered all available treatment medications for treating opioid-use disorders. Interestingly, since 1994, the FDA has approved use of oral naltrexone for treating alcohol dependence, and preliminary research suggests that it may also be useful in treating impulse control disorders like compulsive gambling, shopping, sexual behavior, and eating disorders, among individuals with Parkinson disease. In 2009, the FDA granted approval of an injectable extended-release naltrexone formulation, which is currently marketed under the trade name of Vivitrol. This particular form only needs to be administered once every four weeks, rather than the oral form, which must be taken daily. The injectable extended-release naltrexone is not yet available in generic formulation, and this may help to explain why it is not listed on more PDLs. Interestingly, the FDA has approved use of naltrexone in treating alcohol dependence, and preliminary research suggests that it may also be useful in treating impulse control disorders like compulsive gambling, shopping, sexual behavior, and eating disorders, among individuals with Parkinson disease. U.S. spending on naltrexone totaled $22.6 million in 2009.

Naloxone is an opioid antagonist that is used to counter the effects of an opiate or opioid overdose. Naloxone was developed in the 1960s by Sankyo and is marketed under various trade names such as Narcan, Narcanti, Nalone, and Evzio. The chemical structure of naloxone is very similar to that of oxymorphone, but with an allyl group substituted for the N-methyl group. Naloxone is poorly absorbed orally and sublingually, but it is well absorbed when administered intravenously, intramuscularly, or subcutaneously. In many countries of the developing world, naloxone is included in emergency overdose response kits, such as those given to emergency medical technicians (EMTs), police, and even abusers of heroin and other related painkiller drugs; it is also typically present in medical settings wherever opiates or opioids are being administered intravenously to help remedy any accidental overdoses. Take-home naloxone training is important not only for the individual opiate or opioid user, but also for their family members and/or significant others, as such has been found to increase both opioid overdose related knowledge and also opioid-related attitudes as well as to increase their competence in administering naloxone. A combination formulation of naloxone and oxycodone, which is marketed under the trade name Tangin, is used for relief of opiate- or opioid-induced constipation. In April 2014, the FDA approved a handheld auto-injector formulation of naloxone for home use by family members, friends, and other caregivers; marketed under the trade name of Evzio, it rapidly delivers a 0.4-mg dose of naloxone that can be administered either under the skin or into muscles. Naloxone nasal spray formulations are also under development.

The half-life of naloxone is about 1 to 1.5 hours. The primary metabolite of naloxone is naloxone-3-glucuronide, which is excreted in urine. When administered orally, naloxone has about 90% bioavailability, but it has a high rate of first pass metabolism, which is in the liver; accordingly, it is sometimes necessary to administer additional doses when used prophylactically. Some of the side effects associated with naloxone use include headache, nausea, dizziness, increased sweating, restlessness, nervousness, vomiting, trembling, sudden chest pain, heart rhythm changes, seizures, and pulmonary edema. There is no evidence suggesting the development of tolerance or dependence to naloxone. Unfortunately, naloxone does not have the ability to reverse the overdose potential that exists for use of buprenorphine.

There are also some mixed agonist-antagonist painkillers. Buprenorphine, butorphanol, and pentazocine are examples of mixed agonist-antagonist painkillers. Their pharmacological properties, particularly with respect to those of buprenorphine, justifies their use as painkillers since they have a lower physical dependence potential than the pure opiate or opioid drugs.

OVERDOSE

An overdose is indeed the most severe adverse side effect associated with many different types of painkillers. There is one overdose death every 30 minutes in the United States, and rates of opioid overdose are on the rise around the globe. An opiate or opioid overdose, such as that from morphine or heroin, is the classic textbook type of drug overdose. Some of the general signs of a painkiller overdose include confusion, cold and sweaty skin, extreme sleepiness, shaking, having blue lips and fingernails, trouble breathing, and possibly even coma and death. Heroin is among the top killers of illicit drug users. About 1 out of 10 heroin overdoses results in a fatality. The majority of individuals who died from heroin stopped breathing. Heroin use can also cause kidney failure and heart problems as well as a substantial drop in blood pressure. Heroin use can also cause pulmonary edema, where the blood backs up in the arteries and flows through the lungs, resulting in a drop in oxygen and, often, death. Fatalities most often occur among long-term users, typically a single male who died at home. Furthermore, prescription opioid overdose is now more common in the United States than illicit opiate and opioid overdose. The risk factors associated with overdose of prescription opioid drugs include male gender, low socioeconomic status, older age, and having a psychiatric disorder.

The National Institute on Drug Abuse (NIDA) reported that in 2011, 4.2 million Americans over 11 years of age had tried heroin at least once. It is estimated that about 23% of those who tried at least once will eventually become addicted. After 20 years of use, the risks of having a fatal heroin overdose increase dramatically. Evidence indicates that after 30 years of use, about 16% of heroin users have died. It is estimated that there have been around 125,000 opioid fatalities over the past 10 years in this country. There are nearly 20,000 unintentional opioid deaths each year in the United States. For example, clandestinely produced fentanyl is occasionally mixed with heroin, and due to its dramatically higher potency, along with the difficulty of cutting it, use leads to clusters of overdose fatalities. Unfortunately, overdoses can result from excessive intake of other painkillers as well. In fact, 45 people die every day in the United States from opioid prescription painkiller use, which is more fatalities than from heroin and cocaine combined.

Although painkiller overdose deaths are more common among men than women, the rate among women has been closing the gap from that of men fast. Fatalities from prescription painkiller overdose among women have, in fact, increased over 400% since 1999, compared to a 265% increase among men. About 18 women in the U.S. die each day from a prescription painkiller overdose; and, further, for every woman that dies of a painkiller overdose, 30 others go to an emergency department for painkiller misuse or abuse. At any rate, in 2011 there were almost 17,000 overdose deaths in the U.S. related to prescription opioid medications.

Over-the-Counter Painkiller Overdose

Acetaminophen is the most commonly used drug in an overdose attempt in the United States, with an estimated 100,000 cases of intentional overdose using acetaminophen each year. Unfortunately, liver damage can result from a less than fatal dose. In fact, acetaminophen is now the leading cause of liver failure in the United States. The primary toxic metabolite of acetaminophen is N-acetyl-p-benzoquinone imine, sometimes referred to as NAPQI, which is produced by the liver's cytochrome P-450 enzyme system. Glutathione, which is stored in the liver, usually breaks down NAPQI. However, in an acute acetaminophen overdose, the reserves of glutathione are depleted. When this happens, the NAPQI builds up, and as it accumulates it can cause hepatocellular necrosis and can also possibly spread to cause damage to other organs like the pancreas and the kidneys.

Measuring the serum acetaminophen level is definitively the most accurate way to diagnose an acetaminophen overdose. Treatment involves the oral or intravenous administration of acetylcysteine, a precursor for glutathione, which helps prevent hepatic toxicity. Activated charcoal is given only if acetaminophen is still probably in the gastrointestinal tract.

An aspirin overdose can be either intentional or accidental; it can also be acute or chronic. Acute accidental overdose is particularly common with children. Symptoms of an aspirin overdose initially include dehydration, abdominal pain, vomiting, tinnitus, and lethargy. More serious adverse symptoms manifest in more severe cases; these include fever, rapid breathing, respiratory alkalosis, low blood potassium, low blood glucose, metabolic acidosis, hallucinations, seizures, cerebral edema, and coma. Cardiopulmonary arrest, usually due to pulmonary edema, is the most common cause of death from an aspirin overdose.

A potentially fatal aspirin overdose is generally considered to occur at levels greater than 500 mg per kg of body mass. Following an acute aspirin overdose, plasma salicylate levels, the primary metabolite of aspirin, can range from 700 to 1,400 mg/L. Treatment is according to individual symptoms presented. Activated charcoal is usually administered for gastric decontamination; intravenous fluids with dextrose help maintain urinary output; sodium bicarbonate may also be administered as it enhances urinary elimination of salicylate; and hemodialysis is used in severely toxic cases as it restores electrolyte and acid-base balances as well as removes salicylate.

Ibuprofen overdose can manifest with blurred vision, ringing in the ears, profuse sweating, slow and difficult breathing, drowsiness, unsteadiness, confusion, diarrhea, heartburn, severe stomach pain, nausea, and vomiting. Ibuprofen overdose can inhibit urine production by the kidneys; probable blood loss in intestines and/or stomach; and occasionally seizures and coma can result, as can tachycardia, atrial fibrillation, and cardiac arrest. Activated charcoal can be given as it can absorb ibuprofen before it enters systemic circulation; gastric lavage is less commonly employed.

Naproxen overdose is characterized by drowsiness, indigestion, heartburn, nausea, and/or vomiting. Seizures have occasionally been reported among those with high levels of naproxen. Naproxen is rapidly absorbed, and overdose is best managed by symptomatic and supportive care. Due to its high protein-binding properties, hemodialysis, forced diuresis, and alkalinization of urine are not helpful.

OTHER PROBLEMS

Other problems, in addition to drug overdoses, can result from the use, misuse, and abuse of painkillers. For example, chronic use of opiates or opioids can result in myoclonus, the uncontrollable twitching or jerking of muscles or muscle groups. If an intervention does not address the myoclonus, it can then progress to delirium with hallucinations and, eventually, can result in grand mal–type seizures. Opiate and opioid misusers have been identified as having high psychiatric comorbidity as well as high all-cause mortality rates. Although one does not generally develop dependence to NSAIDs, after prolonged use, there can be adverse consequences to stopping their use abruptly. If someone takes NSAIDs to reduce swelling and inflammation for an extended period of time, then cessation of use would likely result in a resumption of those symptoms. Feelings of anxiety often typically manifest as well as a consequence of developing pain sensations. There are many other risks associated with the use of painkillers—including an increased risk of bone fractures and the potential of having a hormonal imbalance.

The number of hospitalizations for treating drug users has escalated tremendously as a consequence of the increased levels of opiate and opioid use in society. In fact, in the United States there has been a 183% increase in hospitalizations for drug use since 2011. Each year users of prescription opiates and opioids account for slightly under 500,000 hospitalizations; oxycodone users alone account for nearly 150,000 of these hospitalizations. These numbers are severely straining our already stressed health care system.

There are about 12 million clinical office visits for headache in the United States each year. In fact, 95% of women and 90% of men in the United States report having experienced a tension headache sometime in their lives, and 1 out of 4 U.S. households has at least one family member who suffers from migraine headaches. The level of pain is probably greatest in those suffering with cluster headaches; these usually focus on only one side of the head and tend to affect more men than women; however, it is estimated that only about 0.2% of the general population is affected by this condition. On the other hand, the estimated prevalence of severe, recurrent headache approaches 25% of the general population. Although there are situations where opiate or opioid painkiller drugs may be appropriate, they should not, in most situations, be the first-line treatment. It is recommended that advanced imaging with MRI be used rather than CT in non-emergent headache for which imaging was considered to be appropriate. Individuals with migraine headache are typically more likely to be prescribed opiate or opioid drugs compared with individuals with non-migraine headache. At any rate, counseling should be provided much more than it routinely is.

A related issue is that of rebound headaches, which are also known as medication overuse headaches. When one has an occasional headache, many might take a short-acting over-the-counter painkiller, such as aspirin, acetaminophen, or ibuprofen. Rebound headaches can also occur with misuse or overuse of opiate or opioid drugs as well as of other medications, including the ergotamines and the tripans. However, if any these products are not used as directed and as intended, then they could actually make the headaches worse. Misuse or overuse of over-the-counter painkillers, frequently involving exceeding label instructions such as taking the drug 3 or more times a week, can cause one to rebound into another headache. As the effects of the painkiller drug wear off, one might experience some withdrawal reactions, which can prompt inappropriate continued use, and this can escalate to a cycle of chronic daily headaches with greater severity and frequency. Further, overuse of painkillers can interfere with pain signaling in the brain, which, in turn, can lead to worsening headache pain. The rebound headache is most common when combination painkiller products that contain caffeine are used, or if the painkiller products are used in combination with caffeine from other sources, such as coffee, tea, chocolate, or soft drinks. The prevalence rate of rebound headache in the general population in this country is estimated to be between 1% and 2%, but their relative frequency is greater among individuals in secondary or tertiary care settings. Discontinuing use of the painkillers or gradually lowering the dosage is the easiest way to get headaches that are more readily controlled; avoidance of caffeine combination painkiller products is also recommended. Simple over-the-counter painkillers can generally be safely discontinued abruptly; however, abrupt discontinuation of some of these substances—such as, for example, butalbital—can even induce seizures in some individuals with abrupt cessation. A wide variety of prophylactic medications can be beneficial in this process of discontinuation of painkillers; these include assorted anticonvulsant, antidepressant, antihistamine, and antihypertensive medications. Specific prophylactic medicines used during discontinuation of painkillers for those suffering from rebound headaches, for a few examples, include amitriptyline, a tricyclic antidepressant; propranolol, a sympathetic nonselective beta blocker; topiramate, an anticonvulsant; and valporic acid, a mood stabilizer and anticonvulsant. Alternative health practices, such as aerobic exercise, biofeedback, and massage, may also be helpful.

The use of painkillers along with other drugs can be a dangerous and even all too often lethal combination. In 2011, the CDC reported that 31% of prescription painkiller overdose deaths were also linked with the use of benzodiazepines, which are antianxiety medications. Alcohol consumption along with use of painkiller drugs, both those available over the counter as well as those available only with a prescription, substantially increases the risks of drunk driving accidents as well as incidences of violence and other negative consequences. Drinking alcoholic beverages while using opiate or opioid painkiller drugs is particularly dangerous and can lead to complications such as dizziness, breathing problems, and even cardiac arrest.

Numerous other problems are routinely found to be associated with the use, misuse, and abuse of painkiller drugs. Some of these problems even result from failed initiatives intended to improve the issue. For example, problematic criminal justice practices have been well associated with interactions, in particular with injection users of painkiller and related drugs; frequently documented instances of police victimization of injection drug users include cases of extortion and physical and sexual violence. Many of the other problems, as well as intended solutions, now associated with the use, misuse, and abuse of painkiller drugs will be explored in subsequent chapters of this work.

DOCUMENT: HOW DIFFERENT MISUSERS OF PAIN RELIEVERS GET THEIR DRUGS

This table is from the Office of National Drug Control Policy, Office of Public Affairs fact sheet "Opioid Abuse in the United States" and illustrates the varied methods and sources used by misusers of painkillers to obtain their drugs. Most interesting is the fact that 41% of the frequent or chronic users obtained their painkiller drugs from a friend or relative for free or without asking, while 66% of occasional users got their drugs from the same source, as did 68% of the recent initiates. This phenomenon alone shows dramatically just how prevalent these powerful painkiller drugs are and that many nonmedical users of these potent prescription medications are obtained directly from family and friends, often without even being asked for. There is a clear underestimation of just how powerful these painkiller drugs are if they are so readily being given to family members and friends.

	Recent Initiates	Occasional Users	Frequent or Chronic Users
Bought from friend/relative, dealer, or internet	9%	13%	28%
Prescribed from 1 or more doctors	17%	17%	26%
Obtained from friend/relative for free or without asking	68%	66%	41%

Source: Office of National Drug Control Policy (2014). *Fact sheet: Opioid abuse in the United States.* Available online at https://www.whitehouse.gov/sites/default/files/ondcp/Fact_Sheets/opioids_fact_sheet.pdf. Data from SAMHSA, Center for Behavioral Health Statistics and Quality, National Survey on Drug Use and Health, 2009–2010.

DOCUMENT: OVERDOSE DEATHS INVOLVING OPIOID ANALGESICS, COCAINE, AND HEROIN

This is a table from the Office of National Drug Control Policy, Office of Public Affairs fact sheet "Opioid Abuse in the United States." The table illustrates the shocking increase in opioid painkiller fatal overdoses from 1999 to 2010. In fact, as the chart says, there was a 21% increase in the number of overdose deaths from opioid painkillers from 2006 to 2010. There was, even more alarming, a 45% increase in the number of overdose deaths from heroin over the same time, while there was a 44% decline in the percentage change of fatal cocaine overdoses over that time. Heroin overdose deaths most often occur when a user either miscalculates the amount of a dose or the purity of that particular batch of heroin. The data presented on this table indicates that the number of deaths from heroin overdoses rose from 1,963 in 1999 to 3,038 in 2010; most of this dramatic increase can unfortunately be attributed to the increase in purity of heroin available on U.S. streets.

	1999	2000	2001	2002	2003	2004	2005	2006	2007	2008	2009	2010	% Change 2006–2010
Opioid analgesic	4030	4400	5528	7456	8517	9857	10928	13723	14408	14800	15597	16651	21
Cocaine	3822	3544	3833	4599	5199	5443	6208	7448	6512	5129	4350	4183	44
Heroin	1963	1843	1784	2092	2084	1879	2010	2089	2402	3041	3279	3038	45

Source: Office of National Drug Control Policy (2014). *Fact sheet: Opioid abuse in the United States.* Available online at https://www.whitehouse.gov/sites/default/files/ondcp/Fact_Sheets/opioids_fact_sheet.pdf. Data from SAMHSA, Center for Behavioral Health Statistics and Quality, National Survey on Drug Use and Health, 2009–2010.

Chapter 7

Production, Distribution, and Regulation

There are many policy issues represented by myriad laws and various strategies that have arisen with respect to control and regulation of painkillers. The clinical trial system has evolved to provide our primary framework for the development and approval of new painkillers and other drugs—not to say that there are not some serious criticisms of the system as it now operates. The Controlled Substances Act of 1970 and its subsequent amendments are the primary legislative approach in force today for directing the production and regulation of painkillers, including opiates and opioids as well as the non-opioid ones and, as a matter of fact, all other drugs and their precursors.

POLICY ISSUES

Painkillers provide a marvelous lens with which to ponder drug policy issues. There were many early initiatives taken within respective societies to try to address this broad area of concern. Several key pieces of legislation were enacted in this country that have shaped the evolution of our policies toward painkillers, a process that continues to this day. The Pure Food and Drug Act was among the earliest of such measures along with several essentially restrictive endeavors, such as the Opium Exclusion Act, the Harrison Narcotics Act, and the Narcotics Drug Import and Export Act. The Porter Narcotic Farm Act was one of the earliest policy approaches that acknowledged the role of treatment, although enforcement initiatives remain dominant for a considerably longer period of time. However, there was eventually a shift toward rehabilitation efforts, while still maintaining a firm control and regulation stance. These historical policy lessons have shaped the discourse of how we deal with painkillers and other drugs and will, hopefully, better inform our future decisions.

Early Initiatives

Various initiatives have been implemented historically in attempts to curb or eliminate the use and abuse of respective psychoactive substances, including opium. In AD 827, a royal decree issued in Thailand prohibited the sale and use of opium. In 1310, Alluddin Khilji banned opium from the city of Delhi, India. In 17th-century courts in Indonesia, the expansion of the influence of Islam was reflected by prohibitions on the use of opium and tobacco similar to those imposed at the same time in Mughal India. In 1729, the emperor Yung-Cheng issued the first Chinese edict forbidding the sale of opium, but it had little effect. By the 1820s, enough opium was being exported to China to support the habits of about a million addicts. In 1868, Britain passed the Poisons and Pharmacy Act, which restricted the selling of opium only by pharmacists and further stipulated that all packages carry a label stating the contents. The Anglo-Oriental Society for the Suppression of the Opium Trade was founded in November 1874 in London as part of a broader social movement against the opium trade. This politically influential organization was heavily supported by Quakers and other Christian denominations. Their efforts also lent support to the Chinese opium suppression movement. Governmental policies to control the use of opium were enacted in many other places, such as was done in the last quarter of the 19th century and the early part of the 20th century in what is now Indonesia.

In 17th- and 18th-century Britain and other Western societies, opium use, whether for medical or nonmedical use, was rampant, despite a long earlier history of familiarity with its effects, and its use continued for the next couple of centuries. Opium was the most widely used medicine in the early American republic. Most addicts at that time were introduced to opiates by means of a physician's prescription and, consequently, tended to be of the middle and upper classes. In fact, by the middle of the 19th century, it was recognized that the "opium-appetite" had spread across the United States and the European continent, where it was reported that England alone consumed more opium than France, Germany, and Spain combined. It was stated that in 1864, 14% of the patients at the New York State Inebriate Asylum in Binghamton were there due to opium use (Calkins, 1871, p. 42). Laudanum, an alcoholic solution containing opium, was the most common form used by the

American populace, while "subcutaneous injection by means of a syringe" (Calkins, 1871, p. 54) was actually considered to be "less hazardous in instances, but not certainly" (Calkins, 1871, p. 55). Laudanum use among upper-class women, in particular, was much more socially accepted than alcohol use. Women in late 19th-century Britain who injected morphine were said to suffer from "morphinomania," which was discussed in very different terms to male opium eating. Similarly, during the middle of the 19th century, most addicts in America were women abusing opiates as part of purported medical treatment, while by the end of the 19th century, males were the more prevalent gender among addicts. Children were widely overmedicated as well. Nevertheless, in 1880, it was reported that 72% of the opium users in Chicago, Illinois, were women; and in 1881, it was estimated that 80% of the opium users in Albany, New York, were women. Prostitutes were identified as a subgroup of women who used opium. At any rate, opium, along with cocaine and marijuana, remained prevalent throughout most of American history, perhaps surpassed only by the pervasiveness of alcohol. American policy responses to opium, morphine, heroin, and related substances have tended to regard use as a criminal justice issue.

Pure Food and Drug Act

Concerns over the widespread use of opium, morphine, and other substances, particularly in patent medicines and nostrums, led to demands for stricter regulation. Consequently, in 1906, the U.S. Congress passed the Pure Food and Drug Act that was signed into law by President Theodore Roosevelt, who had advocated for it, as Public Law 59-384 (34 Stat. 768). The act created the U.S. Food and Drug Administration (FDA), which was given the authority to regulate aspects of food and drugs. For example, it stipulated that products be labeled identifying the contents and dosages of opium, morphine, and other substances; it further prohibited interstate commerce in adulterated or mislabeled drugs. The efforts leading to the passage of this law were part of the broader Progressive reform movement, notably including the Woman's Christian Temperance Union. Passage of the act was part of the Progressive trend of having so-called experts directing more health and social decisions, purportedly through active application of the scientific method, to counter trumped-up fads. Progressive leaders in the drug manufacturing sector saw it as in their own self-interest to pass such a law. Interestingly, various religious institutions, such as those affiliated with Protestant missionaries, seem to have been associated with several campaigns against drugs.

Opium Exclusion Act

Public alarm in late-19th- and early-20th-century America over opium smoking led to a response that essentially considered opium smoking as a contagion spread by Chinese immigrant laborers; this led to political pressure to exclude both Chinese and opium from the United States. On February 9, 1909, the U.S. Congress, at the urging of Theodore Roosevelt's secretary of state John Milton Hay, following a request signed by the boards of 21 American Chinese missionary societies, passed the Opium Exclusion Act, which made it illegal to import opium for other than medical purposes. The Opium Exclusion Act was intended to promote the gradual global reduction of opium production and an eventual ban on its smoking. The International Opium Commission met in Shanghai from February 1 to February 28, 1909, also at Roosevelt's urging; representatives from 13 nations met at Shanghai to conduct discussions in an international context on problems related to opium and other narcotics. The political response to this concern was useful in helping consolidate several U.S. power bases, including the medicalization of opiates by allopathic doctors (Aurin, 2000). During the Progressive Era, from about 1870 to 1930, numerous reforms were crafted in the United States based on purported scientific and social bases intended to address addiction. America, in fact, has gone through several cycles of tolerance and restraint with respect to measures to control narcotics.

Harrison Narcotics Act

In an effort mainly to address the issues of opium abuse in the Orient, including China, the Hague Convention of 1912 was settled upon. American politicians recognized the irony of their waging an international moral crusade against opium while having no domestic legislation regulating it. Accordingly, on April 8, 1913, Francis Burton Harrison, a congressman from New York State, introduced two bills to ban the importation and use of nonmedical opium and to control the production of opium for smoking within the United States; these bills received popular support, including that of then secretary of state William Jennings Bryan. Harrison had previously been personally embarrassed by an incident of opium smuggling that occurred during his 1913 arrival in the Philippines as the new U.S. governor-general.

In attempting to implement the terms of The Hague Convention, the U.S. Congress therefore passed the Harrison Narcotics Act of 1914, this was signed into law on February 14, 1914, by President Woodrow Wilson as Public Law 63-223 (38 Stat. 789), under which morphine, heroin, and other drugs became controlled substances in the United States such that possession without a prescription became a criminal offense. Modeled after the Boylan Law, which the New York State legislature passed in 1904 to strictly control narcotic dispensation by physicians, the Harrison Narcotics Act had originally been intended to regulate the marketing of opium, morphine and other drugs, particularly as a matter of international relations. It required that anyone who imported or otherwise sold or distributed narcotics had to be registered with the federal government; they also had to pay a small tax, and they were further required to keep detailed records of all transactions, which had to be available for inspection at any time. Unregistered individuals who were caught possessing narcotics were then presumed guilty of violating the law and could, accordingly, be fined and imprisoned for up to five years.

The Harrison Narcotics Act effectively curtailed the supplying of drugs by physicians to addicts. It thus prohibited the distribution of narcotic drugs and effectively criminalized the prescription and use of opiates in America. Enforcement, in effect, became the primary strategy to address narcotics. The subsequent Dangerous Drugs Act of 1920 prohibited all legal use of heroin in the United States, and by 1924, the production of heroin was prohibited. A similar criminal justice approach to these substances prevailed in other countries, including Canada.

United Kingdom and the League of Nations

The United Kingdom developed a different strategy. During World War I, opiate and other drug use, primarily cocaine, was characterized as anti-British since it was believed to weaken soldiers' ability and will to fight. After seeing the consequences of drug regulations in the United States, physicians and pharmacists in the United Kingdom lobbied for the exclusive rights, respectively, to prescribe and to dispense drugs, particularly opiates. It must also be recognized that in the UK, as elsewhere, there are economic foundations for drug policies.

After World War I, the League of Nations was founded. Article 23 of the Covenant of the League of Nations stipulated that the League would have "general supervision over the execution of agreements with regard to . . . the traffic in opium and other dangerous drugs" (Willoughby, 1925, p. 43). Under this provision, the League assumed supervision of the Hague Convention of 1912. The UK along with other countries, including China, France, the Netherlands, Portugal, and Siam, became members of the Advisory Committee on the Traffic in Opium and other Dangerous Drugs of the League of Nations; this organization then served as the major international drug control body.

Narcotics Drug Import and Export Act

The Narcotics Drug Import and Export Act (42 Stat. 596) of 1922, also known as the Jones-Miller Act, restricted the importation and use of morphine and other drugs. It was intended to eliminate the use of narcotic drugs except, of course, for legitimate medical uses. At that time, most drug manufacturers were located in Europe, the United States, and Japan. The act, enacted by President Warren G. Harding, created a rigid control system designed to assure the exportation of manufactured drugs and preparations for medical needs only in the country of destination. It required drug exporters to acquire an appropriate certificate from the importing nation. This act established the U.S. policy of favoring the importation of narcotic raw materials for conversion in the United States into finished drug products, rather than the domestic production of raw materials. This policy also favored the importation of narcotic raw materials over processed narcotic materials as well as over the importation of finished products. This drug policy has been reflected in subsequent legislation and continues today under Section 952: "Importation of Controlled Substances" of the Controlled Substances Act (21 U.S.C. 952(a)).

In 1929, the League of Nations appointed a Commission of Enquiry into the Control of Opium, which estimated that there were then over a million opium smokers in just the 15 colonies studied, which included Burma, Brunei, Formosa, French Indonesia, Hong Kong, Malay, the Netherlands Indonesia, and Siam; and that, due to the intractability of opium smoking, it should be legalized and supplied through governmental monopolies. It was felt that immediate cessation of opium use would be difficult due to the numbers of confirmed addicts, but that gradual suppression might be possible. At any rate, as the British Empire restricted the availability of opium from India, it was replaced by opium from other sources, primarily China and Persia, as well as by heroin and other substances.

Porter Narcotic Farm Act

The Porter Narcotic Farm Act (Public Law 70-672) was passed unanimously by Congress on June 19, 1929, during the administration of President Calvin Coolidge. This act created two hospitals in federal prisons to hold and treat narcotic addicts under the U.S. Public Health Service in Lexington, Kentucky, and Fort Worth, Texas. It was early recognition for the role of treatment, rather than mere incarceration, in addressing opiate and opioid use and abuse.

Enforcement Initiatives

The Porter Narcotic Farm Act initiated the federal responsibility for providing treatment of narcotic addiction. In 1932, the Uniform State Narcotic Act was passed during the administration of President Herbert Hoover to encourage states to establish uniform state drug laws that matched federal ones, including those covering opium, morphine, and related substances. The 1932 act was drafted by the National Conference of Commissioners on Uniform Laws and subsequently adopted by all states; it remained in effect until 1970 with the passage of the Comprehensive Drug Abuse Prevention and Control Act.

Opium was prevalent elsewhere, and efforts to curb its prevalence met with varied success. For instance, in India, which had a very long history of opium use, efforts were fairly successful in prohibiting use after India's independence from Great Britain in 1947.

Certain factors, from a historical perspective, seem to have been related to respective substance use and abuse policy approaches. Symbolism, such as that associated with racism, has been a significant factor behind many substance-related policy issues, such as the anti-Chinese fears that led to the creation of myriad anti-opium laws. Racism, likewise, was a moving force behind the first opium prohibition legislation in 19th-century Australia. Similarly, fear of racial intermarriage was a factor behind the appearance of "dope girls" in the early 20th century, which facilitated the emergence of the British drug underground.

Not surprisingly, a familiar rhetoric has been used historically in calls for drug reforms. Counter-subversion, for instance, was a common theme used in anti-narcotic campaigns in the United States from the 1920s through the 1940s. Moral, economic, political, and other agendas, rather than informed debate, have frequently shaped the shift in public discourse and resulting legislation on various drugs.

Harry Jacob Anslinger, who had been working to enforce alcohol prohibition, became the first American federal commissioner of narcotics in 1930 and strove throughout his career to make the Bureau of Narcotics an agency dedicated to the enforcement of laws pertaining to drugs. He advocated for a uniform national set of drug laws that would better permit enforcement efforts by federal and state governments). Among the driving forces behind the establishment of the Bureau of Narcotics was public concern over issues like opium dens and the fear of drug habits spreading among American women. This gender-based concern was not new, as Dr. Harry Hubbell Kane wrote in 1882: "females are so much excited sexually by the smoking of opium ... many innocent and over-curious girls have thus been seduced" (Kane, 1882, p. 8).

In the late 1940s and 1950s, reformers openly called for a reversal of the reliance upon the criminal justice system to handle the U.S. drug problem. In 1947, Alfred Lindesmith, a leading sociologist, advocated for reform of the U.S. criminological approach to narcotic control. Rufus King and other like-minded lawyers called for such reforms and for ending the incarceration of medical professionals for treating addicts. Some physicians also supported more medical, rather than criminal, management of narcotic addiction. Articles even appeared in popular magazines with compatible themes, such as one in 1952 by Alden Stevens titled "Make Dope Legal." Nevertheless, the prevailing trend was that of repressive legal sanctions for the possession and sale of narcotics.

Boggs Act

In the 1950s and 1960s, researchers recognized and examined what appeared to be a postwar heroin epidemic. Many studies then postulated socioeconomic and/or psychosocial causes for heroin addiction. For example, one study observed that most heroin addicts "are frequently overcome by a sense of futility, expectations of failure, and general depression" (Chein, Gerard, Lee, & Rosenfeld, 1964, p. 14). Policy makers, in the face of such studies, tended to assume that severe criminal penalties could effectively dissuade use. In fact, criminal penalties for drug possession were then widely regarded, even by medical authorities, as helping those with weak moral wills remain abstinent from drugs. Accordingly, in 1951 during the administration of President Harry S. Truman, the U.S. Congress passed the Boggs Act, which was intended to strengthen enforcement efforts; it established both minimum and maximum penalties for the sale or possession of narcotics. No distinction was made by the Boggs Act between users and sellers; first-time offenders received from 2 to 5 years; 5 to 10 years for second offense; and 10 to 20 years for more than two offenses.

Treatment Initiatives

The Narcotics Control Act of 1956 (70 Stat. 567) was passed during the administration of President Dwight D. Eisenhower, with sentiments similar to those behind the Boggs Act; this new act further increased minimum sentences for narcotics possession and distribution. However, with a subsequent federal drug policy ideological change, the Narcotic Addict Rehabilitation

Act of 1966 (Public Law 89-793; 80 Stat. 1438) was passed during the administration of Lyndon B. Johnson; it was intended to provide treatment for narcotic addicts as an alternative to incarceration. The Narcotic Addict Rehabilitation Act significantly enhanced federal efforts for the treatment and rehabilitation of narcotic addicts. This act had provisions for voluntary drug treatment commitment and for pretrial civil commitment. Critics of the act suggested that offenders only went into narcotic treatment programs hoping to obtain an earlier release date, and also that there was too much opportunity for manipulation.

United Nations Conventions

International drug policy initiatives were conducted as well to help control narcotics and other drugs. In 1961, the United Nations adopted the Single Convention on Narcotic Drugs, which attempted to simplify the maze of different national approaches to control narcotics with one overall international agreement. This sweeping initiative advocated, for instance, paying farmers not to cultivate crops of opium poppies, which was ultimately a failed strategy. Opium control policies were part of a broader international control movement. In this vein, in 1968, the United Nations established the International Narcotics Control Board (INCB). The INCB was charged with implementing the drug policies of the UN, including the Single Convention on Narcotic Drugs of 1961 and the 1988 United Nations Convention against Illicit Traffic in Narcotic Drugs and Psychotropic Substances. Interpol's Criminal Organization and Drug Sub-Directorate (CODSD), in cooperation with the UN, monitors international drug trafficking. The UN thus serves a major role in the formulation of policies and strategies to address opiates and opioids on a global scale. It must, of course, also be recognized that the U.S. Congress has considerably greater influence over international drug trafficking than its counterparts in other nations. Congress appropriates funds for and maintains some degree of oversight for international narcotics control efforts. In the 1970s and 1980s, it was claimed that there were integral linkages between trafficking in heroin and other illegal drugs and U.S. security interests.

Rehabilitation Shift

The Narcotic Addict Rehabilitation Act of 1966 helped shift the response to narcotic addiction from incarceration to treatment, but considerable additional legislative efforts were regarded as necessary to promote this change of focus. In 1968, the Alcoholic and Narcotic Addict Rehabilitation Act was enacted by President Lyndon B. Johnson as Public Law 90-574 (82 Stat. 1006), as an amendment to the Community Mental Health Centers Act of 1963. In 1970, Congress passed the Comprehensive Drug Abuse Prevention and Control Act, enacted as Public Law 91-513 by President Richard M. Nixon, Title I of which, among other things, provided for the treatment of substance abusers. The Narcotic Addict Rehabilitation Amendments of 1971 were also enacted by President Nixon as Public Law 92-420 to expand treatment services. Congress passed the Drug Abuse Office and Treatment Act on March 21, 1972, enacted by President Nixon as Public Law 92-255, part of which established the National Institute of Drug Abuse (Costello & Van Vleck, 2009). Similarly, in 1974, the Narcotic Addict Treatment Act (Public Law 93-281; 88 Stat. 124) was enacted to allow medical practitioners to dispense narcotic drugs for detoxification and other treatment purposes.

The practice of providing drug treatment under civil commitment, which was the cornerstone of the Narcotic Addict Rehabilitation Act, declined during the 1970s. On January 2, 1980, the Drug Abuse Prevention, Treatment and Rehabilitation Act was enacted by President Jimmy Carter as Public Law 96-181; it was intended to expand prevention and treatment programs. In 1986, Congress passed the Anti-Drug Abuse Act enacted by President Ronald Reagan as Public Law 99-570, which enhanced block grant funding for substance abuse treatment as well as included funding for research, particularly AIDS research. Admission of voluntary patients to the Lexington, Kentucky, and Fort Worth, Texas, narcotics hospitals ceased in 1988. In 1988, the Omnibus Anti-Drug Act was passed by Congress and enacted by Reagan as Public Law 100-690 (102 Stat. 4181), to increase federal funding for prevention, treatment, and rehabilitation; it also established the Office of National Drug Control Policy under the Executive Office of the President. The mandate for that office was expanded during the administration of President William J. Clinton with the Office of National Drug Control Policy Reauthorization Act of 1998. The Children's Health Act of 2000, enacted by Clinton as Public Law 106-310, repealed the Narcotic Addict Rehabilitation Act of 1966. Nevertheless, that act served as a major drug treatment policy vehicle.

Historical Policy Lessons

Respective policies regarding substances have certainly altered the development of various addiction problems. This was clearly the case regarding attempts to deal with the so-called "French connection" as it was with those recommending methadone treatment; both sets of policies heavily impacted the course of the modern heroin epidemic. In fact, history has repeatedly taught us that there are often unintended consequences to policies. For example, opium use became recognized as a social problem in Turkmenistan in the late 18th century when informal social controls were weakened; but when formal controls were then introduced through policies in the late 19th century, there were both intended and unintended outcomes, the latter including both a shift in the demographic patterns of users as well as of the social and medical consequences of use. In a similar manner, when the British attempted to eradicate opium in China, from about 1880 to World War II, they created instead a demand for heroin, morphine, cocaine, and other substances. Prior to this British "war on drugs," opium use in China was largely associated with complex rituals, and there was little excessive use. Chinese attempts to prohibit opium met, not surprisingly, with considerable resistance, particularly from opium farmers and traders. In fact, up to the late 1980s, opium was still the main substance used by drug abusers in China. Other forms of drug abuse then reemerged with the increasing modernization and Westernization of China. Opiate abuse, mainly of heroin, is now the most widespread drug problem in China. Likewise, when various Asian governments enacted anti-opium laws, heroin use escalated and rapidly and addiction to heroin surpassed opium within ten years. Accordingly, it is recognized that caution should be exercised in efforts to establish opposition to traditional cultural attitudes toward the use of respective substances.

During the 1990s, it was recognized that heroin had moved from urban centers into mainstream culture, particularly popular culture, and American policy makers pondered alternatives to drug policies that seemed to lack effectiveness. At that time, narcotic drug smugglers typically refined raw opium into bricks of morphine that were easier to transport. South American drug traffickers began using Caribbean island nations for systematic money-laundering operations in the 1970s. It also appears that there were minimal barriers against entry to the higher levels of narcotics trafficking. It was widely recognized that other strategies had to be developed. Interdictionist approaches, for instance, have been shown not to succeed in stopping this international narcotics trade. There are, of course, limits to international efforts to control drugs, particularly in a globalized world where national borders are less meaningful.

More Recent Moves

Late in the 20th century, the Netherlands, Switzerland, and then Spain were among the countries that adopted a system based on policies that had existed in the United Kingdom of providing prescription heroin to addicts. Despite claims such as reductions in criminal behavior, these programs tended to maintain if not increase the numbers of individuals actually using opiates. Heroin is still legally used for medical purposes in the UK, which accounts for nearly 95% of the world's legal heroin consumption. Certainly many clinical and ethical issuers are raised by programs that provide injectable heroin and other opiates or opioids, and even supporters of such acknowledge limitations of the approach. Further, U.S. federal regulatory policies have hindered access to treatment for opiate addiction.

Long-term opioid therapy has become increasingly prescribed and, at the same time, fatalities from opioid poisoning have increased. Research suggests that those who receive higher doses of opioid therapy for chronic pain have nearly a ninefold greater risk of overdose compared to those who receive the lowest doses. It has also been noted that more overdoses are reported among those diagnosed as having substance abuse or depression or who were prescribed sedative hypnotics.

Contemporary policies toward drugs have focused primarily on supply-side approaches, like interdiction and eradication. Unfortunately, based on the apparent lack of the effectiveness of these types of strategies, it is difficult to support continued exclusive reliance upon such policies. Further, it must be recognized that decisions regarding implementation of drug policy are commonly made below the level of the nation-state. On the other hand, globalization appears to have lowered the price of heroin and other illicit drugs, but it may also offer opportunities to increase the effectiveness of drug control policies intending to reduce demand. At any rate, many drug policy issues pertaining to opiates and opioids remain unresolved and will continue to be debated for some time.

CLINICAL TRIALS

Clinical trials are research tools intended to evaluate how effective medical techniques are. Each clinical trial has a protocol, or plan of action, for conducting the particular test. This plan fully describes what will be done in the specific study and how each step will be implemented, along with a justification of why each step is necessary. Every clinical trial has a specific set of conditions as to who can, and who cannot, participate in it. Clinical trials can provide useful information about which pharmaceutical products or other medical devices or interventions should be further investigated in better-designed studies.

The origins of clinical trials goes back to the 18th century, when comparison groups were used to evaluate different treatment approaches, such as the eating of citrus fruits to treat scurvy as developed by British physicians. Following an outbreak of fatalities resulting from the use of a di-ethylene glycol solution of sulfanilamide, the Federal Pure Food and Drug Act was amended in 1938 requiring toxicity studies, as well as approval of a New Drug Application (NDA) before a new drug could be marketed and distributed in the United States. In 1962, the Harris-Kefauver Amendment to the Federal Pure Food and Drug Act was enacted, which requires both extensive pharmacological and toxicological research before any drug can be tested in human beings; this established the modern clinical trial system in the United States. The 1992 Prescription Drug User Fee Act and the Food and Drug Administration Modernization Act of 1997 have accelerated the drug approval process under the supervision of the Center for Drug Evaluation and Research.

Clinical trials are generally used to evaluate the effectiveness and safety of a new medical treatment compared to the existing treatment or current standard of care for a particular condition, including pain. These scientific studies typically involve active participation by human subjects to test the safety and effectiveness of new medical approaches. Before a new drug can be released for use in the United States, and in most of the rest of the developed world, it must undergo a rigorous clinical trial process to determine if it is both effective and safe for use. However, not all clinical trials are intended to assess the safety and efficacy of a new pharmacological agent like a painkiller. There are clinical trials, for instance, which are primarily diagnostic in nature and created to try to determine better ways to diagnose a serious illness or disorder; this could, for example, include a symptom like severe chronic pain in a particular part of the body, such as neck pain, lower back pain, and so forth. There are screening trials intended to find the optimal approach to detect a particular disorder or condition; preventative trials examine approaches to prevent specific diseases or conditions, like acute dental pain following surgery. There are also clinical trials intended to find ways to improve the quality of life for those experiencing respective conditions, naturally including pain and so forth. Clinical trials with different purposes would, of course, have different research designs.

Clinical trials are publicly and privately supported research studies. Examples of industry sponsors of clinical trials include pharmaceutical, biotechnology, and medical device companies. Each year, about 80,000 federal and industry sponsored clinical trials are conducted in the United States, utilizing as many as 5,000 to 6,000 research protocols. These trials are conducted at myriad types of sites, actually totaling over 10,000 different locations throughout the country, including universities, independent research centers, doctor's offices, and private and public hospitals and medical centers. Millions of people participate annually as subjects in these clinical trials, and about 200,000 research professionals manage and conduct these studies each year. Clinical trials are, of course, also conducted in many other countries around the world. Unfortunately, the results of clinical trials from different countries or continents are generally not pooled, which would easily and cheaply provide a larger database than any one political entity could generate, and this would provide opportunities for more informed decision-making across the board.

A clinical trial usually investigates a particular intervention or set of interventions, and may even be referred to as an interventional study. The intervention may be a drug or medical device; it may involve different doses of a medication and/or different ways to administer the substance, like a painkiller administered as a transdermal patch rather than as an injection; or it may involve lifestyle changes on the part of the subjects, such as changes in diet, tobacco use, or exercise pattern. An alternative type of research approach to an interventional study is an observational study; variations of these types of clinical trials include case-control, case-crossover, case-only, cohort, community, and ecological studies. A critical characteristic is that clinical trials are prospective in design, not retrospective; they can posit an effect, establish conditions to test this potential relationship, and, in the future, they can accordingly evaluate the results, whether they turn out to be positive, unclear, or negative.

Clinical trials are controlled research studies that are designed according to strict scientific methods. As many variables as possible must be controlled for to determine the effects of a specific drug or other treatment alternative being examined. The independent variable is that variable in the clinical trial that is manipulated by the investigators, such as whether the new drug being tested was given to a particular part of the study sample. The dependent variable is the outcome of the study, such as the effects of a particular medication on a specific disease or disorder. When researchers are selecting samples of mentally ill patients for clinical trials, whether of new drugs or other therapeutic approaches, it must be recognized that they are not a very homogenous population. Attention, accordingly, must be directed to sampling procedures employed to construct a representative sample. Further, certain subgroups may need to be excluded to obtain maximally representative and more generalizable results. For instance, individuals with the anxious and hostile variants of depressive disorder have been found to be poor subjects in clinical drug trials as they have excessively high placebo response rates. On the other hand, individuals with the withdrawn and disorganized variants tend to be poor subjects in clinical trials of neuroleptic drugs as they tend to respond poorly to both placebo and the active drug. The removal of such subjects from clinical trial samples, of course, means that the observed results may not be generalizable to persons with those particular types of conditions.

Phase I Clinical Trials

It is estimated that it may take 20 years and about $800 million to bring one new drug from its discovery through to the final market stage. It takes about 10 years of testing in test tubes and on animals before it might be ready for initial testing on human subjects. It is thought that only about 1 drug out of 50 that undergo preclinical testing will eventually be considered safe and effective for human testing. These preclinical investigations are generally carried out before Phase I studies can begin, and they are usually conducted as in vitro studies and/or as animal studies. There is then an extrapolation of preclinical safety data to humans. The results of laboratory and animal testing, along with detailed study protocols, must be submitted in an Investigational New Drug (IND) application to the FDA. If the application is not rejected by the FDA, then the actual clinical trials can begin. Of the new drugs that enter clinical trials, it is estimated that only about 1 in 5 will eventually prove sufficiently safe and effective to receive FDA approval. About 120 new medical approaches get FDA approval each year. The European Medicines Agency (EMA) is the general regulator of drugs, and thus by default of clinical trials relating to them, in Europe; it is somewhat analogous to the FDA in the United States. The EMA, of course, has its own guidelines and policies pertaining to the conduct and utilization of clinical trials and their results.

Clinical trials that are conducted in the United States for FDA approval are usually divided into four phases. Phase I studies usually involve a small group, perhaps between 20 and 100 individuals who are typically normal, healthy subjects, such as college students, and these studies may last up to one year. Baseline data are generally collected on subjects at the beginning of a clinical trial. Demographic data, such as age, gender, ethnicity, racial background, and so forth, are usually collected. However, different baseline characteristics are gathered depending on the nature of the study. For instance, a study on pain management is likely to record history of injuries, prior use of both prescription and over-the-counter painkillers, alcohol intake, weight, body mass index, and so forth. The primary purpose of Phase I studies is to evaluate safety, such as the dosage ranges, methods of administration, rate of absorption, and distribution of the drug in the body as well as any possible toxicities. A major objective of Phase I clinical trial testing is to determine safe dosage levels before minor side effects, like headaches or nausea, are experienced by users. Subjects in Phase I studies are usually financially compensated, particularly due to the likelihood that they may experience undesirable side effects. Phase I clinical trials are primarily concerned with estimating the maximally tolerated dose of the drug under study as well as determining its pharmacodynamics and pharmacokinetics. About 70% of new medical approaches are able to pass Phase I testing.

Phase II Clinical Trials

Phase II clinical trial studies are concerned with both safety and efficacy issues for particular types of subjects. These, like those in Phase I, are relatively small studies, typically incorporate from 100 up to several hundred subjects who have the disease or condition being investigated for the particular intervention. Phase II clinical trial studies usually take between 1 and 3 years to conduct. Participation requirements are most often stricter for Phase II than for Phase I studies, and subjects are generally randomly assigned to either a control group or a treatment group. The control group may receive a placebo or the standard treatment. There may be several different types of treatment groups being utilized in a particular clinical study. Frequently, neither the subjects nor the investigators will know who gets the treatment and who does not; this procedure is referred to as a double blind study, which is intended to eliminate as much bias as possible. Different dosages of a drug are often examined during Phase II studies. The primary purpose of Phase II clinical trial testing is to determine if the new drug, device, or treatment regimen has sufficient biological activity or efficacy against the particular disease under study to warrant more extensive research and development efforts. About a third of all the drugs under development that enter clinical trials pass Phase II and then are able to move on to Phase III testing.

Phase III Clinical Trials

Phase III clinical trials are usually larger and more expensive to conduct than the Phase I or Phase II studies. Phase III studies typically involve several hundred and up to several thousand subjects and usually last from 2 to 4 or 5 years. The Phase III studies are often conducted in doctor's offices and usually involve a more diverse range of subjects than only those for whom the treatment is intended. Investigators are likely to examine safety and efficacy, as well as cost benefits, in different demographic subsets of subjects, such as younger and older, male and female, various ethnic and racial groups, and individuals with mild, moderate, or severe forms of the particular disease or disorder under study. Different dosage levels are often tried to determine maximum effectiveness while having the fewest side effects. About 80 percent of drugs that undergo Phase III testing will be able to pass this stage.

Once clearing Phase III studies, the research sponsor can submit a New Drug Application (NDA) to the FDA. This application usually takes a review period of about 1 year to be considered; and of these NDAs about 60% are eventually approved by the FDA. If the principal investigator made an agreement with the sponsor of a clinical trial that they would not discuss the results of the study or publish them in any academic or scientific journal then, according to Section 801 of the Food and Drug Administration Amendments Act (Public Law 110-85), a certain agreements document must be completed. At this point, an acceptable package insert must also be prepared through a cooperative effort between the manufacturer and the FDA; it includes precautions, warnings, approved indications, contraindications, adverse reactions, and so forth. The drug can then finally be produced and marketed, but it is only under conditional approval.

Phase IV Clinical Trials

Phase IV studies are conducted post marketing after the FDA has granted approval for, say, a pharmaceutical company to market the new product. It is generally understood that there may be numerous unanticipated adverse as well as potentially beneficial effects that would be detectable only after the drug has been widely distributed, which is why the FDA often urges that Phase IV clinical studies be conducted. However, the release of the new drug is closely monitored by the FDA, and patients are under specified supervision. These Phase IV studies usually involve several hundred to several thousand subjects; usually they are conducted at selected medical centers and administered by qualified physicians, and they typically take from 2 to 10 years to conduct. All physicians who agree to participate in Phase IV clinical trials agree to participate in organized reporting, with close attention directed to both the efficacy and the toxicity of the particular pharmacological agent. However, it must be recognized that studies of certain types of interventions, such as those focusing on lifestyle or behavioral changes or on new surgical or other medical approaches, might not fit into the Phase I through Phase IV clinical testing model. There is also an accelerated approval process for drugs used to treat serious illnesses that lack satisfactory treatments, such as HIV/AIDS. Nevertheless, since January 2004, the FDA continues surveillance through the Adverse Event Reporting System (AERS) on approved all drugs and other therapeutic products.

Meta-analysis

Results from several clinical trials can be pooled for a meta-analysis. When evaluating the safety and efficacy of a particular treatment for a specific condition, an individual clinical trial usually has its own inherent limitations. A meta-analysis can incorporate the heterogeneity of treatment effects by reviewing data from several studies in the analysis of overall efficacy. Relevant covariates can also be included that would further reduce the heterogeneity and permit more specific therapeutic recommendations than would be possible from any one clinical trial.

CRITIQUES OF THE CLINICAL TRIAL SYSTEM

Critics have claimed that many clinical trials are profoundly flawed and that the system within which they currently operate is essentially broken. Substantial reforms have been called for. The crux of the problem, from this perspective, is that the pharmaceutical or other related industries have been allowed to overly control and influence too much of the process. An example of a commonly employed flawed research design for conducting a clinical trial is that of comparing the new drug under development against a placebo when there is, in fact, a perfectly good drug already being used to treat the issue. In such a skewed clinical trial, many drugs would, of course, demonstrate greater efficacy than a placebo, which by definition should have no actual therapeutic effect. Something, almost anything, is bound to have a greater effect than nothing, which is fundamentally what a clinical trial against a placebo is designed to test. Another ploy commonly utilized in crafting a flawed research design for a biased clinical trial is to administer either an abnormally high or an unusually low dosage of a commonly used competing pharmacological agent, thus engineering a much greater likelihood of "finding" either more severe side effects or lack of therapeutic efficacy.

Sample Selection

Another frequently raised critique of clinical trials is related to issues of the sample population used. Most clinical trials are characterized as having a limited number of participants, which is usually rationalized for by asserting the costliness of selecting much larger sample sizes. Further, the subjects selected for many clinical trials may not be very representative of the actual population to whom a particular pharmacological agent or other medical approach will actually be administered. It is, in fact, not uncommon for a young and relatively healthy pool of participants to be sought for a clinical trial, even though the approach under study will ultimately be used, if approved, with a far different population. The unrealistic nature of selecting such samples for the approach under study is more likely to result in approval, but less likely to find potential problems that might become apparent only after wider distribution to populations with more diverse attributes.

Publication Concerns

It is not very surprising that pharmaceutical or other similar industry-sponsored clinical trials might be designed to make it more likely to yield positive results for their medical products under development. What might be somewhat less apparent is the full extent to which the pharmaceutical and related industries control or excessively influence the publication and dissemination of the results of clinical trials, such that they can, and routinely do, withhold negative results and can otherwise manipulate factors that are generally assumed to be more neutral.

The selective publication of only clinical trials that indicate positive findings for medical products produced by a respective pharmaceutical or other related company is very commonplace. The overarching problem is that pharmaceutical and similar companies need not publish all the data from all the clinical trials they conduct on a specific approach. The missing data could well indicate that pharmacological agent or similar product under review is actually no better, or even worse, than other products or approaches already being used. This, unfortunately, can result in the respective research literature on the subject being overly represented with misleading and perhaps even false positive findings. Although rules exist holding that the results of all clinical trials should be released and listed, there is no regulatory body or organization that oversees that such in fact is done. Those who have looked into the matter have actually found that clinical trials with negative results or even those that are just unflattering toward a potential pharmaceutical product are still likely to become available and declared. However, the techniques and strategies employed by the pharmaceutical and related industries to promote the image of their own products go far beyond this level of control.

There are actual publications designed by and, of course, paid for by pharmaceutical and related companies that have the superficial appearance of being an academic research journal, but alas are not. Copies of these so-called "publications" are widely distributed by pharmaceutical representatives or mailed directly to physicians, who may then read them assuming they are legitimate scholarly, and allegedly independent, journals but that are tools that exist solely to market particular pharmaceutical or related products. The pieces contained in these glossy "publications" typically purport to report on objective clinical trial data; but, of course, the entire process has been created by and for the respective company and will therefore naturally extol its products.

There are also indirect pressures that the pharmaceutical or similar industry applies upon the editors and publishers of seemingly independent medical research journals. It is acknowledged that pharmaceutical and similar companies will routinely purchase, for somewhat exorbitant fees, numerous (e.g., hundreds of thousands) reprints of articles in prestigious journals that extol the virtues of one of their respective products. These costly reprints are regularly and widely distributed to physicians and researchers at no charge under the guise of professional education or of simply spreading research knowledge, but this practice is essentially overt advertising. The financial incentive of publishing such favorable articles is substantial, particularly upon smaller academic journals, whose editors are frequently part timers while typically maintaining full-time academic positions and duties. Further, pharmaceutical and related companies also have been known to hire ghost writers to actually prepare glowing draft articles for submission to academic journals and to then find a doctor or researcher willing to submit the manuscript under his or her own name. If accepted and published, the designated author will often then be hired to present those findings at professional conferences and at industry-sponsored continuing medical education venues. These presenters are often supplied with talking points from the pharmaceutical or similar company on the exceptional merits of the particular medical product being discussed. These trainings and related events will influence what pharmacological agents the attendees will prescribe to their patients in the future as well as what products they will spontaneously promote to colleagues and trainees.

Thus, the overall results of perhaps a less-than-well-designed clinical trial could easily become the genesis of what may come to be seen as the state-of-the-art approach for treating a particular medical problem, including acute or chronic pain. This practice of permitting industry-sponsored clinical trial data to remain largely under their control and for uses they see fit to apply it to, regrettably, could and apparently has in some cases already resulted in the cessation of effective medical approaches with their replacement by more expensive and less, if not even harmful, approaches.

ROLE OF THE CONTROLLED SUBSTANCES ACT

The Comprehensive Drug Abuse Prevention and Control Act of 1970 contained, under Title II, the Controlled Substances Act (84 Stat. 1242), which established schedules for manufacturing, possessing, using, importing, and distributing certain substances, including opiates and opioids, as well as many of the chemicals used in the making of these and other controlled substances. The act also established procedures to examine new drugs by evaluating their potential medical uses as well as their likely side effects, particularly their potential for one becoming dependent and addicted.

The Controlled Substances Act was created during the administration of then president Richard M. Nixon under the direction of then U.S. attorney general John N. Mitchell. It was a time when there were growing concerns over drugs in the country and related social issues, in particular the crime rate. An important factor was the concern that soldiers returning home from the Vietnam War, where heroin and other drugs were readily and cheaply available, would overrun America with a tidal wave of addiction. The Controlled Substances Act itself replaced more than 50 other separate pieces of drug legislation. It repealed both the Harrison Narcotics Act of 1916 and many of the 1965 Drug Abuse Control Amendments, many of which were formulated to eliminate the illicit drug trade. There was also mounting concern that lack of coordination and cooperation between numerous agencies was hampering efforts to address aspects of drug control and regulation.

The Controlled Substances Act, which was enacted as part of the Comprehensive Drug Abuse Prevention and Control Act of 1970, provides most of the legal foundation for the so-called federal war on drugs and other related precursor substances. On May 1, 1971, the Controlled Substances Act took effect and was initially enforced by the U.S. Justice Department's Bureau of Narcotics and Dangerous Drugs; that agency was then replaced in 1973 by the Drug Enforcement Administration (DEA). The Controlled Substances Act, under Title 21, Chapter 13, Subchapter 1, Part B, puts drugs into one of five schedules, which serves as a drug classification system for the purposes of enforcement and regulation. These schedules are supposedly based on the differing potentials for abuse and dependence, generally accepted medical uses, and concerns with safety and efficacy for specific controlled substances. The schedule in which a particular substance is placed determines how it will be regulated and controlled.

Scheduling of Drugs

Schedule I substances are for drugs considered the most dangerous. Schedule I substances are those drugs that have a high abuse potential, that do not have any generally accepted medicinal uses in treatment, and that lack an acceptable level of safety such that even under medical supervision they cannot be used safely. Heroin and many synthetic opioids as well as lysergic acid diethylamide (LSD), mescaline, peyote, psilocybin, and other hallucinogens, and marijuana, which some endorse as a painkiller, are all listed as Schedule I drugs.

Schedule II substances are drugs that also have a high potential for abuse, but they currently have some generally accepted medical uses for treatment even with severe restrictions, although it is recognized that these substances can still lead to either severe psychological or physical dependence. Schedule II substances require a prescription for legal use. Methadone and fentanyl, as well as cocaine, amphetamines, and methamphetamine are currently listed as Schedule II drugs.

Schedule III substances are drugs that have less potential for abuse than Schedule I or II drugs, and thus their use may lead to the development of low to moderate risks for physical dependence and/or to high risk for psychological dependence, but they currently have some generally accepted medical treatment uses. Schedule III drugs all require a prescription for legal use. Nalorphine, anabolic steroids, and ketamine are listed as Schedule III drugs.

Schedule IV substances are drugs that are regarded to have a have a low potential for abuse as compared to those substances in Schedule III, but it is acknowledged that limited psychological dependence and/or physical dependence can still develop to these drugs, and they currently have some accepted medicinal treatment uses. Schedule IV substances also require a prescription for legal use. Phenobarbital, chloral hydrate, meprobamate, benziodiazepines (e.g., Librium, Xanax, Valium), and barbital are listed as Schedule IV drugs.

Schedule V is used for those substances that are considered to be the least dangerous. Schedule V substances are drugs that are considered to have a lower potential for abuse than Schedule IV ones, although their use can still lead to the development of psychological and/or physical dependence; and these drugs currently have some accepted medicinal treatment uses. Lomotil and Robitussin A-C, for example, are listed as Schedule V products. Many Schedule V drugs do not generally require a prescription, while those on Schedules II, III, and IV do usually require prescriptions.

The U.S. Department of Justice and the Department of Health and Human Services, including the FDA, control painkillers and other drugs under these five schedules. The Controlled Substances Act prohibits an array of drug offenses and lists a range of penalties for potential violations, including forfeitures and/or fines that can be imposed upon those convicted.

The Controlled Substances Act, as part of the Comprehensive Drug Abuse Prevention and Control Act, recognizes the possibility that there may, from time to time, be a need for the addition, deletion, or transfer of drugs from one schedule to another and has established a framework to do so. Any new drug or concerns over an existing substance can be scientifically and medically considered under its provisions. The Drug Enforcement Administration can consider any substance for inclusion into these schedules based upon information from the FDA and the National Institute on Drug Abuse (NIDA), as well as that from criminal justice agencies, pharmaceutical companies, laboratories, or other external sources. This process of review will determine if the drug or related substance should or should not be controlled under one of the five schedules or removed from them entirely.

The Controlled Substances Act considerably impacted the day-to-day operations of the pharmaceutical industry, including areas from how new drugs are developed, to how all drugs are manufactured, stored, and distributed, including importing and exporting. For example, the act maintained and expanded regulations that require how substances are to be identified with specific stipulated symbols, primarily intended for the use of pharmacists. Each year under the act, the U.S. attorney general is charged to determine and establish annual production quotas for specific controlled substances in Schedule I and in Schedule II, which limits their pharmaceutical production. It also requires the pharmaceutical industry to keep selected drugs physically secure, such as by establishing rigorous standards for maintaining accurate inventories and other associated records. Provisions in the act also regulate and control some of the operations of physicians, nurse practitioners, physician assistants, pharmacists, wholesalers, distributors, and others whose respective scope of services and practice involve the dissemination or use of varied controlled substances. For example, prescriptions for drugs and other medications, including many painkillers, must list the physician's DEA license number. The DEA registration system enables manufacturers, researchers, and medical professionals to potentially access controlled substances on Schedules I, II, III, IV, and V, albeit with severe restrictions at times.

The Comprehensive Drug Abuse Prevention and Control Act, along with its assorted later amendments, significantly changed how the United States deals with abusers of painkillers and other drugs by combining together myriad separate pieces of drug legislation into one broad federal statute that could more effectively address varied aspects of drugs. It broadened the definition of who a "drug dependent person" was and, accordingly, made substantive increases to drug addiction treatment programs by creating more federally sponsored addiction treatment centers. These centers were then able to serve not only narcotic addicts, but also abusers of non-narcotic drugs. It established better ways to regulate the pharmaceutical industry and to better coordinate drug trafficking interdiction initiatives. It endeavored to combine all previous federal drug laws into one statute. It further coordinated and expanded all enforcement efforts related to drugs. The act was amended by Congress to allow the United States to meet all of its obligations under the UN Convention on Psychotropic Substances, which was signed in Vienna, Austria, in February 1971; it did the same after the United States became a signatory to the UN Convention against the Illicit Traffic in Narcotic Drugs and Psychotropic Substances, which was adopted in Vienna on December 20, 1988, and also later amended. The Comprehensive Drug Abuse Prevention and Control Act also amended the Public Services Act, as well as other related laws, to promote additional research on drug addiction, on the use and abuse of controlled substances, and on addicts, and to encourage more prevention research. The Comprehensive Drug Abuse Prevention and Control Act still functions as the primary legal foundation regulating the manufacturing and distribution of drugs, like painkillers, as well as guiding drug enforcement efforts; it significantly changed federal drug policies.

OPIATES

Opium plants are grown in many places around the world. This includes commercial-scale production of opium crops in places like Afghanistan, Burma, China, Colombia, Iran, Laos, Mexico, Pakistan, Thailand, and Turkey. However, India alone grows more than enough opium each year to satisfy the entire legitimate global demand. Unfortunately, most of the rest of the opium poppies produced each year around the world end up in the illicit drug trade. In fact, illicit opium cultivation exists in a small scale in over 30 other countries.

Opiates and opioids, of course, continue to be an area of concern. In this regard, it has been estimated that about 5,240 tons of illegal opium entered the global drug market in 2003, of which about three-quarters, or 3,960 tons, came from Afghanistan. The Taliban certainly benefited substantially from opium trafficking. Indeed, opium production in Afghanistan has permitted the continuance of disparate political factions, such as the Northern Alliance, and thus needs to be understood with respect to both forces of globalization and state fragmentation. According to the UN Office on Drugs and Crime (UNODC), opium cultivation in Afghanistan expanded to 553,000 acres in 2014, a 7% increase over the previous year. Afghanistan now accounts for more than 80% of the global illicit opium supply—much of which, by the way, helps to fund insurgency efforts like those of the Taliban.

The United States continues to support efforts, particularly law enforcement initiatives, in opiate-source countries to reduce supply. These include anti–money laundering measures, capacity building, information sharing, and interdiction operations as well as mentoring and training programs. Opium crop eradication commitments have been vigorously engaged in by government forces in Colombia and Mexico. Nevertheless, almost all heroin in the United States now come through Mexico and South America. In fact, half of the heroin in the United States now comes from poppy fields grown in Mexico. The United States has sponsored opium crop substitution programs in Guatemala, Pakistan, Thailand, and Turkey that have considerably reduced illicit cultivation.

It is very difficult and expensive, although possible, to synthesize morphine in the laboratory. Therefore, most of the morphine used by doctors is still derived from opium. Morphine sulfate is widely marketed under brand names such as Avinza, Duramorph, Infumorph, Kadian, MSIR, MS-Contin, Oramorph, and Roxanol. The average oral dose of morphine is 30 to 60 mg, which typically is taken every 4 to 6 hours.

In the United States, morphine is legally classified under the Controlled Substances Act (21 U.S.C. 801-886) of the 1970 Comprehensive Drug Abuse and Prevention Act as a Schedule II drug by the Drug Enforcement Agency (DEA Number 9300). Schedule II drugs, such as morphine, are so classified because they are considered to have a high potential for causing severe dependence; but they can also be useful medically, as is clear for morphine and its very effective painkilling effects. Morphine is listed internationally as a Schedule I drug under the UN Single Convention on Narcotic Drugs. Other opiates, besides morphine, are produced as well. The average oral dose of codeine is 32 to 65 mg, which typically is taken every 4 to 6 hours.

The semisynthetic opioids, such as hydromorphone, hydrocodone, oxymorphone, oxycodone, dihydrodesoxymorphine, nicomorphine, and nalbuphine are also manufactured and distributed as painkillers. Hydromorphone is manufactured under trade names like Dilaudid, Exalgo, Hydrostat IR, and Palladone; these include tablets and capsules, some of which are in extended-release formulations, as well as a liquid and an intravenous form. The average oral dose of hydromorphone is 4 to 8 mg, which typically is taken every 4 to 6 hours. Hydrocodone is marketed under several trade names including Anexsia, Dicodid, Hycodan, Hycomine, Lorcet, Lortab, Norco, Tussionex, and Vicodin. The FDA approved the marketing and sale of Vicodin in 1984. In a rather controversial move, the FDA in October 2013 approved production and sale of Zohydro ER, a hydrocodone extended-release, long-acting formulation, even though an FDA advisory committee on Zohydro voted overwhelmingly against approval. Oxymorphone is marketed under various trade names such as Numorphan, Opana, and Opana ER. Oxymorphone can be administered through intravenous, intramuscular, and subcutaneous routes, as well as by rectal suppositories or orally as tablets, which also come in an extended-release formulation. The average oral dose of oxymorphone is 1 to 2 mg, which typically is taken every 4 to 6 hours. Oxycodone is marketed under several trade names including Endocet, Endodan, OxyContin, Percocet, Percodan, Roxicet, and Roxiprin. The FDA approved the marketing and sale of OxyContin in 1995 and of Percocet in 1999. The average oral dose of oxycodone is 5 to 10 mg, which typically is taken every 3 to 5 hours. Dihydrodesoxymorphine, also known as desomorphine, was first synthesized in 1932, was patented in 1934, and is marketed under trade names such as Permonid, and as a generic Desomorphine; in 1998, it was declared an illegal narcotic painkiller in Russia, where it is called *krokodil*. Nicomorphine is marketed as Morzet by Apothecon in the Netherlands, as Vilan by Lannacher in Austria and Denmark, and as Synmedic in Switzerland. Nalbuphine is manufactured under the trade name Nubain; it is also marketed as Raltox by Opsonin Pharma Ltd. in Bangladesh and as Kinz by Sami Pharmaceuticals in Pakistan. The average oral dose of nalbuphine is 10 mg, which typically is taken every 4 to 6 hours.

SYNTHETIC OPIOIDS

Synthetic opioids are usually created in a laboratory for the purposes of making a drug that will have similar pharmacological effects of an opiate but that, hopefully, will have less liability for abuse, dependence, and addiction. Some of these synthetic opioids are painkillers like meperidine (Demerol), methadone (Dolophine), and propoxyphene (Darvon).

Phenylpiperidine Group

The phenylpiperidine group of synthetic opioids includes drugs such as meperidine, ketobemidone, and prodine. Meperidine (1-methyl-4-phenyl-piperidine-4-carbolic acid), which essentially is a synthetic opium derivative, was first made in 1939 by O. Eisleb and O. Schaumann of I. G. Farbenindustric in Hoechst, Germany; they called it dolantin. Meperidine, which is also known as pethidine and marketed as Demerol, was first thought to have less potential for leading to dependence than morphine; however, its propensity for leading to addiction was soon very evident. Meperidine, when compared to morphine, has a shorter duration of action as well as less pronounced antitussive and antidiarrheal effects. Meperidine has a shorter half-life—about 3 to 4 hours—and it also is broken down into a toxic metabolite, normeperidine. Therefore, it should only be used for acute dosing, not for chronic painkilling, and it should also be avoided in the elderly and for those patients experiencing renal failure. The average oral dose of meperidine is 50 to 100 mg, which typically is taken every 3 to 5 hours. Under the Controlled Substances Act (21 U.S. 801-8886) of the Comprehensive Drug Abuse Prevention and Control Act of 1970 and its subsequent amendments, meperidine is listed as a Schedule II drug that is regulated and controlled by the Drug Enforcement Administration (DEA No. 9230).

Meperidine was thus the first totally synthesized opioid, and its discovery led to the subsequent synthesizing of a series of many other phenylpiperidine-derived drugs. For instance, diphenoxilate was one such drug created to help decrease intestinal hypermobility. Ketobemidone (1-methyl-4-(3-hydroxy-phenyl)-4-propionypiperidine) was first synthesized during World War II, also by O. Eisled and others at I. G. Farbenindustric in Germany. Ketobemidone is a powerful synthetic opioid painkiller, similar to morphine in its analgesic effectiveness. Unfortunately, the results of experimental research on recovering narcotic addicts indicated that use of ketobemidone could be even more addictive than use of other opiates and opioids. Accordingly, in 1954, the United Nations' Economic and Social Council passed a resolution that called upon member states to cease the manufacture and use of ketobemidone. Thus, ketobemidone is presently mainly used in Scandinavian nations, most prevalently Denmark. The United Kingdom is currently the only manufacturer and exporter of ketobemidone. Under the Controlled Substances Act, ketobemidone is listed as a Schedule I substance (DEA No. 9628). Ketobemidone is also included under Schedule IV of the 1961 UN Single Convention on Narcotic Drugs.

Prodine ((1,3-dimethyl-4-phenylpiperidine-4-yl)propanate) is a synthetic opioid painkiller that is a chemical analogue of meperidine. There are two main isomers of prodine, alphaprodine and betaprodine. Betaprodine is the more potent painkiller of the pair, but it is metabolized more rapidly than alphaprodine; thus only alphaprodine has been developed for medical uses, where it is mainly used during childbirth and in dentistry. Alphaprodine has similar painkiller effects to meperidine, but with a much faster onset and also a shorter duration of action, from 1 to 2 hours. Under the Controlled Substances Act, alphaprodine is listed as a Schedule II drug (DEA No. 9010), and it is marketed primarily as Nisentil or Prisilidine. Other substances belonging to the phenylpiperidine family of synthetic opioids include allylprodine, MPPP (1-(-2-phenethyl)-4-phenyl-4-acetoxypiperidine), and PEPAP (1-methyl-4-phenyl-4-propionoxypiperidine). Allylprodine (DEA No. 9602), MPPP (DEA No. 9661), and PEPAP (DEA No. 9663) are all listed as Schedule I drugs under the Controlled Substances Act. They are also all included in Schedule I of the 1961 UN Single Convention on Narcotic Drugs.

Diphenylpropylamine Derivatives

The diphenylpropylamine derivatives include methadone, levo-alpha-acetylmethadol, propoxyphene, piritramide, bezitramide, and loperamide. Methadone was developed around 1939 by Max Bockmuhl and Gustav Ehrgart, who were working for I. G. Farbenindustric at Hoechst-am-Main in Germany. Methadone (4,4-diphenyl-6-dimethylamino-3-heptanone) was first called Hoechst 10820, and then it was referred to as polamidon; after World War II, Eli Lilly, an American pharmaceutical company, called it Dolophine. Soon after its introduction, it was recognized that methadone had a very high potential for becoming an addictive substance. Methadone was first used by German soldiers during World War II for painkiller purposes as a substitute for morphine that was in short supply. Use of methadone hydrochloride, when administered chronically, leads to the development of tolerance, lethargy, sedation, and edema. However, onset of the acute abstinence syndrome is slower to methadone than that produced by heroin or morphine. The long-term use of methadone also appears to impede learning and immediate recall. Nevertheless, methadone is commonly used to treat opiate and opioid addiction. The average oral dose of methadone is 5 to 20 mg, which typically is taken every 8 hours. Under the Controlled Substances Act, methadone is listed as a Schedule II substance (DEA No. 9250). The United States is the leading global producer of methadone, as it is of many other synthetic opioids. Levo-alpha-acetylmethadol, or LAAM, is a synthetic opioid developed in the 1940s that has a slow onset of action and a long duration that made it unsuitable for pain management. At first, LAAM seemed to be an appropriate drug for treating those chronically dependent on narcotics; LAAM was, accordingly, formerly being given to some patients who were on methadone maintenance. LAAM was, in fact, approved in 1994 by the FDA for treating narcotic addiction. LAAM has a relatively long duration of action varying from 48 to 72 hours, which permitted longer times between office visits than methadone. However, beginning in 2003, the availability of buprenorphine, which does not cause heart problems, led to the sudden discontinuation of the administration of LAAM for treating narcotic addicts. Propoxyphene ((1S,2R)-1-benzyl-3-(dimethylamino)-2-methyl-1-phenylpropyl propionate), also known as dextropropoxyphene, is another synthetic opioid in the diphenylpropylamine derivative family. Propoxyphene hydrochloride, a mild painkiller with similar effects to codeine, was first marketed as Darvon in 1957, and its abuse potential subsequently has been well established. Nonmedical use of propoxyphene was, for example, rather prevalent among American soldiers stationed in what was then West Germany. Many fatalities, unfortunately, have been attributed to the use of propoxyphene. Propoxyphene is a mu narcotic receptor agonist, and it is sometimes used to ease withdrawal symptoms in opiate and opioid addicts; it is also useful in relieving symptoms associated with restless leg syndrome. Propoxyphene napsylate was introduced with the hope that it would be less likely to be abused since it is insoluble in water and, as such, it cannot readily be injected. The United States is the largest producer of propoxyphene, led by Eli Lilly and Company, with India as the second leading producer. The average oral dose of propoxyphene is 65 to 130 mg, which typically is taken every 4 to 6 hours. Propoxyphene itself is listed under the Controlled Substances Act as a Schedule II substance (DEA No. 9273), while preparations containing propoxyphene are listed under Schedule IV (DEA No. 9278). Propoxyphene is also included under Schedule II of the 1961 UN Single Convention on Narcotic Drugs. Propoxyphene, levo-alpha-acetylmethadol, and methadone are all derivatives of diphenylheptane. It is important to note that because they are not chemically related, neither propoxyphene nor methadone will be detected in standard drug urinalysis tests that are focused on more standard opiates and opioids. Piritramide is a synthetic opioid that was first synthesized in Belgium at Janssen Pharmaceutical and that has been marketed under trade names such as Piridolan, Pirium, and Dipidolar, which are used mainly in Europe to treat postoperative pain. Piritramide is listed as a Schedule I substance (DEA No. 9642). Bezitramide is another synthetic opioid that in 1961 was also created at Janssen Pharmaceutical in Belgium and has since been marketed in Europe as Burgodin. Loperamide is another synthetic opioid also created at Janssen Pharmaceutical; it is a derivative of piperidine, which is used widely to treat diarrhea. Other drugs belonging to the diphenylpropylamine derivative family of synthetic opioids include dextromoramide (DEA No. 9613), difenoxin (DEA No. 9168), and dipipanone (DEA No. 9622), all of which are listed as Schedule I substances under the Controlled Substances Act; and diphenoxylate (DEA No. 9170), which is listed as a Schedule II substance.

Benzomorphan Derivatives

The benzomorphan derivatives, which are also known as the benzazocines, include phenazocine and pentazocine. Under the Controlled Substances Act, phenazocine (DEA No. 9715) is listed as a Schedule II substance, while penta-zocine is classified as a Schedule IV substance. Pentazocine was initially intro-duced in 1967 and marketed as Talwin. Pentazocine in combination with tripelennamine was soon commonly being used in the illicit drug market. In an effort to reduce this prevalent illicit abuse, another formulation, mar-keted as Talwin Nx, was created by adding naloxone, a narcotic antagonist, with the intent of countering the narcotic effects of pentazocine when used by injection. The average oral dose of pentazocine is 50 to 100 mg, which typ-ically is taken every 4 to 6 hours. Other drugs in the benzomorphan derivative family include cyclazocine and dezocine.

Anilidopiperidine Family

The anilidopiperidine family of synthetic opioids includes fentanyl, alfenta-nil, beta-hydroxyfentanyl, carfentanil, and sufentanil. In 1959, Paul Janssen initially synthesized fentanyl at a pharmaceutical company he started in Belgium. Fentanyl (1-phenethyl-4-N-propinoylanilinopiperidine) is a syn-thetic opioid that is much more potent than either heroin or morphine. Fentanyl is actually estimated to be approximately 100 times more potent than morphine. It has been found that fentanyl interacts preferentially with the mu opioid receptor sites. Since fentanyl has such a high clinical potency, and as it is not very difficult to synthesize, adulterated heroin is occasionally cut with fen-tanyl. Unfortunately, because of this high potency, the use of this heroin-and-fentanyl mixture has resulted in many fatal drug overdose cases. An increas-ingly popular way to administer fentanyl is by means of controlled-release patches, but even these have been subject to abuse. Fentanyl is classified as a Schedule II under the Controlled Substances Act.

Alfentanil   (N-[1-(2-(4-ethyl-4,5-dihydro-5-oxy-1H-tetrazol-1-yl)ethyl])) and sufentanil (N-(4-(methoxymethyl)-1-[2-(2-thienyl)ethyl]-N-phenylprop-anamide)) are two other synthetic opioid painkillers closely related to fentanyl. Alfentanil is much faster acting, but sufentanil is more potent than fentanyl. Beta-hydroxyfentanyl is another fentanyl analogue that was sold in the early 1980s prior to the passage of the Federal Analog Act, which was enacted to regulate and control entire families of drugs with similar chemical structures rather than scheduling each substance as it appeared. Beta-hydroxyfen-tanyl (N-[1-(2-hydroxy-2-phenethyl)-4-piperidinyl]-N-phenylpropanamide) is listed as a Schedule I substance (DEA No. 9830). Fentanyl, alfentanil, beta-hydroxyfentanyl, and sufentanil are all included under Schedule I of the 1961 UN Single Convention on Narcotic Drugs. Another fentanyl analogue that is much more potent than fentanyl is carfentanil; it is, accordingly, approved for use in veterinary medicine, where it is used to sedate large animals.

Fentanyl was first introduced clinically as a transdermal patch and is now available in many formats, including as a buccal tablet, inhaler, lozenge, and sublingual spray, as well as being made in intranasal and intravenous formulations. It is marketed under brand names such as Abstral, Actiq, Duragesic, Durogesic, Fentora, Haldid, Instanyl, Lazandra, Onsolis, and Sublimaze.

Fentanyl and its several synthetic analogues have unfortunately been abused. However, none of these potent painkiller drugs typically are detected by standard urine drug-screening tests that are focused on morphine-like substances; this is due to the fact that fentanyl and its closely related structural analogues are not chemically related to morphine and other opiates or opioids. Other drugs belonging to the anilidopiperidine family of synthetic opioids include alphamethylfentanyl, ohmefentanyl, and remifentanil. Fentanyl and its many analogues have been sold illicitly with street names such as Apache, China White, Goodfella, and TNT, as well as Tango and Cash. These sorts of drugs include, but are not limited to, alpha-methylfentanyl, alpha-methylthiofentanyl, beta-hydroxyfentanyl, beta-hydroxy-3-methylfentanyl, 3-methylfentanyl, 3-methylthiofentanyl, and thiofentanyl. These fentanyl analogue drugs are relatively more resistant to being metabolized, which results in a longer duration of action, and consequently are known for creating a longer "high." All of these drugs have been listed as Schedule I substances under the Controlled Substance Act and are, in fact, banned under the Federal Analog Act (21 U.S.C. 813) of January 22, 2002.

Oripavine Derivatives

The oripavine derivatives include buprenorphine, dihydroetorphine, and etorphine. Etorphine (tetrahydro-7 alpha-(1-hydroxy-1-methylbutyl)-6,14-endo-ethenooripavine) was first synthesized by K. W. Bentley and D. G. Hardy in the 1960s in Edinburgh, Scotland; it is used primarily as a sedative in veterinary medicine. Etorphine was the synthetic narcotic used in one of the three independent studies that in 1973 simultaneously discovered the narcotic receptors. Etorphine, but not its hydrochloride salt, is classified as a Schedule I substance under the Controlled Substance Act (DEA No. 9056). Etorphine is listed in Schedule IV of the 1961 UN Single Convention on Narcotic Drugs. Buprenorphine is a derivative of thebaine that was approved in 2002 by the FDA for treating narcotic addiction. U.S. physicians can complete a specialized training program authorized by the Drug Addiction Treatment Act of 2000 in order to be able. to prescribe buprenorphine products. Buprenorphine is used outside the United States as well, such as in France for maintenance treatment of narcotic addicts. Buprenorphine is also being used along with methadone for the treatment of opiate and opioid dependence. Drug interactions must, of course, always be an area of concern. There are, for instance, clinically significant drug interactions between buprenorphine and methadone. There are also considerable interactions between buprenorphine and various antiviral medications. Buprenorphine is typically administered as a sublingual tablet. In addition, a buprenorphine transdermal patch is being considered as an alternative way to conduct narcotic detoxification. Since the use of buprenorphine alone has the potential for abuse, it is also produced in a formulation combined with naloxone that is known as Suboxone, which is hoped to reduce the probability for substance abuse. Under the Controlled Substances Act, buprenorphine (DEA No. 9064) is classified as a Schedule III substance.

Dihydroetorphine is another member of the oripavine derivative family; it is actually a derivative of etorphine. Dihydroetorphine (7,8-dihydro-7 alpha-[1-(R)-hydroxy-1-methylbutyl]-6,14-endo-ethanotetrahydrooripavine) is mainly used in China as a powerful painkiller but also occasionally as a substitute for narcotic maintenance therapy. Under the Controlled Substances Act, dihydroetorphine (DEA No. 9334) is classified as a Schedule II substance. Dihydroetorphine is also included under Schedule I of the 1961 UN Single Convention on Narcotic Drugs.

Morphinan Derivatives

The morphinan derivatives include levorphanol and butorphanol. Morphinan (1,2,3,9,10,10a-hexahydro-10,4a(4H)-iminoethan) is the base chemical structure for this family of synthetic narcotics. For example, levorphanol ((-)-3-hydroxy-N-methylmorphinane) is the laevorotary stereoisomer of morphinan; it is a pure narcotic agonist that binds to the delta, kappa, and mu receptors. In fact, it was the substance used in one of the pioneering studies that simultaneously discovered the receptor sites. Levorphanol was initially synthesized in 1946 in Germany, and then it was introduced as a powerful orally active painkiller. Levorphanol is marketed under the trade name Levo-Dromoran. The average oral dose of levorphanol is 2 to 4 mg, which typically is taken every 4 to 6 hours. Under the Controlled Substance Act, levorphanol is listed as a Schedule II substance. Butorphanol (17-cyclobutylmethyl-morphinan-3,14-diol) can also be synthesized from the opiate thebaine, but it is typically totally synthesized. Butorphanol tartrate was initially generically manufactured as an injectable preparation for medical purposes, and it was also sold for use in veterinary medicine; it was then subsequently marketed under names like Butorphic, Torbutrol, or Torbugesic. Butorphanol is more effective as a painkiller in women than it is in men; it can be used to control labor pains. It was then manufactured as a nasal spray, marketed as Stadol, which resulted in greater illicit use. The average oral dose of butorphanol is 2 mg, which typically is taken every 4 to 6 hours. Since 1997, butorphanol was listed under Schedule IV of the Controlled Substance Act (DEA N0. 9720) and is no longer sold in the United States under the brand name Stadol. The International Federation for Equestrian Sports considers it to be a class A drug. Other drugs in the morphinan derivative family include levomethorphan and nalbuphine.

Tramadol and Others

There are several other types of synthetic opioids that do not belong to any of the respective families discussed here. Tramadol, for instance, is one of these. Tramadol is a synthetic opioid analogue of the opiate codeine. Tramadol was developed by the German pharmaceutical company Chemie Grunenthal of Stolberg-am-Rhein in the late 1970s. Tramadol hydrochloride, marketed as Ultram, is another synthetic opioid that has been diverted for purposes of abuse. Tramadol is yet another drug in the very long history of narcotics—natural, semisynthetic, and synthetic—that was introduced with the hoped-for promise of being an alternative substance with a low abuse potential. It was initially thought that tramadol would be effective in treating pain, but that it would probably tend not to be abused. However, increasingly greater numbers of cases of abuse, dependence, and withdrawal were reported among users in different countries, and thus treatment approaches had to be developed, including those based on the administration of methadone. At any rate, it now seems that there is less abuse and dependence on tramadol than there is for hydrocodone. However, the U.S. FDA recently added a warning of suicide risk to the labels of tramadol. Tramadol can also be produced in other formulations in combination with other drugs, such as an acetaminophen-and-tramadol product marketed as Ultracet. Some other synthetic opioids not included in the families listed here include lefetamine, meptazinol, and tilidine.

Work on the design, synthesis, and testing of new synthetic opioids is an ongoing effort. New analogues of various synthetic opioids continue to be introduced from time to time. Much of this continuing research is directed toward developing more effective painkiller drugs without the undesired side effects of earlier synthetic opioids. A vast array of synthetic opioids has, in fact, been created. Many of the synthetic opioids, however, are listed as Schedule I substances under the Controlled Substance Act, which means that they do not have any currently accepted medical use in the United States. Nevertheless, revenues from opioid painkillers has more than doubled over the past decade; this now amounts to over $9 billion annually.

NON-OPIOID PAINKILLERS

· There is actually a wide array of non-opioid drugs that are also used as painkillers. Clonidine, for example, is typically used as an antihypertensive drug that is sometimes used for managing neuropathic pain; it can be administered by means of an implantable pump, which is mostly used to administer morphine. Zinconotide is a non-opioid painkiller that is derived from the toxins of a cone snail; it was approved in 2004 by the FDA for treating severe and chronic pain and is marketed as Prialt. At any rate, we will explore some of the more commonly, and a few of the less commonly, used non-opioid painkiller drugs, such as aspirin, ibuprofen, acetaminophen, ketoprofen, ketorolac, flurbiprofen, diclofenac, and naproxen.

Aspirin

Aspirin is one of the most popular drugs in the United States. Over 16,000 tons of aspirin are made and sold annually in this country. This amounts to about 80 billion pills, which will be sold for around $2 billion each year. Nevertheless, aspirin amounts to less than a third of the over-the-counter sales of painkillers each year in the United States.

Aspirin is available in several different dosage concentrations, ranging from 60 to 650 mg. The average oral dose of aspirin is 650 mg, which typically is taken every 4 to 6 hours. It is typically used in tablet form, but is also available as capsules, caplets, liquid elixirs, powder, and suppositories. The ingredients needed to make an aspirin tablet are acetylsalicylic acid, the active ingredient, along with corn starch, a lubricant, and water. Corn starch, with purified water added, serves as a binding agent, to hold the tablet together, as well as a filler. The mixture is compressed into tablets, which are bottled and packaged for distribution. Quality control tests include tablet hardness, friability, and disintegration. Aspirin is widely sold as a generic drug, and it is also marketed under trade names such as Ascriptin, Bayer, Ecotrin, and St. Joseph.

Ibuprofen

Ibuprofen is derived from propionic acid. Ibuprofen tablets are produced similarly to those of aspirin. Microcrystalline cellulose can be used as a filler, and it has high compressibility; pre-gelatinized starch and sucrose are also used as fillers. Magnesium stearate can be used as a lubricant as it increases blending attributes. Crospovidone can be used as a disintegrant, as can sodium benzoate. Tablets can be coated with a pharmaceutical glaze that includes polyethylene glycol and titanium dioxide and can be labeled with pharmaceutical ink. The average oral dose of ibuprofen is 200 to 400 mg, which typically is taken every 4 to 6 hours. Ibuprofen is widely sold as a generic drug, and it is also marketed under trade names such as Advil and Motrin.

The FDA permitted the sale of ibuprofen over the counter beginning in 1984, prior to which a prescription had been required. Ibuprofen is listed as an FDA pregnancy category D drug. It should not be taken during the last trimester of pregnancy as it can harm the developing fetus.

Acetaminophen

Acetaminophen, or n-acetyl-p-aminophenol, also referred to as APAP, is manufactured beginning with phenol as the starting material. Phenol is nitrated with sodium nitrate, and then the oxygen isomer is removed by means of steam distillation. The result is reduced by hydrogenation to form 4-aminophenol, which is acetylated with acetic acid to produce acetaminophen.

Acetaminophen is contained in over 100 products that are sold over the counter. These include many cough and cold preparations and are produced in an array of forms. Acetaminophen is also contained in many prescription product formulations, sometimes along with other painkillers. Acetaminophen is produced in capsule, effervescent, intramuscular, intravenous, liquid suspension, suppository, and tablet form. Tablets typically contain, in addition to the acetaminophen active ingredient, corn starch as a binder; purified water; magnesium stearate and talc as lubricants; croscarmellose or carboxymethyl starch as a disintegrant; methyl paraben and/or propyl paraben as a preservative; silicon dioxide colloidal as an anti-adherent; and talc antisticking microcrystalline cellulose, gelatin glycerin, or pre-gelatinized starch as a filler. Acetaminophen is widely sold as a generic drug, and it is also marketed under trade names such as Tylenol and Arthriten. The average oral dose of acetaminophen is 650 mg, which typically is taken every 4 to 6 hours.

Other Analgesics

Many other types of painkillers have been identified for their analgesic properties. These include the NSAIDs like ketoprofen, ketorolac, flurbiprofen, diclofenac, and naproxen, although there are many more examples.

Diflunisal, etodolac, fenoprofen, indomethacin, nabumetone, and piroxicam are a few examples of some of these other NSAIDs, all of which are available in the United States only with a doctor's prescription. Diflunisal is marketed in the United States under the trade name Dolobid; the average oral dose of diflunisal is 500 to 1,000 mg, which typically is taken every 8 to 12 hours. Etodolac, which was first approved by the FDA in January 1991 and is marketed under the trade name Lodine, is available in 200-mg and 300-mg capsules; 400-mg and 500-mg tablets; and in 400-mg, 500-mg, and 600-mg extended-release tablets. Fenoprofen is marketed under the trade name Nalfon; the average oral dose of fenoprofen is 200 to 400 mg, which typically is taken every 4 to 6 hours. Indomethacin was first approved by the FDA in January 1965; is marketed under the trade name Indocin; and is available in several formulations, including 25 mg and 50 mg capsules, a 75 mg extended-release capsule, a 25 mg/ml suspension, 50 mg suppositories, and a 1 mg dose of powder that can be mixed in solution for injection. Nabumetone is marketed under the trade name Relafen; the average oral dose is 500 mg or 750 mg tablets. Piroxicam is marketed under the trade name Feldene; the average oral dose of piroxicam is 20 to 40 mg, which typically is taken every 8 to 12 hours. The recommended maximum daily pediatric dose of piroxicam for pain is 15 mg, and the recommended maximum daily adult pain dose is 20 mg. All three of these last-mentioned NSAIDs are listed as FDA pregnancy category C drugs and have demonstrated fetal toxicity in laboratory animals such that risk cannot be ruled out.

Ketoprofen, or 2-(3-benzoylphenyl)-propionic acid, is an NSAID that is available only by prescription. It was formerly available over the counter in a 12.5 mg coated tablet marketed as Actron or as Orudis KT, but this formulation has been discontinued. Ketoprofen is manufactured by Teva Pharmaceuticals in capsules that contain either 50 mg or 75 mg of the active ingredient. The 50-mg dose comes in a light-blue body capsule with a blue cap; it is imprinted "93" over "3193" and is distributed in bottles of 100 capsules. The 75-mg dose comes in a white body capsule with a blue cap; it is imprinted "TEVA" on the cap and "3195" on the body and is distributed in bottles of either 100 or 500 capsules. The capsules also contain lactose as a diluent, magnesium stearate as a lubricant, and sodium starch glycolate as a filler. The capsule shell consists of a mixture of gelatin, red and blue dyes, and sodium lauryl sulfate and is coated with printing ink and titanium dioxide.

It is available in other formulations as well; it is commonly used as a topical plaster for musculoskeletal pain and is produced in cream, ointment, liquid, gel, and spray formulations.

Ketoprofen is listed, in the first and second trimesters, as an FDA pregnancy category C drug and has demonstrated fetal toxicity in laboratory animals. It should only be used in pregnancy if the potential benefits justify the potential risks to the developing fetus; in the third trimester of pregnancy, ketoprofen is classified as a category D drug and should be avoided since it may cause premature closure of the ductus arteriosus. It is commonly used in treating horses and other equines.

Ketorolac tromethamine is a dihydropyrrolizine carbolic acid that is in the heterocyclic acetic acid derivative family. It was first approved by the FDA on November 30, 1989, and introduced by Syntex as Toradol, which is available in tablet and capsule formulations; on November 9, 1992, the FDA approved use in an eye-drop formulation, which was first marketed as Acular by Allergan, under a license from Syntex; an intranasal formulation was approved on May 14, 2010, and introduced as Sprix Nasal Spray by Daiichi Sankyo. It is also available for intravenous administration. Ketorolac is listed as an FDA pregnancy category C drug and has demonstrated fetal toxicity in laboratory animals.

Flurbiprofen, or (RS)-2-(2-fluorobiprofenyl-4-yl) propanoic acid, is a member of the phenylalkonic acid derivative family. Flurbiprofen is marketed by Pfizer as Ansaid and by Abbott Laboratories as Froben. It is available as a 50 mg pill taken orally, with 100 mg as the maximum recommended single dose, and the maximum daily dose should not exceed 300 mg. Flurbiprofen is also used as the active ingredient in some throat lozenges, such as Strepfen (formerly called Strepsils "Intensive") which is manufactured in the UK by Reckitt Benckiser at an 8.75 mg dose.

Flurbiprofen is listed as an FDA pregnancy category C drug, and as a B2 pregnancy drug in Australia. It should not be taken during the last trimester of pregnancy as it can harm the developing fetus.

Diclofenac, or 2-(2,6-dichlorophenylamino) phenylacetic acid, is produced in many different formulations, usually as a potassium or sodium salt, and can be administered through oral, intramuscular, intravenous, rectal, and topical routes. In most formulations and in most countries, it is available only by prescription. For example, it is marketed under various trade names, such as Voltaren or Pennsaid, which is a minimally systemic prescription topical lotion that contains diclofenac sodium and is approved for osteoarthritis of the knee, while it is marketed under the trade name of Flector Patch when used as a topical patch for acute pain from minor sprains, strains, and contusions. In some countries, it is prepared as an eye-drop formulation that is used for acute and chronic inflammations to the anterior regions of the eyes, such as sometimes occurs after eye surgery. It can be taken several times a day as a 50 mg dose or once daily in an extended-release 100 mg tablet; the total daily dose should not generally exceed 150 mg. Diclofenac is listed as an FDA pregnancy category C drug for the first and second trimesters, and as a category D drug in the third trimester; it is also listed as a category C pregnancy drug in Australia. It should not be taken during the last trimester of pregnancy as it can harm the developing fetus.

Naproxen, or (S)-6-methoxy-alpha-methyl-2-naphthalene, also known as DL-Naproxen, is a relatively new painkiller. Phenlacetic acid is converted to naproxen by esterification, C-alkylation, and, finally, hydrolysis. The production of naproxen tablets is similar to that of other nonprescription painkillers, like aspirin and ibuprofen. Tablets or capsules typically contain, in addition to naproxen sodium as the active ingredient, which is a member of the arylacetic acid family of NSAIDs: anhydrous citric acid or lactose as a diluent; corn starch as a binder; purified water; talc microcrystalline cellulose as a filler; polyethylene glycol as a tablet binder and as a lubricant; magnesium stearate as a lubricant; and crospovidone as a disintegrant. Formed tablets can be coated with a mixture of hydroxypropyl methylcellulose, polyethylene glycol, and titanium dioxide and can be labeled with pharmaceutical ink. Naproxen can be sold as a generic drug, and it is also marketed under trade names such as Aleve, Anaprox, and Naprosyn. The average oral dose of naproxen is 250 to 500 mg, which typically is taken every 8 to 12 hours.

DOCUMENT: HOW DRUGS ARE DEVELOPED AND APPROVED

This fact sheet, "How Drugs Are Developed and Approved," is from the U.S. Food and Drug Administration (FDA). It summarizes part of the process by which new drugs are developed and approved in the United States to ensure that they are safe and effective as well as of standard quality. From the beginning of submitting a new drug application (NDA) to the FDA through to the hopeful eventual marketing of the drug product, there are an intensive series of regulatory processes. Initial laboratory studies must be submitted that provide evidence of the safety and efficacy of the new drug product. The FDA's Center for Drug Evaluation and Research (CDER), which includes a team of specialists such as chemists, doctors, pharmacologists, statisticians, and other scientists, reviews the laboratory data, as well as the proposed labeling of the drug. If deemed promising in the laboratory studies, then the drug developers must submit an Investigational New Drug (IND) application.

After this the clinical trial process can begin, which has its own extensive set of regulations and guidelines. If the evidence from the clinical trials is convincing, initial FDA approval for marketing can begin, but the review process continues with monitoring and other concerns. This regulatory process exists to protect the American public and hopefully prevent dangerous painkillers and other products from reaching consumers.

The mission of FDA's Center for Drug Evaluation and Research (CDER) is to ensure that drugs marketed in this country are safe and effective. CDER does not test drugs, although the Center's Office of Testing and Research does conduct limited research in the areas of drug quality, safety, and effectiveness.

CDER is the largest of FDA's six centers. It has responsibility for both prescription and nonprescription or over-the-counter (OTC) drugs. For more information on CDER activities, including performance of drug reviews, post-marketing risk assessment, and other highlights, please see About the Center for Drug Evaluation and Research. The other five FDA centers have responsibility for medical and radiological devices, food and cosmetics, biologics, veterinary drugs, and tobacco products.

Some companies submit a new drug application (NDA) to introduce a new drug product into the U.S. Market. It is the responsibility of the company seeking to market a drug to test it and submit evidence that it is safe and effective. A team of CDER physicians, statisticians, chemists, pharmacologists, and other scientists reviews the sponsor's NDA containing the data and proposed labeling.

The section below entitled *From Fish to Pharmacies: The Story of a Drug's Development,* illustrates how a drug sponsor can work with FDA's regulations and guidance information to bring a new drug to market under the NDA process.

FROM FISH TO PHARMACIES: A STORY OF DRUG DEVELOPMENT

Osteoporosis, a crippling disease marked by a wasting away of bone mass, affects as many as 2 million American, 80 percent of them women, at an expense of $13.8 billion a year, according to the National Osteoporosis Foundation. The disease may be responsible for 5 million fractures of the hip, wrist and spine in people over 50, the foundation says, and may cause 50,000 deaths. Given the pervasiveness of osteoporosis and its cost to society, experts say it is crucial to have therapy alternatives if, for example, a patient can't tolerate estrogen, the first-line treatment.

Enter the salmon, which, like humans, produces a hormone called calcitonin that helps regulate calcium and decreases bone loss. For osteoporosis patients, taking salmon calcitonin, which is 30 times more potent than that secreted by the human thyroid gland, inhibits the activity of specialized bone cells called osteoclasts that absorb bone tissue. This enables bone to retain more bone mass.

Though the calcitonin in drugs is based chemically on salmon calcitonin, it is now made synthetically in the lab in a form that copies the molecular structure of the fish gland extract. Synthetic calcitonin offers a simpler, more economical way to create large quantities of the product.

FDA approved the first drug based on salmon calcitonin in an injectable. Since then, two more drugs, one injectable and one administered through a nasal spray were approved. An oral version of salmon calcitonin is in clinical trials now. Salmon calcitonin is approved only for postmenopausal women who cannot tolerate estrogen, or for whom estrogen is not an option.

How did the developers of injectable salmon calcitonin journey "from fish to pharmacies?"

After obtaining promising data from laboratory studies, the salmon calcitonin drug developers took the next step and submitted an Investigational New Drug (IND) application to CDER. The IND Web page explains the need for this application, the kind of information the application should include, and the Federal regulations to follow.

Once the IND application is in effect, the drug sponsor of salmon calcitonin could begin their clinical trials. After a sponsor submits an IND application, it must wait 30 days before starting a clinical trial to allow FDA time to review the prospective study. If FDA finds a problem, it can order a "clinical hold" to delay an investigation, or interrupt a clinical trial if problems occur during the study.

Clinical trials are experiments that use human subjects to see whether a drug is effective, and what side effects it may cause. The Running Clinical Trials Webpage provides links to the regulations and guidelines that the clinical investigators of salmon calcitonin must have used to conduct a successful study, and to protect their human subjects.

The salmon calcitonin drug sponsor analyzed the clinical trials data and concluded that enough evidence existed on the drug's safety and effectiveness to meet FDA's requirements for marketing approval. The sponsor submitted a New Drug Application (NDA) with full information on manufacturing specifications, stability and bioavailablility data, method of analysis of each of the dosage forms the sponsor intends to market, packaging and labeling for both physician and consumer, and the results of any additional toxicological studies not already submitted in the Investigational New Drug application. The NDA Web page provides resources and guidance on preparing the NDA application, and what to expect during the review process.

New drugs, like other new products, are frequently under patent protection during development. The patent protects the salmon calcitonin sponsor's investment in the drug's development by giving them the sole right to sell the drug while the patent is in effect. When the patents or other periods of exclusivity on brand-name drugs expire, manufacturers can apply to the FDA to sell generic versions. The Abbreviated New Drug Applications (ANDA) for Generic Drug Products Webpage provides links to guidances, laws, regulations, policies and procedures, plus other resources to assist in preparing and submitting applications.

BRINGING NONPRESCRIPTION DRUG PRODUCTS TO THE MARKET UNDER AN OTC MONOGRAPH

OTC drugs can be brought to the market following the NDA process as described above or under an OTC monograph. Each OTC drug monograph is a kind of "recipe book" covering acceptable ingredients, doses, formulations, labeling, and, in some cases, testing parameters. OTC drug monographs are continually updated to add additional ingredients and labeling as needed. Products conforming to a monograph may be marketed without FDA pre-approval. The NDA and monograph processes can be used to introduce new ingredients into the OTC marketplace. For example, OTC drug products previously available only by prescription are first approved through the NDA process and their "switch" to OTC status is approved via the NDA process. OTC ingredients marketed overseas can be introduced into the U.S. market via a monograph under a Time and Extent Application (TEA) as described in 21 CFR 330.14. For a more thorough discussion of how OTC drug products are regulated visit FDA laws, regulations and guidances that affect small business. Information is also provided on financial assistance and incentives that are available for drug development.

CDER SMALL BUSINESS AND INDUSTRY ASSISTANCE (CDER SBIA)

Drug sponsors which qualify as small businesses can take advantage of special offices and programs designed to help meet their unique needs. The CDER Small Business and Industry Assistance (CDER SBIA) Webpage provides links to FDA laws, regulations and guidances that affect small business. Information is also provided on financial assistance and incentives that are available for drug development.

Source: U.S. Food and Drug Administration. (2015). Fact sheet: How drugs are developed and approved. Available online at http://www.fda.gov/Drugs/DevelopmentApprovalProcess/HowDrugsareDeveloped andApproved/

Chapter 8

The Social Dimension
of Painkillers

Pain is an important public health problem that negatively impacts the quality of life of those individuals affected and that also carries a substantial socioeconomic cost. Unfortunately, the social dimensions of pain and of painkillers are highly profound and not very well understood. Researchers have noted that there are substantial cultural differences in how human beings respond to pain. For example, northern Europeans, in general, are relatively non-expressive and frequently even stoic with respect to dealing with pain. Individuals from Mediterranean cultures, on the other hand, tend to be extremely expressive in response to painful experiences. Significant gender differences in pain thresholds and pain tolerance as well as in other related demographic variables have been observed. An examination of some of the social reform pressures over time and of the various approaches taken in treating those who have abused painkillers and similar drugs can all help in fleshing out a slightly broader understanding of some of the social dimensions surrounding this area.

SOCIAL REFORM PRESSURES

Pressure for social reform led to dramatic policy changes and legal restrictions upon the availability of painkillers and related substances. Further, empirical experience as well as numerous experimental studies confirmed the addictive nature of opiate and opioid use. It is generally agreed by most researchers in this area that there were about 250,000 morphine addicts in the United States in 1898, which is a per capita narcotic addiction rate almost double what it is today. At the same time in the UK, opium use was also rather widespread, particularly in East Anglia, where from at least the 1930s through the early 1970s, many liberal reformers called for return of the earlier policy of providing maintenance doses of opiates to addicts. This approach of providing opiates to addicts is often referred to as the British model. In addition, the use of opiates and opioids by the U.S. general population was generally considered legal until the 1940s; thereafter, increased risks of criminal prosecution, and even of the possible loss of their licenses to practice medicine if these substances were misused, led to dramatic declines in the prescribing of such painkiller medications by physicians and other health care providers and, consequently, resulted in a state where there was, in general, a pervasive lack of adequate pain management.

20th Century

It has been estimated that at the beginning of the 20th century, the United States had about 300,000 opiate addicts, many of whom initially began to use opium or morphine in order to relieve the pain and suffering of various medical illnesses; most of these opiate addicts were of either White or Asian background, and many were actually upper-class women. However, by the late 1960s, the situation had changed; there were an estimated 500,000 narcotic addicts in the United States, most of whom were primarily addicted to heroin, and a high proportion of whom were African American or Hispanic members of the urban underclass. It was commonly perceived that the United States was experiencing a heroin epidemic from the mid-1960s through the 1970s. Several studies of opiate use were conducted among incarcerated populations, including those of African Americans and of Mexican Americans. In fact, many studies were conducted attempting to estimate the historical and more recent patterns of opiate addiction. There were widespread associated calls for tougher criminal justice enforcement measures and for related social reforms.

In the early part of the last century, there were pressures to restrict and to nearly eliminate treatment services for drug addicts. For example, in 1914, the U.S. Congress passed legislation that required registration for all doctors who prescribed opiates or opioids, even to those who were dependent. In 1919, the U.S. Supreme Court ruled that the prescribing of opiate drugs to an addict in such a way as to maintain their addiction was contrary to the limits of proper professional practice and thus constituted a violation of the Harrison Narcotics Act of 1914. Restrictive measures increased, and as a consequence, services decreased to the point where imprisonment was practically the only treatment alternative in this country.

The extreme availability of inexpensive and very potent heroin to U.S. troops stationed in Vietnam resulted in high levels of use and addiction during the war. However, when most of the same Vietnam veterans returned to the United States in the early 1970s, where its price was comparatively high and its potency significantly lower—such that it had to be injected rather than smoked—the use of heroin was, somewhat surprisingly, readily discontinued by those veterans. These findings, and related studies, remind us that we must be cautious in generalizing from studies of substance use and abuse based solely on treatment populations. Other populations, in fact, have very different experiences from use of these same substances.

There were also dramatic increases in the prevalence of heroin addiction in other places around the world. In 1971, it was estimated that there were about 12,000 heroin addicts in Western Europe, including Great Britain; by 1976, it probably exceeded 108,000 addicts; and by 1978, the DEA estimated that there were around 200,000 heroin addicts in Western Europe. In 1975 in Singapore, it was estimated that there were 2,000 heroin addicts, 3,000 to 4,000 morphine addicts, and 7,000 to 8,000 opium smokers; this amounts to between 12,000 and 14,000 narcotic addicts out of a total population of 2.2 million.

Almost any substance containing an opiate or opioid painkiller drug has the potential for abuse. For example, paregoric, a camphorated tincture of opium, was first prepared by Le Mort, a chemistry professor at the University of Leyden in the early 1700s, and it has for centuries since been used as a cough sedative, to relieve diarrhea, and for other medicinal purposes. It was a popular household remedy during the 18th and 19th centuries. There were, not surprisingly, several reported instances of outbreaks of paregoric abuse—for instance, in the late 1950s and early 1960s, it was reported that narcotic addicts in Detroit, Michigan, were abusing paregoric. Other cases of paregoric addiction have been noted in other places and at other times.

During the 20th century, developments in pain therapy were closely linked with those in the field of anesthesiology. In the 19th century, it had been widely hoped that general anesthesia could be used to overcome pain. After World War II, surgical approaches like lobotomy and leucotomy were endorsed as ways to separate the psychological processing of pain from the actual experience of pain. Anesthesiological research, such as that conducted by Henry Beecher, endeavored to separate the psyche from the physiology of pathological pain. In the 1950s, John Bonica pioneered an approach to pain based on regional anesthesia, which introduced multidisciplinary teamwork into the treatment of chronic pain. By the late 1970s, the biopsychosocial approach, such as that developed by George Engel, rose to the fore by defining chronic pain as an illness rather than as a disease. Patient-controlled painkilling was introduced in the 1970s and 1980s. Hospitals established acute pain services beginning in the 1980s with the continuous release of opioid drugs.

The study of history is not limited exclusively to the distant past; even relatively contemporary topics are within the legitimate prevue of modern historians. In fact, as substance use and abuse patterns change, new issues may easily arise that lend more or less to varied forms of historical analysis. For example, issues around legal and illegal substances and their licit or illicit use have raised many criminal justice and related societal concerns around the globe. The awareness of this relationship has been well known and widely studied for some time. There have also been substantial changes in the patterns of narcotic addiction in various places at various times, such as notably occurred in Britain in the 1960s. There were certainly mounting concerns in the United States around the association between drugs and crime in the late 1960s and early 1970s, including examination of the significance of the role of ethnicity. For example, the issue of the effects of drug use on criminal responsibility was then a hotly discussed topic of interest. As a consequence over the focus on the nexus between drugs and crime, the Nixon administration's policies toward treatment and law enforcement resulted in a shift for many addicts from heroin to methadone. This kind of thinking, after all, resulted in the passage of the Comprehensive Drug Abuse Prevention and Control Act of 1970. As noted earlier, another area of concern leading to the formation of this act was the fear, fueled by poorly designed studies that were subsequently refuted, that American soldiers returning from tours of duty in Vietnam, where heroin and other drugs were readily available, would return addicted. These fears, it turned out, were largely unfounded, but nonetheless they were very significant at the time.

In the 1970s, researchers examined factors that influenced the cost of purchasing heroin, while other investigators calculated the economic consequences of heroin dependency as well as of other myriad, related issues. These types of studies led to a series of other studies that calculated the costs and benefits of addiction generally and of addiction treatment specifically. At any rate, it has been observed for some time that changes occur in patterns of opiate and opioid addiction. In fact, many varied theories have been explored in attempts to explain the changes in the use of heroin and related substances at varied times. Many additional theories have also been advanced to explain the causes of opiate and opioid addiction, such as those based on the family of the addict and the stepping stone theory, as well as the always popular self-medication hypothesis. In addition to changes over time, ethnic, gender, and other demographic differences have also been examined among narcotic addicts.

Stigma

There, unfortunately, is a consistent societal tendency to stigmatize opiate and opioid addicts in general and females in particular, as well as methadone clients and abusers of painkillers. Stigma tends to discredit and damage the reputation of, or even the identity of, individuals viewed as different or deviant, frequently rejecting and isolating them from mainstream society; it is also referred to as negative stereotyping. Perhaps one of the most salient features of stigmatization is the devaluation of those regarded as "others." Other members of society have continually tended to distrust or dislike those who are addicted to painkillers and related substances.

Members of dominant social groups in most societies have repeatedly perceived drug abusers as members of less powerful groups as part of the collective others, which is not necessarily where most actual abusers of painkillers come from. This has resulted in conditions of widespread discrimination of painkiller abusers and other addicts, such as in areas of finding gainful employment, avoiding high rates of incarceration, and encountering barriers of access to needed services, including addiction treatment and related social services. These stigmatizing attitudes toward people who abuse painkillers are not conducive to a therapeutic interaction and could easily result in a treatment failure. In fact, stigmatized individuals, like addicts, frequently internalize the perspectives of others who regard them in a contemptible manner. This can manifest in a fear of becoming labeled as an addict that can block efforts to pursue access to appropriate treatments. Unfortunately, we still have a long way to go in this area. Nevertheless, public health efforts to counter the perceived dangers of painkiller abuse will likely help ease the social stigma placed on this phenomenon. Further, efforts that emphasize the issues of the treatability of these conditions would be helpful, but probably less so than the former strategy of reducing stigma by emphasizing commonalities rather than divergences.

Injection heroin users are particularly stigmatized by society. This phenomenon is underscored by the fact that some of the common signs of heroin use actually help to reinforce the notion that heroin users are really different from nonusers; thus it can be perceived of as appropriate to stigmatize them. Heroin users, for example, tend to withdraw from situations that they once enjoyed and can be characterized by their personal and social isolation. Their observed behaviors further help to identify them as being of the "others"; these behaviors include excessive sleeping, lack of interest in food, stealing, paranoia, and/or hostility. Heroin addicts often even bear more blatant signs of being a user, specifically having needle marks on their arms and legs. These signs serve only to enhance the likelihood that heroin users will be stigmatized by other members of society.

Based on reviews of many experimental and clinical studies, most experts in the area of addictions medicine now would recommend that individuals who have an opiate or opioid use disorder should be offered medication-assisted treatment on a routine basis. Unfortunately, there is considerable resistance to this treatment approach from many professionals in the field of addiction treatment. An opioid use disorder diagnosis still carries substantial social stigma, at least to the degree that such bias can affect not only the individuals receiving the diagnosis, but also those addiction treatment professionals and other health care providers to whom these individuals may turn to seek care. The suggestion by several studies that medication-assisted treatment can be effectively integrated into general medical practice by physicians and other appropriate health care providers who are not trained addiction specialists has also added to the resistance to these approaches. In fact, the general con-sensus is that about 80% of those individuals who have an opioid use disorder do not receive treatment, due not only to the social stigma, although that should not be ignored, but also to the limited availability of treatment, to financial obstacles, and to other barriers to health care. Conversely, some researchers have suggested that perhaps the destigmatization of heroin has actually contributed to its dramatic increases recently.

21st Century

Historically, many physicians and other health care providers had generally underprescribed painkillers due to legitimate concerns over the potential for patients becoming addicted. This practice came to be known as "opiophobia" and resulted in many individuals not being provided with adequate relief from the pain they were actually suffering. The prevalence of chronic pain is experi-enced by about 30% of individuals following surgery, for example, and some surgical procedures (e.g., thoracic surgery) can lead to as many as 50% of the total number of individuals involved experiencing chronic pain after surgery. The burden of inadequate pain control affects the speed of recovery, raises the likelihood of developing chronic pain, and increases health care costs. However, this century we have seen a dramatic and very intentional reversal of this earlier practice, largely the result of the prompting of the pharmaceuti-cal industry. Over the first decade of this century, from 1999 to 2010, we had a threefold increase in the number of opioid prescriptions written; while there were 76 million opioid prescriptions in 1999, the number rose to 210 million by 2010. Opioid prescriptions have, in fact, quadrupled over the past 15 years in the United States. In 2010, for instance, enough opioid prescriptions were written to medicate every adult American 24 hours a day, 7 days a week for a month. In addition, it is estimated that about 9% of the general U.S. population is believed to misuse opiate or opioid drugs, whether obtained by licit or illicit means, at some time over the course of their lifetime.

Prescription opiates and opioids are very effective at relieving pain for those suffering with a terminal illness at the end of their lives. They are also very useful for short-term treatment for pain. On the other hand, it should be recognized that non-pharmacological approaches should be the first line of treatment for long-term chronic pain at least. The United States currently consumes over 80% of all the opioid drugs produced globally. Twice as many painkiller prescriptions per person are written in the United States as in Canada. In fact, with only 4% of the world's population, the United States currently accounts for around 84% of the world's oxycodone prescriptions and 99% of the world's hydrocodone prescriptions. On the other hand, Australia, Canada, France, and Germany, collectively, account for only about 13% of global oxycodone consumption.

At the opening of the 21st century, awareness of the diversion and abuse of oxycodone, also known as dihydrohydroxycodeinone, a powerful opioid analgesic, visibly surfaced. The opiate thebaine, by the way, is identified as the precursor for oxycodone. The semisynthetic opioid oxycodone was first synthesized in 1916 by Martin Freund and Edmund Speyer, two chemists at the University of Frankfurt in Germany; it was first used clinically in 1917. It was first introduced to the U.S. market in May 1939. Oxycodone was further developed by Purdue Pharma and first marketed as OxyContin in December 1995 as a time-release formulation with an intended misuse-resistant polymer to inhibit its drug release mechanism. It has been manufactured in a reformulated version since August 2010 that makes it nearly impossible to crush, snort, or dissolve and inject. Other trade names for oxycodone include Endone, Oxecta, OxyIR, Oxynorm and Roxicodone. Initial public concern was that this phenomenon might herald the onset of a new wave of drug addiction; however, a closer examination of the evidence indicated that most nonmedical users of oxycodone had prior abuse histories. A better sociocultural understanding of oxycodone diversion and abuse has been called for, as has the need for greater communication between addiction treatment and pain management communities. Oxycodone is metabolized, in part, by a cytochrome P-450 dependent process in the liver that is highly individualized due to metabolic issues, which also make it highly vulnerable to drug interactions; thus some individuals may metabolize it more quickly or slowly than others. Oxycodone is presently the most frequently prescribed medication in the United States, and its abuse has increased as a direct consequence.

Other opioids have increased in popularity as well in this century, due at least in part to the reformulations of oxycodone. Hydrocodone abuse, for instance, has also dramatically increased in this country. In this regard, 19,221 emergency room visits resulting from hydrocodone were reported in 2000; by 2009, the number had risen to 86,258, a 449% increase. In 2006, Endo Pharmaceuticals introduced a time-release formulation of oxymorphone, which is also referred to as 14-Hydromorphinone, marketed under the trade name of Opana. Oxymorphone has replaced the reformulated oxycodone as a substance of choice among injection drug users.

The proliferation of opioid prescription painkillers has become a serious public health issue. Since 2009, painkiller overdoses helped drug fatalities surpass traffic accidents as a major cause of death in the United States. Each day, an average of 46 individuals die from an overdose of prescription painkillers. For U.S. women, 7 out of 10 prescription drug deaths included use of painkillers. In 2009, the Drug Abuse Warning Network (DAWN) reported that over 343,000 emergency department visits were attributed to prescription opioid pain relievers, a rate more than double that of five years earlier. More than 240 million opioid prescriptions are currently written each year in the United States; in fact, opioid prescriptions have risen 300% in the past decade. It thus should not be very surprising that the number of people receiving treatment for prescription painkiller abuse and addiction quadrupled from 2004 to 2010. In 2010, there were about 164 million visits to U.S. doctor's offices for individuals seeking relief from non-cancer-related pain. In 2000, about 26% of individuals visiting doctors for pain were given non-opioid painkiller prescriptions, while in 2010, 29% were given opioid painkiller prescriptions. There was a far more pronounced increase, however, in the number of prescriptions written for opioid painkiller drugs over the same decade; specifically, opioid painkiller prescriptions rose from about 11% to about 20%, or nearly a doubling over 10 years.

The pharmaceutical industry has garnered substantial profits from the rise of prescription painkiller drugs, even while abuse has dramatically escalated. In fact, over the past 10 years, pharmaceutical company profits from opioid prescription painkillers have more than doubled. For example, prescription opioids alone accounted for $9 billion in profits in 2012. The Centers for Disease Control and Prevention (CDC) reported a fourfold increase in opioid sales from 1999 to 2010; this, of course, coincided with a dramatic increase in opioid painkiller overdoses as discussed in Chapter 6. In fact, from 1999 to

2012, the age-adjusted mortality involving opioids tripled, from 1.4 cases to 5.1 cases per 100,000 population.

According to findings from the 2010 National Survey on Drug Use and Health (NSDUH) each year, about 2.4 million Americans use prescription drugs for nonmedical purposes for the first time. This amounts to around 6,600 additional prescription drug misuse initiates each day. About a third of these new misusers were between 12 and 17 years old, and more than half were female. Further, each month, 5.9% of young adults 18 to 25 years of age reported nonmedical prescription drug abuse. In addition, the elderly, those 65 years of age and older, account for more than a third of total outpatient spending on prescription drugs in the United States. In 2011, over 52 million Americans over the age of 12 reported using prescription drugs at least once in their lifetime, and 6.2 million did so in the past month.

According to findings from the 2013 National Survey on Drug Use and Health released by the Substance Abuse and Mental Health Services Administration (SAMHSA), the situation with respect to diversion of prescription painkillers for improper uses is getting even worse. In 2012 and 2013, nearly 55% of individuals who misused prescription painkillers got them for free from a relative or friend, while around 20% received their drugs through a physician or other health care provider's prescription. It is now estimated that each month 4.5 million Americans engage in the use of painkillers for nonmedical use; and, that each year that 1.5 million individuals used prescription painkillers for the first time nonmedically. Further, about 1.9 million Americans each year meet the criteria for opioid use disorder due to their nonmedical use of prescription painkillers. The average age for the first-time use of prescription painkillers was 21.7 years from 2002 to 2012; while nonmedical use of painkillers within the last year among adults 18 to 25 years old has hovered around 12%. On the other hand, the results of the National Institute of Health's (NIH) 2014 Monitoring the Future survey of high school students indicated that prevalence data on prescription and over-the-counter drug abuse suggest a positive downward trend, at least for that segment of the population. Use of narcotics other than heroin in 2014, which includes all opioid pain relievers, was reported to be 6.1% for high school seniors, compared to 7.1% in 2013 and 9.5% in 2004. Nevertheless, lifetime prevalence of narcotics other than heroin was reported by 9.5% of high school seniors in 2014. There was a significant 5-year decrease in the use of Vicodin, an opioid painkiller, with 4.8% of high school seniors reporting use of Vicodin for nonmedical purposes in 2014; this is half of the level reported 5 years before, that is, 9.7%. Heroin use was relatively stable, with 1% of high school seniors and

0.9% of juniors indicating that they had used heroin at least once in their lives. OxyContin use within the past year was reported by 3.3% of the high school seniors. The states with the highest reported rates of narcotic painkiller abuse are all located in the west, specifically Arizona, Colorado, Idaho, Nevada, New Mexico, Oregon, and Washington.

People who abuse prescription painkillers frequently engage in "doctor shopping." This involves intentionally going to many different doctors for the purpose of trying to get as many painkiller prescriptions as they can, and also looking for those doctors who more readily write such prescriptions. This practice usually also involves the abusers taking their prescriptions to many different pharmacies to be filled. Such individuals often engage in other deceptive practices including overreporting the pain they actually experience, denying histories of substance abuse, reporting injuries and accidents that never actually occurred, and even intentionally hurting themselves for the express purpose of being prescribed painkillers.

The rise in prescription opioid abuse has resulted in a dramatic concomitant rise in the abuse of heroin. The natural history of prescription painkiller abusers typically progresses from swallowing, to snorting, to injecting prescription painkillers and then moving on to heroin. According to the findings of the 2013 National Survey on Drug Use and Health, 4.8 million Americans have used heroin at some point in their lives. It was reported that in 2012, around 669,000 Americans used heroin. In 2003, 314,000 Americans admitted to using heroin that year; by 2013, 681,000 Americans reported using heroin within the past year. This is more than a doubling of heroin users in a decade. The annual heroin use rate has been steadily rising even more dramatically since 2007. By the 2010s, heroin users in the United States were reported to be 90.3% White and only 9.7% non-White, a dramatic shift from the late 20th century. Further, about 51.6% of heroin users are now female, which represents a 34.4% increase from the 1960s. This upward trend is largely attributed to the dramatic increases in heroin use reported among young adults. It was reported that 169,000 individuals aged 12 years and older in the United States had used heroin for the first time within the past 12 months; and, that among those between the ages of 12 and 49 years old, the average age of first use of heroin was 24.5 years. The number of individuals using heroin for the first time in 2012 was reported as 156,000 persons; this is a rate nearly double that reported for 2006. Similarly, the number of Americans meeting the criteria for heroin dependence or abuse, as defined by the *Diagnostic and Statistical Manual of Mental Disorders*, 4th edition (DSM-IV), that was then in effect, more than doubled, with the 214,000 people reported for 2002 rising to 467,000 in 2012. In fact, around 300,000 Americans in the past month were regular users of heroin. Further, in 2013, 517,000 users of heroin were reportedly physically dependent upon the drug, which accounts for more than 75% of the total users and supports the understanding of the addiction potential of heroin.

Those individuals who have abused prescription painkillers are much more likely to use illicit heroin. In fact, it has been documented that heroin abuse goes up as access to prescription painkillers goes down. Further, it should also be acknowledged that nearly all of most contemporary heroin users began with prescription opioid use and abuse. Heroin use has actually doubled in the past 5 years in this country. It is now recognized that at least 4 out of 5 current users of heroin in the United States moved to this status from first using prescription opioids like oxycodone and hydrocodone. Economics alone can explain much of this. On the streets of America today, each opioid painkiller pill can sell for between $60 and $100 each, while a single dose of heroin can be purchased for about $10.

These phenomena are being observed in many other countries around the world. In this regard, the UN estimates that there are between 15 million and 21 million global heroin users between the ages of 15 and 64 years old. Many factors have been examined to explore their relationship to heroin use on a global scale. Transnational migration, for example, is but one of these factors currently being examined.

TREATMENT APPROACHES

There are a variety of approaches available for treating painkiller abuse and addiction. These include both behavioral and pharmacological approaches, all of which endeavor to help restore a degree of normalcy in brain function and behavior. This restoration will hopefully permit a recovery of life activities, such as higher employment rates, less criminal behavior, and better overall health. The most effective strategies appear, not surprisingly, to involve an integration of both behavioral and pharmacological approaches to treatment.

Opiate and opioid addiction is a chronic disease characterized by relapse, which offers substantial challenges for treatment providers. Unfortunately, research on narcotic treatment approaches is considerably influenced by political rather than scientific or medical considerations, and it must be recognized that moral belief systems, or ideologies, often underlie this arena.

Early Treatments

Different systems of treatment for opiates have also been developed at various times and places. In 1700, a British physician, John Jones, described how to treat opium addicts and cautioned against abrupt withdrawal, rather advocating a gradual weaning off process. Of course, not all treatment approaches were necessarily equally effective. In 1884, for instance, inhalation of amyl nitrite was reported as a treatment for opium poisoning. In 1885, Sigmund Freud treated a close friend, Von Fleischl, who was a morphine addict, with cocaine. During the era of patent medicines, various elixirs and panaceas were widely available for "curing" opiate addiction; for example, in 1902, one could order through the Sears Roebuck catalog a "Cure for the Opium and Morphia Habit" available for the price of $0.67 per bottle. After passage of the Harrison Narcotics Act of 1914, a wave of court decisions prohibited the maintenance of addiction by physicians; some doctors were arrested for prescribing such substances and, consequently, most stopped treating addiction. In 1910, at the annual meeting of the British Medical Association, a report was made on the use of hypnotism to cure the morphine habit. The Modinos treatment system, which constituted the application of blister serum, was lauded as a form of opium treatment during the 1930s in Burma and contemporaneously was unsuccessfully attempted using incarcerated addicts in Ireland. These are but a few examples of the misguided—from our modern perspective—approaches to treating opiate and opioid addiction. At any rate, after 1962, when in *Robinson v. California* the U.S. Supreme Court ruled that criminal conviction for narcotic addiction violated both the Eighth and Fourteenth Amendments to the U.S. Constitution, addiction treatment initiatives were reestablished in this country.

Substitution

Administration of opiates and other drugs to treat opiate addiction was becoming increasingly unpopular during the early 20th century. At the opening of the 20th century, for example, an opiate treatment regimen including administration of belladonna was advocated. A few narcotic clinics were established in the early 20th century, but their successes, despite early acclaims, were limited, and most were soon closed. By the 1920s, at least 20 U.S. states passed laws that prohibited physicians from giving morphine to addicts, usually specifying that they go to hospitals for treatment. At any rate, on June 19, 1929, the U.S. Congress unanimously passed the Porter bill, which provided for the creation of two prison hospitals that would provide medical treatment, psychiatric counseling, and vocational training for addicts. Thus in the 1930s, the U.S. Public Health Service established federal treatment programs at Lexington, Kentucky, and Fort Worth, Texas, to treat narcotic addicts. In the late 1960s, the so-called British system of heroin addiction treatment was popular. Accordingly, since 1968, under the Dangerous Drugs Act, heroin addicts in the United Kingdom could obtain legal prescriptions for either heroin or methadone as long as they were patients at Drug Dependence Clinics. Through historical analysis, it is evident that there is a gender perspective with respect to the British system, as there is, of course, with most similar topics.

Diversion—that is, individuals who share or sell their medications—is a reality in any substitution treatment program. Rather than focusing mostly on stricter control measures, diversion is more likely to be reduced by focusing mainly on expanded access to drug treatment and on psychosocial and lifestyle-changing interventions.

Detoxification

Detoxification is a useful, and often physically necessary, first step in a painkiller treatment regimen. Detoxification is essentially designed to eliminate toxins, basically abused drugs, from the body of someone who is physically dependent on those substances. Several medications have been shown to be helpful in easing the craving and various physical symptoms of withdrawal, such as diarrhea, nausea, vomiting, and pain. These withdrawal symptoms are typical when an individual first stops using opiate or opioid drugs.

The goal of detoxification for an opiate or opioid drug addict is to minimize the withdrawal effects of the drugs in a safe and effective manner. This may, as just mentioned, entail the administration of various pharmacological agents, including full opioid agonists, partial opioid agonists, and opioid antagonists. This approach is commonly known as medical detoxification, which consists of medically supervised and controlled withdrawal of addictive drugs. This involves both treatments to counter the physical effects of abrupt cessation of use as well as those to remove metabolites and other toxins left as a result of the abusive drug consumption. There are also outpatient medical detoxification approaches; these might utilize buprenorphine and naloxone combination medication, or clonidine, or these in combination with naltrexone. These outpatient approaches typically can complete detoxification in 1 to 2 weeks.

Various other methods of detoxification have been developed for treating individuals with opiate and opioid dependence, including those dependent upon methadone. There is clearly no one single detoxification approach that will be suitable for treating all addicts. Acupuncture, for example, has been used for heroin detoxification. There is, consequently, a history to the treatment of narcotic withdrawal. In Egypt, for instance, insulin is given by injection to help opium addicts who are going through withdrawal. There are also detoxification programs based on social models; these types of programs tend to focus on psychological and social support of the recovering individual, usually with minimal or no use of medication. Social detoxification was a popular approach based on maintaining a calm, supportive environment that was widely used during the 1960s and 1970s, particularly on college campuses. On the other hand, there are many detoxification programs based on a medical model that rely heavily upon the use of medications to minimize physical withdrawal symptoms. The use of methadone with a gradual reduction of dosage is by far the most common detoxification approach in use today for this problem; this generally can be accomplished in between 3 and 12 weeks. Theoretically, any opiate or opioid drug could be used to reduce withdrawal symptoms, but the most commonly used medications for detoxification include clonidine, levo-alpha acetyl methadol (LAAM), methadone, and buprenorphine. Clonidine is used for rapid opioid detoxification; although it reduces most physiological withdrawal symptoms, it does not decrease some of the more subjective symptoms, such as irritability and cravings. Methadone requires a longer period of detoxification with doses gradually decreased; withdrawal from methadone can last from 7 to 180 days; that means it can range from 1 week to 6 months. LAAM is another medication that was formerly used for detoxification purposes, but due to its health risks, it has been discontinued. Use of LAAM was associated, in particular, with prolonged QT intervals and cases of heart arrhythmia and even fatalities. In addition to the black box warning by the FDA and its removal from the market, LAAM has also been removed from the market in the European Union (EU). If a patient overdoses, buprenorphine is a much safer alternative than either LAAM or methadone. There is a clear decreased potential for physical dependence to buprenorphine compared to other detoxification medications.

Rapid detoxification usually occurs in the intensive care unit (ICU) of a hospital. The patient is typically asleep under general anesthesia and is intravenously given substances to block the effects of the opiate or opioid drugs; these can include naltrexone, naloxone, or nalmefene. Other medications, such as antinausea medications like metoclopramide or prochlorperazine, antidiarrheal medications like loperamide, or muscle relaxants, may also be injected. With these procedures, rapid detoxification can be accomplished in 4 to 8 hours, with the patient asleep and thus not having to consciously experience the pain and discomfort of withdrawal. Variations of this approach include stepped rapid detoxification, which is somewhat longer, and ultrarapid detoxification, which is substantially faster; the latter technique involves administering naltrexone to a patient under general anesthesia and can be accomplished in 5 to 30 minutes.

Detoxification programs are usually staffed by a team approach, which includes a combination of medical and social support specialists such as counselors, doctors, nurses, social workers, and other clinical staff. Some programs are set up as inpatient programs, typically in a hospital or in a residential treatment center, while others are operated on an outpatient basis, such as from a counseling center or clinic.

Opiate or opioid detoxification during pregnancy is a particular area of concern as withdrawal has been associated with preterm delivery, impaired fetal development, and even fetal death. Newborns are generally observed for symptoms of neonatal abstinence syndrome.

Elsewhere

There are, of course, also various culture specific approaches to treating opiate and opioid dependence. For instance, members of certain Laotian hill tribes who are opium addicts "make offerings to the opium goddess and take sacred vows to abstain" (Tseng, 2001, p. 525) as part of traditional treatment. Several Buddhist temples in Thailand, for instance, provide indigenous treatment for drug dependence conducted by priests and includes the taking of a vow to the Buddha for "a pledge of abstinence for life from opium, morphine, heroin, ... and other drugs that cause dependence" (Poshyachinda, 1980, p. 122). Herbal medicines are used in China to treat heroin dependency. In Egypt, attempts have been made to integrate the mosque and Islamic clergymen into therapeutic treatment. The Malaysian government is currently transitioning from compulsory drug detention centers to Cure and Care centers that are voluntary drug treatment programs that embrace a holistic treatment based approach to drug addiction rehabilitation.

Many other narcotic treatment approaches have been developed and examined. In 1976, Indonesia passed a severe narcotics law that regulated the distribution of drugs for medical purposes, which resulted in medically trained general practitioners becoming the primary treatment providers. General practitioners certainly played a crucial role in the "British system" of narcotic treatment. In many countries, like France, general practitioners as well as specialized addiction treatment centers provide alternative treatment approaches; the general practitioner typically offers a less structured approach. However, in other countries, such as Nigeria and Pakistan, general practitioners generally play less of a role in narcotic treatment. In Israel, opiate addicts have been treated with methadone since the early 1970s. The rate of heroin addiction in Israel has increased significantly since the 1970s as has the need for methadone treatment programs. Similarly, in Australia, methadone maintenance was introduced in 1969, but there was a substantial increase in the number of programs in the 1990s. Challenges exist in providing methadone maintenance treatment in other places, such as Iran, China, and the Ukraine.

Treatment approaches anywhere should be informed by findings related to changes in the brains of addicts. For instance, cerebral blood flow changes representing a blood perfusion defect have been identified in the brains of opioid-dependent individuals, but these appear to be at least partially reversible with short-term abstinence. However, cerebral perfusion abnormalities appear to be present during withdrawal. At any rate, chronic exposure to opiates is associated with structural changes in dopaminergic neurons, and treatment approaches should endeavor to address this phenomenon.

Behavioral Approaches

Several behavioral approaches have been employed in treating painkiller abuse and addiction. A general commonality to these behavioral approaches to treatment is to provide the social and psychological supports intended to help the individual cease abuse of these substances.

Cognitive behavioral therapy (CBT) focuses primarily on an individual's thoughts and behaviors and is based on the premise that drug abusers have both positive and negative drug-related beliefs that stem from inaccurate thought processes. CBT has been used in addiction treatment programs since the mid-1980s, and it is designed to help patients to acquire specific skills that can be used to resist drug use, along with learning various coping techniques to help reduce problems associated with drug abuse. Individuals are taught to avoid high-risk situations and to better understand how those decisions made can result in positive or negative consequences. Rational Emotive Behavior Therapy, formerly called Rational Therapy and then Rational Emotive Therapy, was developed by the late Albert Ellis; it is a form of CBT focused on resolving behavioral and emotional problems. Rational Emotive Behavior Therapy attempts to reduce pain catastrophizing, which is a negatively distorted perception of pain, such as regarding pain as an awful, horrible, and unbearable condition. The catastrophizing of pain, by the way, is heavily associated with depression. Interestingly, the likelihood of pain catastrophizing appears to change during the life span; younger adults seem to have a higher engagement with emotional compared to sensory processing of pain than do older adults.

The contingency management approach to substance abuse treatment utilizes a system based on vouchers for which patients earn points based on having clean, or negative, drug screening tests. These vouchers can be used to obtain items that promote a healthy lifestyle. This approach uses motivational incentives that hopefully serve as positive reinforcers to encourage abstinence from drugs.

Dynamic psychotherapy is based on the premise that all symptoms come from underlying unconscious psychological conflicts. The major goal of dynamic psychotherapy is to help an individual to become more aware of such conflicts and to foster the acquisition of adaptive coping mechanisms as well as developing healthier ways to resolve intra-psychic conflict.

Group therapy can be particularly effective in painkiller treatment as it targets the social stigma associated with the loss of control typically experienced by addicts. Group members benefit from hearing other group members who admit to having similar issues.

Multidimensional family therapy, also known as multimodal family therapy, is another technique that can be used in preventing and treating painkiller abuse. Multimodal therapy is a therapeutic approach pioneered by Albert Lazarus that is grounded in social learning theory; it is a technically eclectic approach to therapy that is theoretically consistent and comprehensive. Multimodal therapy focuses on 7 discrete but reciprocally interactive modalities, or dimensions, of personality: Behavior, Affect, Sensation, Imagery, Cognition, Interpersonal relationships, and Drugs/biology (represented in the acronym BASIC ID). This psycho-educational framework encourages addiction counselors to improvise and to tailor brief therapy to the individual client. Family therapy involves working with members of a family to explore and improve family relationships and processes to promote the mental health of the individual members and of the collective family unit. Multidimensional family therapy was created by Howard Liddle as a multiple systems–oriented way to integrate an array of developmentally focused therapeutic techniques emphasizing the relationships between cognition, affect, behavior, and environmental inputs. It is believed that these factors all contribute to addiction, and that this multifaceted approach is an effective way to address so many areas. Multidimensional family therapy recognizes and embraces the concept that the "family" of a painkiller abuser does not necessarily consist of only the nuclear family of origin, but can be constituted in myriad other ways. Research into the family configurations of opiate and opioid addicts suggests that a common pattern is that of having inconsistent, overindulgent, and rejecting mothers along with passive if not entirely absent fathers. Further, many addicts appear to have experienced neglect or abuse as children, and perhaps at least one-third come from substance abusing homes.

Many other modalities can be used by behavioral counselors in assisting individuals with painkiller abuse issues. For example, prolonged exposure is a therapeutic technique that involves repeatedly revisiting a traumatic event, such as an accident that precipitated a pain condition. This is done with the hope that prolonged exposure can help normalize the event and reduce symptoms. Relaxation exercises and habituation to traumatic settings are frequently incorporated over time in this approach, and imagery or other techniques can also sometimes be helpful. Eye movement desensitization and reprocessing (EMDR) therapy is another approach that is intended to reduce stress by processing the meaning of events in the context of the individual's autobiographical memory. It relies upon eliciting distressing memories but distracting the individual with physical stimuli, such as instructing the individual to follow the counselor's fingers or gaze. Once the memory is expressed, the individual is immediately prompted to note any feelings or ideas that came up; positive associations, along with eye movements, are encouraged and practiced.

There are also various self-help groups that can be incorporated into painkiller treatment. Narcotics Anonymous (NA) was formed in 1947 in Lexington, Kentucky. NA is a self-help fellowship based on 12 steps of recovery similar to the 12-step fellowship of Alcoholics Anonymous (AA). SMART Recovery is a non-12-step, secular, and scientifically based self-help approach that utilizes techniques of cognitive behavioral therapy, particularly Rational Emotive Behavior Therapy, and motivational interviewing to help individuals seeking abstinence from addictive behaviors; SMART is an acronym for Self Management and Recovery Training.

Therapeutic Communities

Therapeutic communities, such as the pioneering programs at Synanon and Phoenix House, are a popular alternative to methadone for treating narcotic addiction. Synanon was established in 1958 in California as a prototypical drug-free therapeutic community (TC) committed to rehabilitating drug addicts by means of a process of resocialization drawing upon systems of authority, the family, and attack therapy groups. Daytop Village began in 1963 in New York City; Phoenix House was formed in 1967, also in New York City; and Integrity House was established in 1968 in Newark, New Jersey. All were nonprofit substance abuse treatment programs based on the TC model, which emphasizes the role of peers in working toward recovery and of holding clients accountable for their behaviors. Therapeutic communities traditionally believed that drug addiction is symptomatic of a character disorder caused by the inadequacies of addicts to handle stress, due usually to either poor self-esteem or immaturity. Early TCs were highly confrontational and felt that addicts needed to be broken down before they could be rehabilitated; however, as TCs have evolved, they have become more similar to other traditional drug treatment centers in their approaches. However, they tend to keep clients in a longer period of treatment than other types of programs with a gradual reentry into the local community, which certainly helps in their successes. However, therapeutic communities and methadone are not, as was once asserted, necessarily mutually exclusive treatment approaches.

Methadone Treatment

Methadone has certainly served as a cornerstone of narcotic treatment for some time. Oral methadone hydrochloride has been used successfully for several decades to treat heroin addicts. Injectable methadone has also been used for some time, particularly in the United Kingdom.

Methadone maintenance treatment was pioneered in 1965 by Dr. Vincent Dole and Dr. Marie Nyswander of Rockefeller University in New York City. This approach is based on the prescribing of methadone as a substitute for heroin primarily, but also as a substitute for morphine and other similar opiate- and opioid-abused drugs. The intent of this approach to treatment is to maintain an addict in treatment indefinitely so that they neither use their illicit drug of choice nor experience withdrawal symptoms. It is a pragmatic strategy intended to stabilize someone who typically engaged in a high degree of risk-taking activities and who usually had a chaotic lifestyle while using heroin or a related drug. The funding that supported this drug habit was frequently financed by means of criminal behavior, particularly burglary and robbery. In 1968, the American Medical Association officially endorsed the use of methadone for maintenance treatment of addicts. By 1971, about 25,000 clients were enrolled in methadone maintenance programs in the United States; and by 1976, the number had increased to about 135,000 clients.

Methadone maintenance has been shown to be a highly cost-effective form of treatment. However, it is also clear that short-run success with methadone treatment does not readily translate to long-run abstinence. At any rate, methadone treatment has been shown in studies, such as those conducted in Sweden and Australia, to markedly reduce the mortality rate compared to those who continue their heroin addiction. Methadone has also been found to be an effective treatment for members of various ethnic groups, such as Chicanos. In fact, ethnic and gender differences have been examined with respect to the effectiveness of methadone maintenance treatment. Further, the Drug Abuse Treatment Outcome Study (DATOS) examined the long-term effects of outpatient methadone treatment and found a reduction in both heroin use and illegal activity. It is estimated that about 250,000 narcotic addicts receive methadone in the United States alone, and that overall, about 320,000 patients are currently receiving methadone in the United States.

Methadone, which is marketed under trade names such as Amidone, Dolophine, Heptadon, Methadose, Physeptone, and Symoron, is administered orally, which results in a slower rate of absorption; since the drug takes longer to get to the brain, the euphoric sensation is dampened compared to other routes of administration. The recommended standard initial dose of methadone is between 30 and 40 mg per day.

Methadone is available only by prescription in the United States through participation in an approved treatment program. These are typically outpatient treatment programs that usually dispense the methadone to patients on a daily basis. However, there has been considerable resistance generated from many communities when methadone maintenance clinics are proposed; there is a prevalent concern expressed over the fear of having large numbers of drug addicts aggregating in residential neighborhoods.

Researchers and practitioners continue to explore ways to optimize methadone maintenance treatment effectiveness. Unfortunately, of course, some patients do continue to use heroin or other substances after completing treatment. This includes the use of alcohol, cocaine, and other drugs. Methadone use actually may enhance some of the physiological effects, as well as some of the subjective effects, of cocaine and other drugs of abuse. Side effects associated with methadone use include constipation, dry mouth, and increased sweating. Methadone diversion is another issue that has been of concern for several decades. Attempts to produce variations to the chemical structure of methadone led to the discovery of opioids such as diphenoxylate and loperamide, which have useful antidiarrheal properties. At any rate, the use of methadone is more widely accepted and socially sanctioned than that of heroin and other opiates. In addition, methadone maintenance treatment appears to have long-term benefits not only of reduced opiate and opioid use, but also of reduced criminal activities.

Agonist and Antagonist Medications

An agonist drug is a substance that binds to a receptor binding site. There are endogenously produced substances produced in the body that function similarly to agonist drugs; these types of substances include hormones and neurotransmitters, like endorphins and encephalins. The agonist drugs produce similar physiological responses to those observed when the endogenous substances bind to their respective receptor sites. The greater the level of an agonist used, the greater the number of receptors that are occupied, and also the greater the magnitude of the resulting response will be. The potency of a particular agonist drug corresponds to its affinity to bind to a receptor and to activate its intrinsic activity—in other words, to invoke its biological response.

Several initiatives have been developed relying on the use of various opiate and opioid agonist and antagonist medications to treat narcotic addiction. For example, treatment approaches based upon the administration of both buprenorphine and naloxone have been implemented. In July 2013, the FDA granted approval of Zubsolv, a buprenorphine and naloxone combined product in a 4:1 ratio, for the maintenance treatment of opiate and opioid dependence. In June 2014, the FDA granted approval of Bunavail, a buccal combination formulation of buprenorphine and naloxone in a 6–7:1 ratio, for opiate- and opioid-dependence maintenance treatment. Buprenorphine maintenance therapy has been found to be superior to buprenorphine detoxification for reducing the use of illicit opioids and for increasing abstinence rates. Maintenance doses of buprenorphine usually range between 12 mg and 32 mg, but should, of course, be individualized. Buprenorphine was the first medication made available for certified physicians to prescribe in accord with the Drug Addiction Treatment Act. Various settings, such as primary care clinics, have been examined in considering how to utilize buprenorphine and similar substances to treat narcotic abusers. Although it should be recognized that considerable barriers still limit the provision of office-based opiate or opioid agonist treatment, such as those that utilize buprenorphine.

An opioid antagonist can be added to a formulation in order to interfere with, reduce, or defeat the euphoria that is sought with abuse. Naltrexone is an opioid antagonist that was initially approved by the FDA in 1984 for treating opiate and opioid dependence; it is a long-lasting antagonist that tightly binds to an individual's opioid receptors for between 24 hours to 30 hours when administered orally and up to 30 days when injected as an extended release formulation. In 2006, the FDA granted approval of Vivitrol, an injectable extended release formulation of the opioid antagonist naltrexone; it only needs to be administered once every 4 weeks, rather than taken daily. In 2009, the United States spent $22.6 million on naltrexone. The advent of these types of agonist- and antagonist-based therapies is changing the landscape of how we treat opiate- or opioid-dependent individuals.

Narcan is the trade name of a pure opiate and opioid antagonist product that has been hailed as an antidote to opiate or opioid overdose deaths. Naloxone hydrochloride, the active ingredient in Narcan, is approved by the FDA for use by means of injection administration; however, nasal spray administration, as commonly employed when administering Narcan, is not so approved but is considered to be an off-label use. This off-label procedure involves 1 mg of naloxone hydrochloride that is administered to each nostril, and it is reported to bring an opiate- or opioid-overdose victim back to consciousness in 45 seconds to 1 minute. Unfortunately, from 2014 to 2015, the price of Narcan nearly doubled, which resulted in considerable profits for its manufacturer Amphastar Pharmaceuticals. Amphastar's stock value has risen 70% since its initial public offering in June 2014. Amphastar has asserted that the price increase is due to the rising cost of raw materials, energy, and labor.

Methadone and buprenorphine treatment programs have been instituted for incarcerated opiate and opioid abusers, both in the United States and elsewhere, including Australia, Puerto Rico, France, and Spain. It is also recognized that prisons are high-risk environments for the initiation and use of heroin and other drugs. Certainly prisoners in many countries are opiate or opioid dependent and have associated treatment needs.

Opioid agonist therapy with either methadone or a combination of buprenorphine and naloxone has become the standard medical treatment for opiate or opioid use disorder. However, these medications are frequently either not well accepted or tolerated by individuals in treatment. Naltrexone for extended-release injectable suspension (XR-NTX), which is typically administered by means of intramuscular injection once every 4 weeks, has more recently been suggested as an alternative treatment modality. Thus far, it appears that this new approach may have greater efficacy in retaining individuals in treatment both by increasing abstinence and by decreasing drug cravings. Challenges, of course, exist for providing these and related services. Reviewing the types of studies covered in this section can be of considerable benefit in expanding our understanding of the historicity of the field of addiction studies and of different treatment best practices approaches.

Overdose Fatalities

Opiate and opioid overdose is a leading cause of death among injection drug users. Consequently, it has been suggested that training opioid users to recognize and manage overdoses could help prevent drug-related deaths. A study of opioid users in St. Petersburg, Russia, for instance, suggested high interest in receiving training for overdose recognition and prevention.

When prescription opioids, such as hydrocodone and oxycodone, are taken by routes other than that prescribed, such as by snorting or injecting crushed tablets, there is an increased risk of respiratory depression, which can result in coma and even death. There have been dramatic increases since the late 1990s in the number of unintentional opioid poisoning deaths, frequently when taken in combination with alcohol or other drugs. In fact, overdoses of prescription painkillers kill 46 people per day, or nearly 17,000 people each year in the United States. This is more than a 400% increase since 1999. Overdose deaths from opioid painkillers in the United States surpassed the number of fatalities from heroin and cocaine combined for the first time in 2008. Opioid overdose deaths was the leading cause of injury death in 2013 in the United States. They remain a serious and growing area of concern.

The pattern of painkiller overdose fatalities, of course, varies somewhat from state to state. For example, a review of overdose deaths for Kentucky in 2011 reveal an interesting situation. In 2010, oxymorphone was identified in the blood of 24 fatal overdose victims, which accounted for 2% of the total number of drug overdoses in Kentucky that year. In 2011, the very next year, oxymorphone overdose deaths accounted for 23% (n = 154) of the drug overdose deaths in Kentucky. That same year, oxycodone accounted for 31% (n = 213) of all fatal drug overdoses in Kentucky; hydrocodone accounted for 27% (n = 187) of all fatal drug overdoses; and alprazolam, a short-acting anxiolytic drug of the benzodiazepine family, accounted for 42% (n = 286) of all fatal drug overdoses in Kentucky. By the way, the percentages add up to more than 100% because the presence of more than one drug was sometimes detected in the bodies of the decedents.

SPECIAL POPULATIONS

There are different issues around the use and abuse of painkillers with various special segments of the population. These special populations include, for instance, the elderly and myriad ethnic groups, but many others as well.

The higher prevalence of pain among the elderly results in a greater number of prescriptions being written for opiate and opioid medications. The prevalence of chronic pain and the duration of chronic pain increases as we age. In fact, the rise of chronic pain in America is a direct consequence of the epidemiological shift in our aging population. One in two individuals who have reached the age of 65 years will experience chronic pain. The unintentional misuse or abuse of these painkiller medications can have dangerous health consequences due to the likelihood of comorbid conditions, including the common phenomenon of having multiple prescriptions, which increases the potential for harmful drug interactions, including fatalities. These issues are exacerbated by the changes in drug metabolism that are typically age related. Furthermore, Americans over the age of 65 years have the highest rates of problems resulting from the abuse of opiate- and opioid-painkiller medications, including overdose deaths. In fact, prescriptions for opiate and opioid medications have increased more than twice as much among older individuals than among their younger counterparts.

Ethnic group affiliation is certainly an important variable to consider when attempting to gain a better understanding of any phenomenon, including the use and abuse of painkillers. Ethnographic research, for example, has indicated that poverty, antagonist race relations, sociocultural political and geographic linkage to Caribbean and U.S. drug trafficking routes, and kinship solidarities all helped poor Puerto Rican neighborhoods position themselves to serve as commercial distribution centers for high-quality, low-cost Colombian heroin. In this vein, there was found to be a significant inverse relationship between the level of Hispanic segregation, particularly high levels of Puerto Rican segregation, and the price of heroin in the United States from 1990 to 2000. However, no such association was found for African American segregation and Colombian-sourced heroin price or prevalence. Therefore, the existence of highly segregated Puerto Rican communities helps to explain how heroin from Colombia was able to enter and spread across the United States, making Colombia the dominant source of U.S. heroin. Further, we have come to recognize that the genetic background of various ethnic groups can influence the sensitivity of individuals to any particular opiate or opioid drug as well as influence the relative efficacies and potencies of respective painkillers within an individual. There are, for instance, ethnicity-specific variation in pain-reduction genes, such as that responsible for guanosine triphosphate cyclohydrolase 1/dopa-responsive dystonia (GCH1), which is essential for the synthesis of dopamine and serotonin. This gene, GCH1, has been found to be protective for pain in White populations, but a risk factor for pain in American Blacks with sickle cell genes. There thus appears to be genetic variation of the pharmacogenetic shaping of painkiller metabolism, or pharmacokinetics, as well as of transport and receptor signaling or pharmacodynamics.

Injection drug users are clearly a special population closely associated with painkiller abuse. The World Health Organization (WHO) and the UN Office on Drugs and Crime (UNODC) estimate that between 8.9 million and 22.4 million people inject drugs globally, with an average of about 12.7 million. Among these injection drug users, about 1.7 million, or 13.1%, are living with HIV; the range of estimates for this group is between 0.9 million and 4.8 million people living with HIV globally. Ukraine, for instance, has one of the highest rates of HIV prevalence in Eastern Europe; it has been reported that 42% of patients in opioid substitution treatment programs in Ukraine are HIV-positive, and that 51% are infected with Hepatitis C, 19% with Hepatitis B, and nearly 17% with tuberculosis.

Researchers have identified numerous other factors that could help identify other special groups with different concerns as relates to pain and painkillers. One study, for example, of smoking status found that men who were current smokers who had unsuccessfully attempted to quit smoking were more likely than current smokers who made no attempts to quit to report pain and frequent depressive symptoms as well as both mental and physical distress. At any rate, more resources are sorely needed for increasing treatment services. In this regard, the United States spends less than a quarter of its drug control funds on treatment.

DOCUMENT: "WHAT EVERY INDIVIDUAL NEEDS TO KNOW ABOUT METHADONE MAINTENANCE TREATMENT"

Individuals on methadone maintenance receive a specific dose of methadone on a regular basis to help maintain their normal physiological state without using other painkillers. The pamphlet "What Every Individual Needs to Know about Methadone Maintenance Treatment" is distributed by the U.S. Department of Health and Human Services (HHS), Substance Abuse and Mental Health Services Administration (SAMHSA) to serve as a general introduction to methadone. It addresses many of the areas of concern to someone considering commencing methadone maintenance treatment (MMT) and provides basic factual information on methadone and its use. For example, a section of the pamphlet addresses the dangers of mixing methadone with other drugs. There is also a listing of important resources for individuals pondering the decision of whether or not to use methadone, including a helpline and a treatment facility locator.

WHAT IS METHADONE?

Methadone is a long-acting opioid medication that is used as a pain reliever and, together with counseling and other psychosocial services, is used to treat individuals addicted to heroin and certain prescription drugs.

WHAT IS METHADONE MAINTENANCE TREATMENT (MMT)?

MMT helps normalize your body's neurological and hormonal functions that have been impaired by the use of heroin or misuse of other short-acting opioids. Opioids are a group of drugs that act on the central nervous system. They include opiates such as codeine, morphine, and heroin as well as synthetic drugs such as oxycodone, oxycontin, hydrocodone, and methadone.

Appropriate MMT provides several benefits:

- Reduces or eliminates craving for opioid drugs
- Prevents the onset of withdrawal for 24 hours or more
- Blocks the effects of other opioids
- Promotes increased physical and emotional health
- Raises the overall quality of life of the patient.

IS METHADONE MAINTENANCE TREATMENT RIGHT FOR YOU?

Have you been through detoxification and found you couldn't feel normal? MMT can allow you to regain a sense of normalcy.

Have you been using opioids such as heroin, codeine, or oxycodone but can't seem to stop? MMT can help you quit using those drugs and focus your life.

Are you pregnant and using heroin? Seek MMT right away to prevent miscarriage and protect your baby from life-threatening withdrawal.

Have you tested positive for HIV or Hepatitis C? If you have tested positive, MMT can allow you to regain your quality of life and begin essential treatment of your viral infection. If you have not tested positive, MMT can help you stop using needles, which is the primary route of infection for drug users.

Beginning MMT can help stabilize and improve your health and can move you toward getting the care you need.

STARTING METHADONE MAINTENANCE TREATMENT

Depending on where you live, you may have a choice of methadone providers, or you may live in an area where methadone treatment is not available. If you have not already made contact with a doctor or clinic that treats opioid addiction, find out whether treatment is available nearby.

- Talk with your family doctor. Generally, your doctor is not authorized to prescribe methadone for addiction treatment or withdrawal management purposes. Ask to be referred to an authorized doctor or a methadone clinic, or ask whether other treatment options such as buprenorphine are available.
- Contact a referral service. To find the treatment provider closest to you, call SAMHSA's National Helpline at 1-800-662-HELP at any time of the day or night, or search online for a treatment facility at www.findtreatment.samhsa.gov.

Assessment

Assessment includes determining your history with drug use as well as a physical examination by a doctor. You should be asked about medical problems that are commonly associated with opioid addictions, and you may be asked to consent to a blood test to check for HIV, Hepatitis, and other infectious or sexually transmitted diseases.

Expect questions. You may be asked about your drug use, your physical and mental health, your home and family, and your employment.

Ask questions. What are you being tested for? What other services are available? Remember, knowledge is power.

You may be assessed again during treatment to review your progress

Dosing

For safety, your first dose of methadone will be low or moderate. New patients usually start at a dose not to exceed 30 to 40 mgs. A larger dose of 60 to 120 mgs a day may be required for long-term maintenance. You and your physician should determine what dose works best for you.

Your dose is right when withdrawal symptoms, drug cravings, drowsiness, and side effects fade. With a correct dose, you should feel more energetic, clearheaded, and able to do the things that matter in your life. Until you have adjusted, make sure not to drive a car or operate heavy machinery.

You should discuss a dose adjustment with your doctor if you still are experiencing drug cravings. The majority of properly dosed patients have no physical desire to use other drugs.

Drug Testing

Routine tests of urine or oral fluids will show whether you have been using other illicit or inappropriate drugs and whether you have been taking your methadone. You may have to give supervised samples to ensure they are yours. With continual negative results, you'll be asked to take drug tests less often.

If you test positive for other drugs, it may hold up your schedule for taking home doses, and your provider may ask that you take drug tests more often.

Some providers expect zero drug use while others are more tolerant.* If you test positive for a drug when you know you haven't used, you can request to be retested.

Methadone Facts

When methadone is taken as directed:

- MMT can improve your health.
- Methadone will not cause euphoria.
- Methadone will not make you sick.
- Methadone will not affect your immune system.
- Methadone does not damage your teeth and bones.
- Methadone does not make you gain weight.

Confidentiality

Drug treatment patients are protected by special Federal confidentiality regulations. No one will be told you are in treatment or what you talk about in treatment, except for certain situations:

- Information about a client often is shared within a treatment team in the clinic.
- You may consent in writing that your information be shared under certain specified conditions—for example, to forward your records to another doctor or clinic.
- If your doctor or counselor has reason to think you might hurt yourself or others, he or she must inform others.
- If you are facing trial, the court may subpoena your treatment records.
- If you test positive for HIV and other communicable diseases, these facts will be shared with public health officials. In certain States, your intimate partners at risk for these diseases may be told that they have been exposed.

LIVING WITH METHADONE

Take Home Doses

At the start of treatment, you will have to go to the clinic daily to take your dose under observation. This daily contact confirms to the staff that you are taking the dose ordered by the physician. It also helps the staff to see if your dose is enough or too much and whether you are experiencing side effects, in which case an adjustment may be necessary. After a few months, your provider may let you take home or "carry" doses for unsupervised use. Ask to find out when and under what conditions you will be given carry doses.

It is likely that you will be asked to sign an agreement claiming responsibility for using and storing the doses safely. Your provider may take away your take-home privileges if you do not comply with the agreement or if your drug tests are positive for drug use.

Safety and Storage

Your maintenance dose of methadone could seriously harm or kill someone who has no tolerance for the drug. Take precautions:

- Never transfer your medication to a container that might make it easier to mistake what's inside.
- Keep your doses in a locked box, such as one sold for fishing tackle or cash.

Hospital Stays

If you are admitted to the hospital, let the staff there know that you are a methadone patient. This is vital so that you can receive your dose and because other drugs can be dangerous if combined with methadone. Urge the hospital staff to talk with your MMT doctor about your medication and care.

Dealing with Side Effects

Methadone maintenance carries some side effects:

- Constipation. Eat foods that are high in fiber and drink plenty of water. You also should avoid foods that are high in fat; they are harder to digest and tend to make your system sluggish.
- Excessive sweating. Adjusting the dose may stop the sweating, and there are other medications available to help control this.
- Changes in sex drive. Some people on methadone have little sex drive and are unable to have an orgasm. You may be taking a medication that affects your sex drive. Talk with your doctor about possible treatments that will improve this side effect.

Methadone and Employment

Once you're on a stable dose of methadone, it shouldn't affect the work you do or how well you do your job. For most jobs, there's no need to mention that you take methadone. Your employer has no right to know.

HIV, Hepatitis, and Methadone

Methadone can be a great benefit if you are HIV/AIDS or Hepatitis B (HBV) or C (HCV) positive. Methadone allows you to lead a "normal" life so it's easier to take care of yourself, to eat better, and to take your medication at the right times. However, prescription drugs for your HIV/AIDS or HBV/HCV may interfere with methadone, and your dose may need to be changed. Talk with the program doctor about other drugs you have been prescribed.

Tips on Taking Methadone

- Methadone usually works best when it's taken once a day at the same time every day.
- You drink your dose of methadone, usually in a mixture with orange juice.
- It takes a few days to feel the full effects of a dose adjustment.
- Taking other drugs may interfere with the adjustment of your dose.
- Taking more opioids won't get you high, but you could overdose.
- Hang in there—give it 2 to 6 weeks to find the right dose.

Patient Rights and Responsibilities

If you are unhappy with your treatment—for example, you feel your dose has not been adjusted correctly—talk it over with your doctor or counselor. If a treatment problem hasn't been fixed to your satisfaction by talking with your doctor or counselor, you may consider changing your provider.

You also can anonymously report problems with your treatment provider to his/her accrediting agency. To learn more about grievance procedures, you can visit the Patient Support and Community Education Project online at www.dpt.samhsa.gov/patient/index.htm.

As a patient in treatment, you are protected by a set of Medication-Assisted Treatment Patient Rights and Responsibilities. You can see the SAMHSA Guidelines for the Accreditation of Opioid Treatment Programs online at www.dpt.samhsa.gov/guidelines.pdf.

Methadone and Pain Relief

Methadone can provide effective pain relief. Yet, once you are on a stable dose of methadone, you may be tolerant to its pain-relieving effects and may require additional pain medication. Some MMT patients need more pain medication than patients who are not a part of MMT.

Mixing Methadone with Other Drugs Can Be Dangerous

Methadone interacts with many medications. This can change the safety of the methadone you are taking and potentially can cause withdrawal. It is important to tell your doctor about all of the drugs you take.

Combinations with Methadone That Can Result in Withdrawal Syndrome

Opiate analogs such as:

- Nubain
- Talwin
- Stadol

Opiate antagonists such as:

- Naloxone
- Naltrexone

Partial agonists such as:

- Buprenorphine
- Alcohol

HOW LONG WILL I BE ON METHADONE?

The longer you've been dependent on opioids, the more likely it is that you would benefit from being on methadone. Those who withdraw from methadone after short-term treatment are more likely to return to drug use than those who stay in treatment until they have obtained the optimal benefits.

Remember the risks that come with drug use: high rates of HIV and Hepatitis C infection among people who inject drugs, greater odds of committing crimes and going to prison, and possible death from overdose.

Recovery to a normal life is possible. You should stay in treatment as long as you are benefiting from it. The length of time you stay in MMT is an issue that should be decided solely by you and your physician. Some people are in MMT only for a few weeks, while others choose to stay in MMT indefinitely.

ENDING TREATMENT

If you are thinking about ending MMT, talk with the doctor at the program. It can be a slow process to taper off of methadone. Though doses are tapered slowly to reduce withdrawal symptoms, you may experience some aching, insomnia, and lack of appetite for a few weeks. You also may feel a sense of loss, sadness, and sleeplessness for months. However, over time this should dissipate.

Long-term withdrawal can take from 6 months up to a year before you can completely taper off of methadone treatment. You should never set time limitations on yourself—taper off at your own pace in cooperation with your treatment provider.

Throughout treatment and after treatment ends, be sure to maintain and extend your support network. You can request to come back to the program every few weeks for the first year and expect to have the same privileges that you did before tapering off. Should you feel that you may relapse, return to your program immediately for re-dosing. You always can return to treatment. Returning to treatment is not a failure—it's a choice about what is best for you.

Important Resources

Substance Abuse and Mental Health Services Administration (SAMHSA)
www.samhsa.gov
SAMHSA's National Helpline
1-800-662-HELP (4357)
SAMHSA's Center for Substance Abuse Treatment (CSAT)
www.csat.samhsa.gov
SAMHSA's National Clearinghouse for Alcohol and Drug Information
1-800-SAY-NOTO (729-6686)
www.samhsa.gov
SAMHSA's Substance Abuse Treatment Facility Locator
www.findtreatment.samhsa.gov
Patient Support and Community Education Project (PSCEP)
www.dpt.samhsa.gov/patient/index.htm

Source: SAMSHA. (2006). *Introduction to methadone: What every individual needs to know about methadone maintenance treatment.* DHHS Publication No. [SMA] 06-4123.

Chapter 9

The Future of Painkillers

This discussion is, in part at least, predicated upon the assumption that a better understanding of yesterday will help provide resources to more fully comprehend today. Similarly, a better understanding of the situation today should better help us plan how to address the issues in the future. With particular respect to opium, morphine, and other opiates and opioids, it is expected that a greater historical awareness will furnish a more informed basis to make choices and decisions regarding how to proceed with areas such as policy, particularly including issues of prevention, treatment, enforcement, and so forth, particularly as concerns opiates, opioids, and other painkillers.

Caution must be exercised, however, in telling the history of these and other substances used to cure pain. There are deeply rooted cultural values that have resulted in many individuals holding preconceived notions as to what the historical examination of this area should reveal. Historians and other scholars have found that telling the truth can be difficult, and that there is often more than one truth pertaining to the history of various substances. Indeed, although historiography may analyze a particular topic one way, those with vested interests will typically interpret and repackage those findings in ways unintended by the historian.

Examining the history of opium, morphine, and other opiate painkillers reveals an all-too-familiar pattern. A new drug is discovered; its use is initially enthusiastically advocated; it is often promoted as a cure for an earlier used substance that is then being demonized; then as the levels of use of this new substance reach sufficient numbers of users, the awareness of problems with its use are recognized; the initial allure of the substance is replaced with the tales of its observed evils. This trajectory is clearly evident from the historical review presented in much of this work. As levels of opium use in society reached levels where it was seen as problematic, morphine was introduced as its safe substitute. Morphine abuse, once recognized as an issue, was seen to be solvable by heroin. After heroin was seen as a scourge, methadone was then accepted as its desired replacement. Methadone detractors are certainly not difficult to find. Further, opioid receptor antagonists, such as naloxone and naltrexone, have been recommended as part of the alternatives to daily methadone maintenance. These approaches are not without their respective problems as well. A better understanding of the historical background behind this area, along with the review of pharmacological properties of the respective painkillers, should be helpful in formulating new approaches to more appropriately address issues of concern.

Issues associated with opium, morphine, heroin, and other related substances, as well as with the numerous unrelated painkiller substances, have significantly shaped policy responses to drugs in respective societies. Certainly drug control policy can be readily understood as essentially an ideological phenomenon. It should therefore not be very surprising that the social attitudes toward these substances have shaped the development of policy responses more than scientific research. Nevertheless, medical authorities have often played a prominent role in the crafting of policies concerning narcotics and related painkiller substances. Unfortunately, public opinion rather than research findings tend generally to direct this evolution.

Painkillers and many other essential medications are often in short supply in many places around the world. In Senegal, for example, morphine could be used as an effective and relatively inexpensive drug for treating severe pain, such as that commonly associated with certain cancers. Unfortunately, however, Senegal imports only about 1 kilogram of morphine every year, which is only enough to treat approximately 200 patients suffering from pain caused by advanced cancer alone. Human Rights Watch reports that about 70,000 Senegalese patients each year need palliative care to manage symptoms related to chronic, potentially fatal diseases. Morphine, in fact, is reportedly available only in the capital city, Dakar; and even there, access is regularly limited due to chronic shortages. In 2013, for instance, Senegal used about 0.084 mg of morphine/capita, which is actually 71 times less than the global average of 5.96 mg/capita. In a similar vein, in Burundi the annual consumption of morphine is 0.011518 mg/capita, fentanyl is 0.021158 mg/capita, and meperidine is 0.300966 mg/capita. Niger reported that their annual consumption of morphine in 2009 was 0.011493 mg/capita, while that for fentanyl was 0.061340 mg/capita, and meperidine was 0.031624 mg/capita. Cote d'Ivoire reported that the annual consumption of morphine in 2010 was 0.00277 mg/

capita and fentanyl was 0.000365 mg/capita. Alarmingly, even lower amounts of painkiller imports are reported for Burkina Faso, where the annual consumption of morphine is only 0.000004627 mg/capita, fentanyl is 0.00002 mg/capita, and meperidine is 0.00167 mg/capita. Thus, many individuals in these and similar countries elsewhere around the world must suffer pain due to a lack of resources available for appropriate pain management.

Risk factors for experiencing pain are numerous and include variables such as female gender, divorce, increased age, low educational attainment, and racial background. In the United States, for example, Whites appear to experience pain for longer durations but with less intensity than Black non-Hispanics or Hispanics. Pain is negatively associated with many various domains of health. Individuals who live with persistent pain are 4 times more likely than those without pain to experience anxiety or depression, and they are twice as likely to have difficulty working. Research has indicated that negative psychological factors and poor coping skills increase one's susceptibility to chronic pain and to impaired pain control. Psychiatric disorders appear to decrease pain thresholds and to increase the degree of functional impairment experienced from pain.

Overdose fatalities are increasing at alarming rates and must, in the immediate future, become an issue that we more comprehensively address. In this regard, opiate and opioid overdose deaths more than tripled from 1999 to 2012; on top of this, opiate and opioid overdose deaths also tripled between 2010 and 2013. Someone dies of a prescription drug overdose, mostly painkillers, every 19 minutes in this country, and thus there are 46 deaths every day from use of opiate or opioid painkiller drugs. We are experiencing a wave of these tragedies and must implement measures as soon as possible to remediate the situation. Promoting greater availability and training in the use of naloxone hydrochloride and related approaches will contribute to reducing this scourge, as would measures already adopted in some states of eliminating any risks of prosecution to first responders, like police and firefighters, and others who administer naloxone hydrochloride or other similar agents in an attempt to prevent a fatal overdose.

Opiate and opioid drugs have been and continue to be the most potent analgesics available. They are certainly among the most effective tools for managing severe acute pain. However, they are less effective with certain forms of neuropathic pain, such as that associated with causalgia and diabetic neuropathy. Further, the increasing prosecution of physicians engaged in pain management has led to greater under treatment of pain. On the other hand, paradoxically, there has also been a surge in the over prescribing and over-medication of patients with painkillers, such as that revealed at some Veterans Administration (VA) hospitals. In 2012, for instance, U.S. health care providers wrote 259 million prescriptions for opiate or opioid painkillers, enough for every adult American to get one bottle of painkiller pills. Extended-release long-acting opioid painkillers, in particular, can be very useful in the management of persistent severe pain in some selected patients. Although there are serious risks associated with the use of opiate and opioid drugs in general, the risks are magnified with the use of the extended-release long-acting painkillers. Inappropriate prescribing and improper use of these pharmacological products are associated with severe negative consequences, including addiction and overdose fatalities. In this vein, educating patients and their caregivers about the proper use of extended-release long-acting painkillers, including proper storage and disposal procedures, can be helpful in reducing the associated problems. Individuals have an intense personal interest in having their pain managed effectively and in being afforded protection from the abuse of prescription or nonprescription painkiller drugs, or of relapse to a preexisting addictive disease. In addition, research suggests that long-term treatment with opiate or opioid medications can induce hyperalgesia, a heightening of pain sensitivity as a direct consequence of chronic administration of these drugs.

Nevertheless, at least for the foreseeable future, opiate and opioid drugs will no doubt remain the most effective and affordable option for the management of pain. However, they do generate considerable undesirable side effects, not the least of which is their addictive potential. Further, unintentional poisoning fatalities, most commonly from opioid pain medications, have recently increased dramatically in the United States. Accordingly, the multimodal approach to the management of pain has become the accepted standard. There are the 4 A's of pain management that are widely accepted and used, consisting, respectively, of Analgesia, Activities of daily living, Adverse effects, and Aberrant drug taking behaviors. There are, of course, many different types of aberrant drug-taking behaviors; examples of some of these include hoarding of medications, seeking early refills, multiple unsanctioned dose escalations, and asking multiple health care providers for prescriptions. Some have suggested that two other issues be added to the 4 A's, namely, Assessment of diagnosis and Action plan. This balanced approach acknowledges the multifactorial nature of pain and generally relies on multiple agents to avoid use of a single drug to reduce the doses of those used.

DEVELOPMENT OF NEW PAINKILLERS

The development of better painkillers is a major public health priority. There is an increasingly aging population with a growing rate of chronic illnesses, many necessitating the use of painkillers. There is also a large number of returning military veterans, many of whom have experienced injuries requiring the administration of painkillers. These and other factors contribute to the crucial need for safer, nonaddicting painkillers.

Research is ongoing into the development of potential sources of future painkillers. Since time immemorial, there has been a search for powerful, non-addictive painkillers. Some researchers suggest that a newly crafted drug may help in this longstanding quest. A mirror-image molecule of naloxone, referred to as (+)-naloxone, looks like it may, when coadministered with opiates or opioids, both block the drugs from producing a high and, at the same time, increasing their painkilling effects, at least in laboratory rats. The (+)-naloxone appears to activate a specific type of receptor, the toll-like receptor 4 that is found on glial cells in the brain, but not on brain neurons. It appears to be part of an immune receptor complex. Activation of these particular receptors on glial cells seems to amplify pain signals by priming the neurons in the pain pathways. The (+)-naloxone appears to suppress the glia, which hinders the development of tolerance and withdrawal symptoms associated with continued use of opiates and opioids. Another drug that also blocks activation of the toll-like receptor 4, ibudilast, was undergoing clinical trial testing in human subjects as of this writing. Another novel painkiller is Aldail, a drug that promotes production of aldehyde dehydrogenase 2, an enzyme that has anti-inflammatory properties. These new types of drugs offer interesting possibilities for combination uses, but it is far too early to conclude that they will actually provide us with safe, nonaddictive, and effective painkillers. New anti-inflammatory painkiller drugs are also being developed that have effects of signal transduction and also function as anti-cytokine agents.

Novel chemical entities may yet be created that can function as safer painkillers. New classes of NSAIDs are being explored in this search; these include nitric oxide (NO)–releasing NSAIDs, also known as CINODs, and hydrogen sulfide–releasing NSAIDs. Nitric oxide, by the way, is a universal transducer molecule that plays a crucial role in pain signaling. These new substances have the potential of serving as alternatives to the traditional NSAIDs and the selective COX-2 inhibitors. For example, naproxcinod is a hybrid molecule generated by coupling nitric oxide to naproxen; it appears to have significantly reduced risk of causing a destabilization of blood pressure control for those individuals taking antihypertensive medications, as well as demonstrating a slight improvement in gastrointestinal tolerability. Nevertheless, lack of outcome studies led to a voluntary withdrawal of its application for FDA approval in May 2011. Another novel hybrid painkiller and anti-inflammatory drug is VA694, a nitric oxide–releasing selective COX-2 inhibitor; it is hoped that the nitric oxide releasing properties of VA694 might help mitigate the deleterious cardiovascular effects associated with traditional selective COX-2 inhibitors. At any rate, research continues on various other hybrids and may yet offer novel chemical entities that demonstrate beneficial effects, such as the release of hydrogen sulfide or by exerting antioxidant effects. Hybrid versions of traditional painkillers are only one potential source of new products that may exert beneficial painkilling effects without the standard adverse side effects.

Scientists are bioengineering genetic material into organisms such as Baker's yeast cells so that they will hopefully produce opioid-like chemicals. Other researchers are studying mambalgins, peptides in Black Mamba venom, that have analgesic properties as they inhibit acid-sensing ion channels in central or peripheral neurons. Investigators are also examining venom and other substances from other snakes, as well as that from centipedes, scorpions, spiders, and other animals and plants as sources of potential painkillers. There is also hope for substances extracted from the skin of poison arrow frogs that appear to be a very potent painkiller but that lacks the negative side effects of opiates and opioid drugs, like addiction and constipation. Research efforts are also ongoing with many of the substances that have been used as painkillers for some time but that may not be fully understood, particularly with respect to mechanisms of action and other related factors. For example, salicylic acid is a phytohormone involved as a key signaling molecule in many plants for inducing defense-related genes and for rapid but localized cell death at the site of pathogen infection; its anti-inflammatory effects have been utilized for a considerable span of time.

More rapid delivery of painkillers would be a very crucial step toward improving the effective management of both acute and chronic pain. One novel technique under development is to administer painkillers and other medications by means of a new transdermal delivery system that utilizes micro-needles attached to an adhesive patch. The tiny needles make micrometer-sized porous channels through the skin. Since the small needles are only about 600 micro-meters long, they do not create any perceivable pain sensations. Further, drug permeation is enhanced as the drug is encapsulated in backing layers that circumvents premature closing of the miniaturized pores opened up by the micro-needles. Experiments with the new type of patch suggest that the new system can deliver lidocaine within 5 minutes of application, while a traditional commercial lidocaine transdermal patch takes about 45 minutes for the painkiller to penetrate the skin. This novel drug delivery system could be highly useful for managing situations such as preoperative pain and chronic pain in those suffering with conditions like cancer and diabetes, as well as in pediatric applications. This approach permits a larger dose of painkillers to be delivered in less time which could also reduce the likelihood of individuals experiencing skin irritations.

Some clinicians are experimenting with switching from intravenous (IV) sedation with painkillers before many invasive pain intervention procedures to use of oral anxiolysis instead; in such a program, oral benzodiazepines, for instance, might be used instead of IV administration of opioid drugs. Heavy sedation, such as is often used with IV sedation, can compromise safety, particularly by preventing patient feedback, which can often help reduce the possibility of earlier interventions when needed.

There are many other approaches currently being examined, and many more not yet presently even imagined, that hopefully may yet yield better ways to control and manage pain. Nutritional approaches, such as those that utilize so-called medical foods like theramine, an amino acid blend, may, for example, prove effective at relief of specific types of pain symptoms, in this case chronic low back pain. Theramine is chemically designed to target specific precursors to neurotransmitters involved in inflammation sand pain, such as acetylcholine, D-serine, histamine, and nitric oxide.

REDUCING ABUSE

The development of opioids that are harder to abuse is a crucial area of concern. Various abuse deterrent approaches are being considered. One of these approaches is the development of altered tablet and capsule formulations that make it more difficult to smash them into powder that can be snorted or injected, or even chewed and swallowed. The approval by the FDA of Hysingla ER is one example of this opioid abuse prevention strategy. This extended-release tablet with a maximum dose of 120 mg of hydrocodone bitartrate is designed to last for 24 hours, as compared to Zohydro ER, also a hydrocodone bitartrate tablet that is designed to last for 12 hours. The Hysingla ER tablet is designed so that if crushed, it forms a thick gel that is extremely difficult to inject or snort.

Certain drug release designs, by their very nature, offer some resistance to drug abuse. For example, a subcutaneous implant or a sustained-release depot injectable formulation of a painkiller can be more difficult to manipulate for abuse purposes. Chemical barriers can also be added to opiate or opioid formulations such that extraction of the active ingredients using common solvents like water, alcohol, or other organic solvents can be resisted. Substances can also be combined in novel ways to produce an aversive, unpleasant effect if the dosage form is manipulated before consumption or if taken in a higher dosage than directed to use. These are but a few of the potential technological modifications to painkillers that could make them more difficult to misuse and abuse.

Physicians and other health care providers can help reduce the risk of addiction to painkillers by better screening their patients prior to use for possible abuse risk factors, such as having a personal or family history of substance abuse or of mental illness. Patients should also be regularly monitored for signs of misuse or abuse of their prescription painkillers as well as of other related substances. Requests for early or frequent refills of prescription painkillers, for example, can indicate the development of tolerance, the beginnings of a substance abuse problem, or even the progression of an illness. It is the responsibility of the physician or other health care provider to determine which of these possibilities is involved with each respective patient and to take appropriate measures to address them.

More effective and appropriate pain management can also go a long way toward reducing the use and abuse of painkiller drugs. Inadequate acute pain management, in particular, can result in several negative consequences. These adverse outcomes include increased hospital stays and/or more frequent treatment readmissions, as well as an overall reduced quality of life, including areas like impaired sleep and other medical complications being more likely. There is also a dramatic decrease in functional recovery being achieved and a substantial risk of clear physical function impairments. Furthermore, there is a much greater probability of progressing to chronic pain if the acute pain is not managed well. By individualizing each patient's pain profile, we are much more likely to more appropriately address their unique needs. Adequate individualized pharmacologic pain management must consider individual differences, such as those with respect to opioid metabolism and drug-to-drug interactions. Synchronized use of 2 or more pharmacologic painkiller agents with different mechanisms of action can provide effective multimodal therapy. We know that fixed dose combinations of an opioid and a non-opioid painkiller, for instance, can provide better pain relief than use of either drug alone. There can also be synergistic actions occurring with use of multiple pharmacologic agents. Accordingly, we can often achieve greater pain relief with lower doses and fewer adverse consequences, which, naturally, results in less abuse of painkillers.

Painkiller efficacy can also be improved by occasional rotation of medications —that is, changing either the specific painkiller used or changing the route of administration. This also can lead to improved physical and/or psychosocial functioning and better quality of life, as well as in reducing the number of adverse experiences. When switching painkiller medications in an opiate- or opioid-tolerant individual, the dose of the new medication is usually calculated by using an equianalgesic dosing table and then reducing the calculated dose by 25% to 50% to permit the possibility of enhanced painkiller efficacy.

Better prescription drug monitoring programs need to be developed and improved. Physicians and other health care providers can monitor for prescription opiate or opioid abuse. Regular follow-ups with reassessment and documentation is an essential component of pain management precautions. Urine drug testing is probably one of the most effective ways to assess medication intake and the use of illicit drugs. Other methods that can be used in clinical practice to monitor an individual's use of prescription painkillers include a written agreement signed by both the health care provider and the patient and included as part of the medical record; pill counts can be conducted at each visit; and use of the respective state Prescription Drug Monitoring Program (PDMP). Clearly, state-level strategies to try to reduce illicit opiate or opioid use should include measures to prevent the overprescribing of painkiller medications by health care providers, while also ensuring access to safe, effective pain management for those individuals who need it. Many factors could be helpful in enhancing respective state PDMPs; these include measures such as active management, including transmission of alerts to prescribers for whom potential problems have been detected, real-time data availability, and universal use of the system by all possible prescribers of all controlled substances.

U.S. states have the primary responsibility for regulating and enforcing prescription drug practices, including those of painkillers. Pain clinics, in particular, have proliferated at alarming rates. Some pain clinics have arisen to be one of the major contributors to our current prescription painkiller abuse epidemic, specifically those that are a ready source of large numbers of prescriptions. Laws to regulate pain clinics can help reduce much of the misuse and abuse of painkiller medications. These include, for example, laws that require state oversight of pain management clinics as well as those that require specific registration, licensure, or ownership requirements for pain management clinics. Pain management clinics are facilities that prescribe and distribute controlled painkiller substances. Any stipulated conditions upon such operations are all potential cases that could possibly be covered by painkiller legislation, such as: inspection and complaint procedures; specified personnel and operational requirements; processes for awarding, denying, renewing, or revoking of licenses; health and safety requirements; billing procedures; and standards of care. Collectively, these types of measures should help at least reduce, if not eliminate, indiscriminate or inappropriate prescribing and dispensing of painkiller medications. By August 31, 2010, three states had enacted pain management clinic laws, and by September 28, 2012, eight states had implemented such laws. For example, states like Florida and Kentucky include provisions on controlling the advertising of pain management services. However, as enforcement efforts have become focused on rogue pain clinics in one state, many simply relocate to a nearby state with fewer regulatory controls. For instance, as many pain clinics were investigated and closed down in Florida, where much of the trend initially flourished, many just moved their operations on to Georgia, and then on to Tennessee, and so forth.

There is, somewhat surprisingly, considerable variability in the rate of prescriptions written for opiate or opioid painkillers among respective U.S. states, despite the relative uniformity of the underlying health conditions acknowledged to cause pain. In 2012, Alabama was the highest prescribing state with a prevalence of 143 per 100 people, which is nearly 3 times the prevalence of painkiller prescriptions per person in the lowest-prescribing state. After Alabama, Tennessee, and West Virginia were the next highest painkiller prescribing states; in fact, 10 of the highest prescribing states were located in the South. Of course, it is recognized that higher prevalence rates of prescribing are associated with more deaths from overdose. On the other hand, per-person prescribing rates for long-acting and high-dose opioid painkiller medications were highest in the Northeast, particularly in Maine and in New Hampshire. However, even in Hawaii, the lowest-prescribing state, there was still an exceedingly high prevalence rate of painkiller prescribing at 52 per 100 people.

It is highly imperative that we establish a series of policies and programs that will increase the number of addicts engaged in drug treatment. This would, of necessity, include measures directed at expansion of the patient capacity of drug treatment programs to make them more appealing and convenient to painkiller abusers. Removal of any barriers to treatment entry is very critical, including those around cost and insurance coverage. It is estimated, for instance, that currently established methadone maintenance clinics can accommodate only about 15% to 20% of the total number of heroin addicts in the United States. Further, some addicts refuse to enroll in methadone maintenance programs because of the fear of stigmatization if they were seen entering such clinics. The need for other treatment options is clearly well established. Buprenorphine maintenance treatment programs have emerged as safer and effective therapeutic alternatives. Since buprenorphine is a partial agonist, there is a "ceiling effect" at which point higher doses do not produce greater effects. This effect creates a wider margin of safety than that associated with use of methadone, larger doses of which can result in fatal overdoses. This greater safety margin is part of the reason that buprenorphine is listed as a Schedule III medication, while methadone is a more highly regulated Schedule II medication. In addition, withdrawal symptoms appear to be resolved more rapidly when buprenorphine is used to taper off individuals than when methadone is used. Furthermore, administration of other medications has been shown to improve treatment effectiveness. For example, in preliminary clinical studies, administration of catechol-O-methyltransferase inhibitors, such as entacapone, has been found to improve patient adherence with buprenorphine main-tenance treatment programs. Similarly, use of beta-blockers, such as the beta-adrenoceptor antagonist propranolol, appears to decrease the risk of relapse after a period of abstinence. There should also be coordination with criminal justice initiatives. Achieving a full capacity and multimodality treatment system is a lofty but worthwhile and attainable objective that would go a long way toward amelio-rating our current painkiller crisis.

There is also the promise of new and emerging pharmacologic agents and other treatments that may, in the future, help manage, if not possibly even cure, some of the health conditions routinely associated with the experience of pain on the part of those afflicted and thereby necessitating the ready use of painkillers. For example, potential advances for addressing rheumatoid arthritis include biological drugs that act as inhibitors to neutralize cytokines and inhibiting inflammation, such as JAK-STAT inhibitors like ABT-494, baricitinib, and filcotinib, which play a role in cytokine-induced signal trans-duction and interleukin inhibiting. Tofacitinib and other JAK inhibitors, for instance, suppress phosphorylation and transformational alterations in the sig-nal transduction and activator of transcription (STAT) pathway of tyrosine kinases preventing downstream pro-inflammatory mediation. Tocilizumab is an interleukin-6 inhibitor that has helped some individuals achieve remis-sion of rheumatoid arthritis symptoms. Many other related pharmacological agents, such as mavrilimumab and surilumab, are under development and may, in the future, serve to effectively remediate pain associated with rheuma-toid arthritis; with similar work being done to address some of the other disor-ders commonly associated with pain and thereby reducing the reliance upon and overuse of painkillers. Furthermore, individuals in treatment programs for opiate and opioid dependency, particularly those in integrated opioid sub-stitution programs, are more likely to be assessed for and be delivered treat-ment services for other associated health problems, such as HIV and hepatitis C virus infections.

Pharmaceutical regulation is a strategy that has long been used to prevent abuse. For example, in London, the Royal College of Physicians endeavored from their founding in 1518 to supervise the professional activities engaged in by apothecaries, who could examine and order destruction of any defective pharmaceutical products, including opium. In 1617, also in London, the Society of Apothecaries was founded as a separate guild that regulated the affairs of its members. In 1851, the Pharmacy Act was passed by the British Parliament, and in 1868, it passed the more important Pharmacy and Poisons Act, both of which regulated the sale of drugs, including painkillers. In 1914, the U.S. Congress passed the Harrison Narcotics Act, which forbid the sale of opiates unless prescribed by a physician and dispensed by a pharmacist. A series of subsequent legislation, as discussed in Chapter 7, further tightened the regulation and control of painkillers and related pharmaceutical products.

Harm reduction strategies are intended to minimize the harmful consequences associated with the use of painkillers and other drugs. Harm reduction considers painkiller use to be a complex, multifaceted phenomenon that ranges along a wide continuum of behaviors from severe addiction to total abstinence. It recognizes that there are some ways of using painkillers that are obviously safer than other ways. Harm reduction proponents hold to a nonjudgmental, noncoercive approach to policies, services, and resources. Needle exchange programs, for example, are a harm reduction approach that are designed to reduce the probability that injection drug users will share their syringes, which, in turn, would help reduce the spread of infectious diseases like HIV and hepatitis C. These needle exchange programs provide clean injection equipment, and most provide additional services such as safe injection sites, information about drugs and related health information, and referrals to drug treatment by request. Substitution therapies, such as those utilizing methadone or buprenorphine, are also a harm reduction approach intended to reduce the harmful consequences of illicit painkiller use; other drugs tried in some countries for painkiller replacement therapy include heroin, morphine, dihydrocodeine, dihydroetorphine, hydromorphone, and piritramide. Many countries also have harm reduction programs that use naloxone to prevent opiate- or opioid-overdose deaths.

The experience of having different types of pain are, of course, interrelated. For instance, we know that the prevalence of preexisting pain, or of chronic pain as well, increases the risk of suffering from severe postoperative pain. Variability in pain experiences is very commonly observed, including an individual's response to a specific painkiller. The inter-individual variability in most pain disorders is only slightly explained by demographic, environmental, psychological, and physiological factors. Pain experiences clearly shape the attentional and emotional processes related to pain. Further, we know that individuals taking preoperative opiates or opioids are more likely to report chronic postsurgical pain than those not taking such drugs. Accordingly, identification and successful resolution of such intervening background variables might be highly effective at reducing, if not even eliminating, the need for the use of painkillers in the first place. These types of preventative initiatives could potentially positively alter the levels of painkiller abuse presently observed.

Genetic testing is a technique that may be incorporated in the management of pain to optimize the efficacy of and to increase the appropriate prescribing of painkillers on an individualized basis. We recognize, for example, that genetics can influence both our sensitivity to a physical pain stimulus as well as alter the potencies of many painkiller drugs. The cytochrome P450 (CYP) family of genes is known to be responsible for the synthesis of at least 57 enzymes, many of which are involved in the metabolism of most currently used painkiller drugs. The CYP2D6 gene is a highly polymorphic member of this family; it is only about 2% of all CYP genes expressed in the human body, but it is responsible for the conversion and metabolism of many drugs; it has more than 80 variants, and these are responsible for, among other things, the metabolism of codeine into morphine. Thus, knowledge of specific CYP2D alleles an individual carries can be predictive of low or high morphine formation from codeine administration. The CYP2C9 gene is responsible for the synthesis of about 50% of the enzymes in this metabolic system, lack of which can lead to poor metabolism and prolonged action of NSAIDs that can cause severe gastrointestinal bleeding. Women, for instance, who have the G allele of the OPRM1 gene experience twice as much pain as men and thus also require higher doses of fentanyl for pain relief. Separately designed genetic testing may, in the future, also be useful for helping to predict the risks for painkiller abuse and addiction in individuals with different genetic backgrounds, such as those associated with the regulation of the dopamine reward system. There are, in this regard, 7 pain reduction genes, including that responsible for guanosine triphosphate cyclohydrolase 1/ dopa-responsive dystonia (GCH1), which is essential for dopamine and serotonin synthesis. The GCH1 gene has been found to be protective for pain in White populations, but not for pain in American Blacks with sickle cell genes. There is a pyrosequencing tool under investigational research that focuses on 11 loci in the DRD2 gene and in the ANKK1 domain of genes that may help screen for risk assessment for opioid abuse and addiction. These are but a few examples to illustrate that there are multiple drug-related genes. There therefore appears to be variation in the pharmacogenetic shaping of painkiller metabolism, or pharmacokinetics, as well as of transport and receptor signaling, or pharmacodynamics. The future of genotype-based selection and dosing of respective painkillers can provide for more targeted and safer pharmacogenetics with fewer adverse side effects, and hopefully, this will then help reduce abuse. Genetic testing might, accordingly, be used in the future to inform clinical decisions on not only the best therapeutic options for an individual patient, but also, perhaps, help to predict outcomes.

The continuum of care concept holds that painkiller and related treatment programs should provide appropriate services to individuals with multiple needs at appropriate times. This is based on a systems-level approach to coordinating health and human services to individuals with multiple needs, such as those with co-occurring disorders, homelessness, and assorted medical conditions on top of their painkiller abuse. Treatment planning within the continuum of care should endeavor to provide seamless services for patient-centered treatment tailored to an individual's needs. This approach should both enhance treatment outcomes as well as improve the quality of life for patients.

CRIMINAL JUSTICE INITIATIVES

Criminal justice initiatives have been and will no doubt in the future continue to be a major component of a comprehensive response to painkiller abuse. In this regard, it has been estimated that about 4,187 tons of opium, or about 418 tons if the total was all converted to heroin, are produced annually around the world for illicit use. Several criminal justice initiatives have been directed at controlling the flow of painkiller drugs, especially the opiates and opioids. The criminal justice approaches employed in this endeavor will, out of necessity, have to be multifaceted and multilayered.

Trade in prohibited painkillers and other psychoactive drugs is arguably the largest illegal market in the world; accordingly, drug smuggling is probably the type of transnational criminal activity that generates the greatest revenues for its participants. Around 13.5 million people around the world are estimated to be consumers of opiate and opioid drugs, about 9 million of whom are primarily heroin users. Across Europe, it is estimated that about 1.5 million individuals are regular consumers of heroin, with about 200,000 individuals in the United States using heroin. This volume of use generates considerable demand, which drug traffickers are readily attempting to satisfy. In fact, sophisticated multinational distribution systems have been created to conduct this illegal trade and, consequently, numerous criminal justice initiatives have been developed to counter it.

Several criminal justice agencies are actively involved in combating these drug-related issues. The Drug Enforcement Administration (DEA) of the U.S. Department of Justice is a leading federal criminal justice agency tasked with combating drug use and trafficking, including that of licit and illicit painkillers. The DEA was established in 1973 during the Nixon administration as part of the so-called War on Drugs. In 1988, the Office of National Drug Control Policy (ONDCP) was established by the Anti-Drug Abuse Act, which was amended in 1996 and reauthorized in 1998 to expand its authority and functions, basically to target drug-related crime and violence, including, of course, that related to painkillers.

The U.S. Department of State Bureau of International Narcotics and Law Enforcement is a federal agency responsible for reducing the entry of illegal drugs by minimizing the impacts of international narcotics trafficking and its associated criminal activities. Efforts of the bureau include modernizing law enforcement and criminal justice systems in other countries. The bureau was initially called the Bureau of International Narcotics Matters as initially created by the U.S. Congress on October 1, 1975, with passage of the Foreign Relations Authorization Act for 1979. On February 10, 1995, it was renamed the Bureau of International Narcotics and Law Enforcement. It has established International Law Enforcement Academies in four geographic areas—Europe, Africa, Asia, and South America. The various academies are designed to protect American citizens and corporations around the world, to help sustain democracy and free markets, and to aid in fostering government legitimacy, as well as improving security and stability by means of reducing narcotics trafficking and associated crime. Other initiatives of the Bureau of International Narcotics and Law Enforcement involve providing training and equipment to criminal justice enforcement operations, as well as oversight and technical assistance for long-term reform of security agencies, corrections systems, and related criminal justice institutions around the world. These efforts help individual countries to improve the interdiction of trafficked drugs, to gather intelligence, and to communicate effectively with other criminal justice organizations. The Bureau of International Narcotics and Law Enforcement also has a Narcotics Reward Program that is able to issue rewards of up to $5 million for information that leads to the arrest and conviction of major narcotics traffickers operating outside of the United States. The Bureau of International Narcotics and Law Enforcement operates the Office of Civilian Police and Rule of Law Programs that help to establish adequate law enforcement, criminal justice, and corrections systems in postconflict societies. The Bureau of International Narcotics and Law Enforcement also operates under its charge an Office of Aviation that provides support for the planning, logistics, and conducting of counter-narcotics aviation initiatives around the world.

There are two major international agencies involved in the policing of international drug crimes—the International Criminal Police Organization, known as Interpol; and the European Police Office, known as Europol. These two criminal justice agencies are poised to provide much of the policing of painkillers and related drugs around the world.

The International Narcotics Control Board (INCB) is a UN agency that is responsible for regulating the global supply of opium as well as that of related painkiller drugs. It does this, as previously mentioned under the discussion of international policies, by means of enforcing the rules of the 1961 Single

Convention on Narcotic Drugs and subsequent conventions. This Single Convention stipulates that a country can purchase opium poppies only in an amount corresponding to its use of opium-derived drugs, such as codeine and morphine. It also empowers the UN policy bodies, the World Health Organization (WHO) and the Commission on Narcotic Drugs, to maintain and update schedules of controlled substances so that newly created drugs, such as synthetic opioids, can rapidly be addressed.

Drug interdiction efforts consist of myriad strategies intended to reduce consumption of specific drugs, such as the opiate painkillers, by making it more risky and expensive for smugglers to conduct their operations. Drug interdiction consists of monitoring, detection, pursuit, and apprehension activities. Drug interdiction has accounted for a substantial portion of spending by the federal government on drug control. Critics have argued that these funds could probably be more effectively spent if allocated to drug treatment programs and other efforts that could help reduce demand rather than supply of illicit drugs.

Nearly all illegal drug sales require some type of money laundering. The Money Laundering Control Act, passed by Congress in 1986, established the criminalization of money laundering in the United States. The 1988 UN Convention against Illicit Traffic in Narcotic Drugs and Psychotropic Substances established the basic accepted elements of criminal money laundering. The Annunzio-Wylie Anti–Money Laundering Suppression Act of 1992 and the Money Laundering Suppression Act of 1994 strengthened the sanctions and enhanced the procedures for referring money laundering cases to criminal justice agencies. Anti–money laundering controls are promulgated by the Financial Action Task Force (FATF) on Money Laundering. The UNODC maintains a website that disseminates information and software programs that can be used for data collection and analysis of money laundering activities; the site is referred to as the International Money Laundering Information Network. The World Bank also maintains a website that provides best practices for governments and private sector organizations on issues related to money laundering.

An extensive and very expensive series of drug eradication efforts have been directed over the years at reducing the cultivation of opium poppies and production of its illicit drug derivatives; most of these eradication programs were conducted in the Golden Crescent, in the Golden Triangle, and in Latin America. Eradication techniques have included aerial spraying of poisons and destroying plants by hand or by machines like tractors, but alternative development programs may, in the future, be the most effective approaches. Since the middle of the 1970s, Mexico has engaged in aerial herbicide spraying of opium and cannabis fields. Crop substitution programs have met with some success. For example, in the early 1970s, Turkey paid farmers to harvest opium poppies early before the opiate containing seed pods developed. Rural development projects have been a related strategy used with some success as well to reduce poppy cultivation. In the early 1980s, joint U.S. and Pakistani development effort resulted in a reduction of poppy production. Similarly, in the early 1990s, the Highland Village Project conducted development activities in northern Thailand that helped convince many members in traditional opium-producing hill tribes to decrease opium cultivation. Over the same time, the international drug control system evolved, mainly by means of a series of international conventions. These types of measures have certainly impacted global opium production, which is currently substantially lower than it was at the opening of the 20th century. For example, in 2002, global opium production was one-sixth the level of production that existed in 1907 to 1908. Seizures of illicit opiate and opioid drugs, mainly opium, morphine, and heroin, have also increased dramatically. This trend noticeably emerged in the 1980s and was expanded even more in the 1990s. Most of the narcotics seized in North America were produced in Mexico and South America, principally Colombia, but from elsewhere around the globe as well. However, opiate seizures in North American accounted for only about 4% of global seizures. Most of the opium, morphine, and heroin—over three-quarters, in fact—trafficked around the world was produced in Southwest and Central Asia, described previously as the Golden Crescent, principally those nations that border Afghanistan. In this vein, in April 2015, the Indian navy seized a boat carrying 200 kg of heroin estimated to be worth almost $100 million, which makes it the largest heroin seizure ever. The so-called Golden Triangle of Southeast Asia, also discussed earlier, is the world's second-largest producer and trafficker of these types of drugs. Myanmar alone accounts for about 18% of all global opium production. However, most of these drugs produced in Southeast Asia are consumed within the region.

An interesting type of criminal justice initiative that has helped with supply reduction, as well as with reducing crime rates, is those designed to reduce drug dealing. Project High Point, for example, is a very successful antidrug program based on a police-community partnership to help identify drug dealers in the community, warn them about the undesirable outcomes if they continued dealing drugs, and provide them with supportive services for rehabilitation and for treatment if needed. Likewise, HOPE Probation is a high-intensity program of criminal justice supervision intended to reduce recidivism by offering rapid and predictable sanctions to probation violators by means of implementing random urine drug testing. These kinds of programs have already demonstrated promising results, including a reduction of local crime rates, and offer hope for similar initiatives in the future.

Criminal justice statistics can furnish a reasonable foundation for those wishing to diminish use of painkillers and related drugs. In this vein, the Bureau of Justice Statistics reported that there has been an increasingly significant trend from 2000 to 2013 in the growing proportion of arrestees testing positive for opiates and opioids in their bodies at the time of arrest. For example, in Sacramento, California, in 2000, 3% of all arrestees tested positive for opiates, 6% tested positive in 2007, and 18% tested positive in 2013 (the most recent year for which data is available). Similarly, in Denver, Colorado, 4% of arrestees were opiate positive in 2000, which doubled to 8% in 2013. In addition, significant increases in heroin use among a younger group of users is indicated by the proportion of users being drawn from the younger ranks of arrestees. The average age at first use for those arrestees who admitted heroin use in the past 30 days dropped in many major cities in this country from 2012 to 2013, such as: from 23.7% to 21.2% in Atlanta, Georgia; from 24.1% to 23.4% in Denver; and from 23.3% to 22.1% in New York City. The increased availability of heroin for sale on the streets of New York City has risen significantly as evidenced by the percentages of arrestees reporting difficulty in purchasing heroin, which dropped from 77% in 2007 to 35% in 2013. In fact, 22% of arrestees in New York City who reported a failed heroin purchase attributed it to greater police activity, while another 12% attributed it to a lack of availability—again attributable, at least in part, to criminal justice initiatives. Further, the acquisition of heroin in the past 30 days by arrestees increased in several major cities from 2012 to 2013, such as: from 10.0% to 15.5% in Chicago, Illinois; from 6.2% to 8.3% in Denver; and from 7.4% to 11.6% in Sacramento. The percentage of adult male arrestees who acquired heroin and reported cash buys in the past 30 days also increased in most cities from 2012 to 2013, such as: from 94.3% to 96.7% in Chicago; from 74.1% to 97.2% in Denver; from 63.3% to 93.5% in New York City; and from 52.3% to 74.7% in Sacramento. Likewise, the average number of purchases of heroin in the past 30 days also increased in most cities from 2012 to 2013, such as: from 11.6% to 14.4% in Atlanta; from 13.7% to 19.1% in Chicago; from 14.0% to 16.0% in Denver; from 16.3% to 16.7% in New York City; and from 7.8% to 16.2% in Sacramento. Very alarmingly, the percentage of arrestees who reported injection drug use at their most recent use increased considerably in several major cities in this country from 2012 to 2013, such as: from 42.5% to 49.4% in Denver; from 39.2% to 42.8% in New York City; and from 56.7% to 66.2% in Sacramento.

In March 2015, the UN Commission on Narcotics Drugs adopted a resolution calling on criminal justice and health agencies to work collaboratively to offer a range of alternatives to incarceration of those affected by a substance use disorder. The resolution was initially proposed by the White House Office of National Drug Control Policy and reflects an emerging global consensus that simply arresting and incarcerating those affected by a substance use disorder will not solve the drug problem. Sustained recovery when achieved would not only promote fairness, but it would substantially help reduce prison overcrowding. Various reforms including reduced or suspended sentences, pretrial and trial diversion programs, home detention, fines, community service, victim restitution, random drug testing, and GPS tracking are some of the potential recommendations suggested as alternatives to incarceration. The first drug court opened in 1989 in Miami, Florida, and today there are nearly 4,000 drug courts operating in all 50 U.S. states and territories as well as in several foreign countries, such as Australia, Canada, New Zealand, and the UK. Decriminalization measures, where addicts are not punished, rather than outright legalization of drugs, may also offer additional promise. For example, decriminalization along with increased drug treatment such as has been implemented in Portugal appears to be a highly effective approach, where over 10 years the level of injection drug use declined by 50%. Effectively combining criminal justice supervision and evidence-based drug treatment can not only lower prison costs, but also promote better health outcomes and effective crime prevention, including a reduction of painkiller misuse and abuse.

Another criminal justice area that has witnessed a considerable array of initiatives has been that of providing substance abuse treatment in jails and prisons. It is generally accepted that there may be compelling reasons that lead an individual to engage in criminal activity. For many individuals, it may be problems with painkillers or related drugs that directly led to criminal behaviors. Accordingly, prisons and jails can serve as appropriate places to begin or continue substance abuse treatment, particularly for the younger-aged offenders whose dependence issues contributed to their involvement in criminal activities. These programs operate along a range of intensity from preventative educational and support group programs to more intensive group therapy–based approaches to various total immersion strategies, such as that of therapeutic communities, which have, in fact, become fairly prevalent in correctional settings.

PATIENT RIGHTS

The rights of patients suffering with pain has a long political history in American society. In 1956, during his first administration, President Dwight

D. Eisenhower signed the Social Security Amendments that ushered in an era
of politicized pain. This legislation and subsequent measures have progressively expanded the scope of pain and disability rights. A liberal pain standard
arose during the 1960s, but there was a conservative backlash during the
Ronald Reagan era of the 1980s. The movement to expand consideration of
pain continued to gain momentum throughout the 1990s. The Affordable
Care Act, which contains measures for pain relief, including end-of-life provisions and fetal pain, continues this trend.

Advances achieved after passage of the Affordable Care Act have helped
enhance marketplace operations in order to make them more patient focused.
The Affordable Care Act, in fact, includes substance abuse disorders as one of
the 10 elements of essential health benefits. Improvements have been indicated in areas such as nondiscrimination, transparency, uniformity, continuity
of care, and enforcement. Qualified health plans are prohibited from discrimi-
nating against individuals with preexisting conditions; this includes those suffering with complex chronic conditions like those associated with some pain
disorders. Benefit design elements such as utilization management techniques,
cost-sharing requirements, and the structure of the formulary could potentially
create barriers to access by imposing unintended or intended restrictions to use
certain newer, and usually more costly, painkillers. With respect to transparency, information about health plans should contain easy-to-find formularies,
including painkillers covered, as well as provider networks covered. As for uniformity, it would be helpful if the federal government required qualified health
plans to use a standard template for formularies, which would make comparison between plans easier; it would also be helpful if the process to appeal
adverse plan coverage determinations was easier to understand and navigate,
particularly with respect to what constitutes a medical necessity. Continuity
of care becomes an issue when individuals elect to transition to new plans, particularly with respect to following prescriptions for painkillers and other medications on which the patient was stabilized. Enforcement to assure that
qualified health plans authorized under the Affordable Care Act have standards
that are uniform across the United States would benefit from broad federal
monitoring.

The fragmented nature of the American health care system exacerbates the
lack of coordination in health care delivery, including that pertaining to pain
care. The processing of prescription payments and management of the preferred drug list or formulary, for just two examples, have imposed inappropriate barriers to reasonable pain care. Hopefully, revisions to the Affordable
Care Act will help remediate these current shortcomings in our health care
system.

As a consequence of provisions in the Affordable Care Act, the Centers for Medicare and Medicaid Services (CMS) have been charged with additional responsibilities. These include administration of program integration initiatives, facilitating greater transparency and increasing data collection and analysis. It is hoped that use of both provider data and data on individual patients can help move these agencies from a fee-for-service-based payer to a value-based purchaser of health care. The charge of greater transparency means that the availability and utility of health care data will be collaboratively available to all interested stakeholders, including nonprofit, private, and public-sector agencies. This will include, for a few examples, Part D prescription drug event data, assessment data, Medicare Advantage encounter data and fee for service claims data, quality data and survey data, such as that from the Consumer Assessment of Healthcare Providers and Systems, the Health Outcomes Survey, the Healthcare Effectiveness Data and Information Set, and the Medicare Current Beneficiary Survey. CMS, for example, has been using its Fraud Prevention System since June 2011 to screen claims; in its second year, the system identified or prevented $210.7 million in inappropriate payments, and administrative action was taken against 938 service providers and suppliers, including several pain clinics. CMS also maintains Physician Compare, a website that allows consumers to search for physicians and other health care professionals who provide Medicare services, including pain management services.

As more health care providers move from paper-based to electronic, real-time, standardized processes, some of the barriers to access that have reduced the use of painkillers and other medications may be eliminated. Further, as these processes become more integrated into health care providers' operations, it could substantially reduce the time required to secure authorizations for coverage.

More patient education activities can increase the likelihood that pain patients will be more active in their health care and, hopefully, reduce the levels of misuse and abuse of painkillers. We know that patient adherence is greater among individuals with positive attitudes. Accordingly, more patient education activities designed to alter attitudes and beliefs about pain management may help achieve greater rates of treatment success. It is, for instance, not uncommon for individuals to equate lack of achieving successful pain management and the associated need for more painkillers with personal failure. Similarly, negative attitudes on the part of health care providers can undermine optimal pain management. Sociocultural factors also can contribute to an individual's attitudes and beliefs about pain management, including their view of patient-provider relationships. However, we must recognize that knowledge alone is not sufficient to improve treatment outcomes, but it can at least help prevent some of the common misunderstandings about pain care. It is thus important to engage patients in shared decision-making and helping them to set realistic and achievable goals. Better-educated patients are much more likely to engage with providers and to adhere to therapeutic guidelines. Successful pain management can help build mutually beneficial and respectful partnerships with clearer communication interactions. This can be done only if the health care providers take the time to understand what is regarded as important to the patient and are able and willing to take the time to listen to them.

Certainly each individual and each family should be actively engaged partners in their pain care. For this to be a reality, individuals must be given access to information and knowledge in order to be able to make better-informed decisions. The importance of patient education is central to this approach to better foster collaboration in which individuals and clinicians can work together to help attain mutually agreed-upon painkiller goals. Individuals joining online pain communities can also be at least a partial solution. Other possible strategies include use of wearable technologies, more pre-visit planning, and incorporation of patient advisory councils, all to lead to improved communication, more affordable health care, and healthier people. This is all within the context of participatory medicine, in which networked individuals take greater responsibility for their health care. This should not only yield better outcomes and increase patient satisfaction, but also generate substantial cost savings and reduced medical errors.

It is estimated that about 8% of individuals living in the United States have a substance use disorder and that between 9% and 14% of Medicaid beneficiaries have a substance use disorder. Unfortunately, despite the significant role that some medications can potentially play in successfully treating these disorders, particularly for the treatment of opiate and opioid dependence, Medicaid programs need to improve the funding and delivery of clinically effective as well as cost-effective approaches available for providing these medications and related counseling services. In this regard, prior authorization, as of 2013, was required in 48 Medicaid programs for coverage of buprenorphine and buprenorphine naloxone combination formulations. However, as buprenorphine and naloxone combined medications have recently become available in generic formulations, we can expect a relaxing of the prior authorization requirements.

The advent of generic drugs has generally resulted in greater access and lower costs for most individuals. In the 1960s, only about 10% of prescriptions were filled by pharmacists with generic drugs, but by 2014, the proportion had risen to over 84%. Currently, generic drugs account for 29% of all pharmaceutical spending and 86% of all drugs dispensed in the United States. As more painkiller medications as well as more medications used in treating painkiller abusers, such as buprenorphine and naloxone, become available in generic forms in the future, we can expect to see even more people having the availability of and the routine using of these substances.

The problems of opiate and opioid drug abuse and dependence will likely remain a serious problem for the near future. There are currently around 700,000 heroin users in the United States, a figure that is double of what it was in 2005. It is generally thought that about 23% of heroin users will eventually become dependent on it. Further, it is believed that 81% of current first-time heroin users first started using prescription opioids. Thus, drug prevention efforts that successfully reduce the use and abuse of prescription opioids should, in turn, also result in substantial reductions in heroin use and abuse.

The Affordable Care Act is encouraging new addiction treatment models and improvements in both the quantity and quality of painkiller treatment options. The safety, efficacy and cost-effectiveness of medication assisted treatments, in particular, offers considerable hope for future improvements and the development of even more painkiller treatment alternatives. Medication assisted treatments have already been shown to have much success in reducing illicit opiate or opioid use and in restoring individuals to healthier lifestyles. Certainly not all painkiller abusers could benefit from medication-assisted treatment, but most probably could. Many pharmacological agents are potentially available to offer various alternatives so that treatment can be tailored to each individual's needs and circumstances.

SUMMARY

Pain control and management should be based on the best evidence available. As research efforts progress, we must be vigilant and continuously measure and close the feedback loops in treating individuals with pain issues. We must make a concerted effort to reduce the unexplained clinical variation with respect to the use of respective painkillers. This may be at least partly dealt with by reducing the rigid constraints of professional domains of autonomy. Further, health care providers need to engage with clients across the continuum of care in order to provide better pain treatment. In this regard, health care workers often serve as an interface between individuals who inject drugs and standard health care services. The use of community health workers can partially help overcome common barriers to access, such as fear of stigma, discrimination, and mistrust. Although pharmaceutical manufacturers, criminal justice authorities, regulatory bodies, and health plans attempt to introduce multiple and more complex countermeasures, the misuse and abuse of prescription opiate and opioid painkillers continues and is increasing.

This consideration of painkillers, such as opium, morphine, and other opiate and opioid drugs, as well as of the NSAIDs and other over-the-counter and prescription analgesics, has revealed much about the background to these substances. However, like many academic endeavors, this examination through the lens of these substances shows us more about ourselves and other societies than it does about the substances themselves.

DOCUMENT: A MODEL POLICY FOR THE USE OF PAINKILLERS

Policy makers are grappling with the drastic need to adopt strategies that will both protect clinical practice while also helping reduce the rising levels of opiate and opioid abuse. Many states have already adopted a model policy for the medical use of controlled substances that was drafted by the Federation of State Medical Boards. The accompanying table, adapted from P. G. Fine and R. K. Portenoy's (2007) "A Clinical Guide to Opioid Analgesia," 2nd edition, and included in Opioid Prescribing: Clinical Tools and Risk Management Strategies *by A. V. Anderson, P. G. Fine, and S. M. Fishman, presents the key elements for such a model policy for the use of controlled substances in the treatment of pain consistent with these guidelines, along with recommendations for the implementation of these strategies in clinical practice. The dire reality is that clinicians must struggle with trying to treat pain patients, while at the same time becoming increasingly fearful of the emerging difficulties involved in managing the provision of opiate and opioid analgesics. These guidelines can serve as the basis for formulating a cogent framework approach to structure and document the delivery of appropriate painkiller therapy.*

Implementing the Model Policy for the Use of Controlled Substances for the Treatment of Pain

Guideline	Criteria	How to Integrate into Practice
Patient evaluation	• Document history and physical examination • Document pain history, comorbidities, history of substance abuse, and indication for opioid	• Make time to listen carefully to patients in pain using a reflective listening approach • Remain mindful of the need for suspicion without a rush to judgment • Look for signs of abuse, but recognize the complexities of presentation and the possibilities of pseudoaddiction • Remember that not treating pain is often not a "safe" option
Treatment plan	• State objectives that determine success (pain relief, improved physical and psychosocial function) • Adjust treatment over time to reflect individual patient needs • Prescribe nonopioid therapies when needed	• Use a function-based paradigm at diagnosis and for treatment plan • Develop list of functional losses and gains to be impacted by care, then track and modify • "Feeling better" without improved function may not reflect quality of life improvement • Modest pain score reductions may reflect significant gains in function
Informed consent and agreement for treatment	• Discuss risks and benefits of controlled substance with patient and/or family/guardian • Use one physician and pharmacy whenever possible • Consider written agreement if risk of abuse is high, including drug screening when requested, number and frequency of all prescription refills, and reason for discontinuing drug therapy (violation of agreement)	• Patients must fully understand potential risks and benefits of any procedure or treatment to be fully informed • Incorporate risk education information into a clear and transparent process, whether or not you are prescribing a controlled substance • Prepare educational materials and develop a process for implementation in advance • Use a written agreement/informed consent process to address key points
Periodic review	• Evaluate progress toward treatment objectives to determine continuation or modification of therapy • Satisfactory response includes decreased pain, increased function, and improved quality of life • Use objective indicators as well as information from family members and other caregivers • Reconsider or change treatment if progress is unsatisfactory	• Closely monitor treatment outcomes and be alert to wide range of adverse effects • Have means of measuring progress toward functional goals and clearly document • Patients bear the responsibility of attaining treatment goals and providing evidence • Assess functional goals and adjust as needed

(continued)

Implementing the Model Policy for the Use of Controlled Substances for the Treatment of Pain

Guideline	Criteria	How to Integrate into Practice
Consultation	• Be willing to refer patients at particular risk for or misuse, abuse, or diversion • Consider consulting an expert for patients with history of substance abuse or comorbid psychiatric disorder	• Build a network of clinical experts to whom you can turn for specialized needs • Be clear with yourself about your expertise and don't hesitate to refer patients early • Remember that the most "difficult" patients may be the ones who need your help the most

Documentation	• Accurate and complete medical records should include:
	  ○ Medical history and physical exam
	  ○ Diagnostic, therapeutic, and laboratory results
	  ○ Evaluations and consultations
	  ○ Treatment objectives
	  ○ Discussion of risks and benefits
	  ○ Informed consent
	  ○ Treatments
	  ○ Medications (date, type, dosage, and quantity prescribed)
	  ○ Instructions and agreements
	  ○ Periodic reviews
		• Documentation is essential at every step of pain care delivery
		• Document assessments, treatment agreements, education, action plans, and patient monitoring activities
		• Be clear and transparent about risk management decision making
		• Include specific information that can be understood by others reading the record

Compliance with controlled substances laws and regulations	• Physician must be licensed in the state and comply with applicable federal and state regulations	• Know regulations on controlled substances issued by state medical board and adhere strictly to them • Know and adhere to federal regulations issued in the Physicians Manual of the US Drug Enforcement Administration

Source: A. V. Anderson, P. G. Fine, and S. M. Fishman. "Table 12. Implementing a Model Policy for the Treatment of Pain." Opioid prescribing: Clinical tools and Risk management strategies. Available online at http://mn.gov/health-licensing-boards/images/Opioid_Prescribing_Clinical_Tools_and_Risk_Management_Strategies.pdf. Used by permission of the American Academy of Pain Management.

Directory of Resources

CENTERS FOR DISEASE CONTROL AND PREVENTION (CDC)

The U.S. CDC is charged with protecting America from health, safety, and security threats. To accomplish its objective, the CDC provides health information, including that related to painkiller use and abuse.

Contact: United States Centers for Disease Control and Prevention
1600 Clifton Road
Atlanta, GA 30329
1-800-CDC-INFO (1-800-323-4636)
http://www.cdc.gov/

DRUG ENFORCEMENT AGENCY (DEA)

The DEA is part of the U.S. Department of Justice. It is the major federal agency responsible for domestic enforcement of U.S. drug policy.

Contact: United States Drug Enforcement Agency
800 K Street, NW, Suite 500
Washington, DC 20001
1-202-305-8500
http://www.dea.gov/

To report illegal painkiller sales/distribution, call: 1-877-792-2873

FOOD AND DRUG ADMINISTRATION (FDA)

The U.S. FDA is responsible for protecting the public health by assuring that foods and drugs, including painkiller medications, are properly labeled and sanitary; with respect to drugs and medical devices, the FDA is responsible for ensuring that they are both safe and effective.

Contact: U.S. Food and Drug Administration
10903 New Hampshire Avenue
Silver Spring, MD 20993
1-888-INFO-FDA (1-888-463-6332)
http://www.fda.gov/

NARCOTICS ANONYMOUS (NA)

Narcotics Anonymous is a 12-step fellowship of men and women seeking recovery from drug addiction.

Contact: NA World Services
P.O. Box 9999
Van Nuys, CA 91409
1-818-773-9999
http://www.na.org

SUBSTANCE ABUSE AND MENTAL HEALTH SERVICES ADMINISTRATION (SAMHSA)

SAMHSA is part of the U.S. Department of Health and Human Services. The primary mission of SAMHSA is to improve the availability and quality of substance abuse prevention, treatment, and mental health services. SAMHSA encompasses the Center for Substance Abuse Prevention (CSAP), the Center for Substance Abuse Treatment (CSAT), and the Center for Mental Health Services, as well as its Office of Applied Studies. Collectively, it is the major federal agency in the United States supporting substance abuse treatment and prevention and mental health initiatives.

Contact: Substance Abuse and Mental Health Services Administration
1 Choke Cherry Road
Rockville, MD 20857
1-877-SAMHSA-7 (1-877-726-4727)

TDD: 1-800-487-4889
http://www.samhsa.gov/

TREATMENT LOCATORS

Buprenorphine Physician and Treatment Program Locator:
http://buprenorphine.samhsa.gov/bwns_locator/

Opioid Treatment Program Directory:
http://dpt2.samhsa.gov/treatment/

Treatment Referral Routing Service Helpline:
1-800-662-HELP (4357)
http://www.samhsa.gov/find-help/national-helpline

Glossary

Abuse: The intentional continued consumption of, in this case, any painkiller drug despite recognition of the harmful consequences of such problems.

Action potential: When a neuron becomes depolarized and as sodium rushes in, a signal is transmitted down the axon; it is an all-or-nothing process either resulting in activation or not firing at all.

Addiction: A primary chronic disease, characterized by relapse, in which compulsive drug seeking and use predominates, even after serious negative consequences are experienced and understood to result from such use; its development and manifestations can be influenced by environmental, genetic, and psychosocial factors.

Afferent: System to transmit pain signals and other neuronal impulses from the periphery into the center, such as from a sensory ending to the central nervous system.

Agonist: A substance that binds to a receptor site and activates it by mimicking the action of other substances that also binds there.

Amygdala: A part of the limbic system of the brain that functions in generating feelings of pain, pleasure, and fear.

Analgesia: The absence of pain sensations in the presence of typically painful stimuli; the body seems to use endorphins and serotonin to block pain stimuli, and painkillers produce a similar effect.

Antagonist: A substance that binds to a receptor site and blocks its action preventing a drug or neurotransmitter from activating it.

Arthritis: Chronic disease that is characterized by inflammation of the joints and its associated pain.

Axon: A fibrous structure that transmits pain signals and other neuronal impulses away from the cell body to neurons or other structures, such as glands or muscles.

Buprenorphine: A mixed opioid agonist/antagonist substance used for treating opiate and opioid dependence.

Central nervous system: That part of the nervous system, specifically the brain and spinal cord, that serves to centrally process information from the sensory systems and to select an appropriate response.

Cognitive behavioral therapy: A treatment approach that helps individuals change the way they think and behave by changing their ways of thinking.

Dendrite: A fibrous structure that transmits pain signals and other neuronal impulses toward the cell body; one neuron can have many hundreds of dendrites.

Efferent: System to transmit pain signals and other neuronal impulses away from the center to the periphery, such as from the spinal cord to a muscle.

Endorphins: Group of neurotransmitters that bind to the same receptor sites that opiate or opioid drugs do and that, consequently, produce similar effects including relief of pain and feelings of euphoria.

Gate control theory: A theory that posits a gate along the spinal cord that either allows pain signals to transmit to the brain or blocks them.

Methadone: A synthetic opioid used in treating opiate and opioid addiction as well as sometimes used as a painkiller.

Misuse: Consumption of, in this case, any painkiller drug in any manner or for any purpose other than that recommended or prescribed by a health care professional.

Myelin sheath: White lipid covering of an axon; provides the white matter for the brain and spinal cord and helps increase the speed of an action potential.

Narcotic: A substance that is used to induce stupor or narcosis, which can include both opiate and opioid drugs.

Neuron: Nerve cell in the brain and nervous system that transmits chemical and electrical impulses.

Neurotransmitter: A chemical substance that enables signal transmission between neurons and related structures, such as acetylcholine, dopamine, and serotonin.

NSAIDs (Non-Steroidal Anti-Inflammatory Drugs): Block the production of prostaglandins, such as acetaminophen, aspirin, and ibuprofen.

Opiate: An opiate drug is a substance that is naturally produced by the opium poppy as a constituent of opium and its derivatives, such as morphine, codeine, and other closely related substances.

Opioid: An opioid drug is a semisynthetic or a synthetic substance that has effects similar to the opiate drugs; heroin is one of the best-known semisynthetic opioids, while drugs like methadone and meperidine are totally synthetic.

Osteoarthritis: A form of arthritis characterized by degeneration of the joint cartilage and its associated pain.

Pain: A subjective warning system that alerts the body to potentially dangerous injuries or conditions manifesting as an unpleasant emotional or sensory experience.

Pain disorder: A somatoform condition characterized by complaints of severe, sometimes constant pain that has no apparent physical cause.

Painkillers: Any substance that when administered helps reduce or manage pain symptoms.

Physical dependence: A physiological state of adaptation that results from chronic use of a drug, where tolerance is generally developed, and one in which withdrawal symptoms manifest when use is dramatically reduced or ceased. It can occur with any type of chronic use, either appropriate or inappropriate, of a drug.

Polydrug abuse: The abuse of two or more drugs at the same general time.

Postsynaptic potential: A change in the potential of a neuron's membrane that received a transmission signal from another neuron.

Prescription abuse: Use of a drug without a prescription, or use in any way other than that prescribed; used interchangeably with nonmedical use.

Receptor site: A structure on the surface of a neuron that allows only specific neurotransmitters or other substances, such as a psychoactive drug or its derivatives, to fit into it and thereby activate it to create an action potential.

Rheumatoid arthritis: A form of arthritis characterized by inflammation of the joints, swelling, stiffness, and associated pain; it can be the most crippling type of arthritis.

Substitution: Practice of administering any substance with the intent of replacing the misuse or abuse of, in this case, any painkiller drug.

Synapse: The minute space between two or more neurons where neurotransmission of signals take place.

Tolerance: A situation of adaptation where, in this case, greater amounts of a painkiller are required to produce a similar effect experienced during earlier use with a lower amount.

Glossary

Use: Consumption of, in this case, any painkiller drug, whether by legal or illegal means.

Vesicle: A small sac-like structure of a neuron that contains a neurotransmitter or its precursor substances produced by the neuron.

Withdrawal: A constellation of unpleasant symptoms that appear when chronic use of, in this case, a painkiller drug is abruptly reduced or stopped.

Bibliography

Acker, C. J. (2002). *Creating the American junkie: Addiction research in the classic era of narcotic control.* Baltimore, MD: Johns Hopkins University Press.

Adams, E. H., Breiner, S. B., Cicero, T. J., Geller, A., Inciardi, J. A., Schnoll, S. H., Senay, E. C., & Woody, G. E. (2005). A comparison of the abuse liability of tramadol, NSAIDs, and hydrocodone in patients with chronic pain. *Journal of Pain and Symptom Management 31*, 465–476.

Agar, M., & Reisinger, H. S. (2002). A tale of two policies: The French connection, methadone, and heroin epidemics. *Culture, medicine and psychiatry 26*, 371–396.

Ahamad, K., Milloy, M. J., Ngyuen, P., Uhlmann, S., Johnson, C., Koethius, T. P., Kerr, T., & Wood, E. (2015). Factors associated with willingness to take extended release naltrexone among injection drug users. *Addiction Science and Clinical Practice 10*, 12.

Ahmadi, J., Sharifi, M., Mohagheghzadeh, S., Dehbozorgi, G. R., Farrashbabdi, H., Moosavinasab, M., Firoozabadi, A., Pridmore, S., Evren, C., Busch, S., & Farash, S. (2004). Pattern of cocaine and heroin abuse in a sample of Iranian population. *German Journal of Psychiatry 8*, 1–4.

Alford, D. P., Compton, P., & Samet, J. H. (2006). Acute pain management for patients receiving maintenance methadone or buprenorphine therapy. *Annals of Internal Medicine 144*, 127–134.

al-Ghazal, S. K. (2003a). Al-Zahrawi (Albucasis)—a light in the Dark Middle Ages in Europe. *Journal of the International Society for the History of Islamic Medicine 2*, 37–38.

al-Ghazal, S. K. (2003b). The valuable contributions of Al-Razi (Rhazes) in the history of pharmacy during the Middle Ages. *Journal of the International Society for the History of Islamic Medicine 2*, 9–11.

Allbutt, T. C. (1869). On the hypodermic use of morphia in diseases of the heart and great vessels. *Practitioner 3*, 342–346.

Allsop, S. J., Ali, R. L., & Edmonds, C. A. (2000). A training, authorization and review process for methadone prescribers. *Journal of Maintenance in the Addictions 1*, 15–25.

Ameke, W. (1885). *History of homoeopathy: Its origins, its conflicts, with an appendix on the present state of university medicine*. London: E. Gould & Son.

American Psychiatric Association (2000). *Diagnostic and statistical manual of mental disorders* (4th ed., text rev.). Washington, DC: Author.

Anderson, A. V., Fine, P. G., & Fishman, S. M. *Opioid prescribing: Clinical tools and risk management strategies* (https://mn.gov/health-licensing-boards/images/Opioid_Prescribing_Clinical_Tools_and_Risk_Management_Strategies.pdf; accessed September 2015).

Anderson, S., & Berridge, V. (2003). Drug misuse and the community pharmacist: A historical overview. In J. Sheridan & J. Strang (Eds.), *Drug misuse and community pharmacy* (pp. 17–35). London: Taylor & Francis.

Angst, M. S., & Clark, D. J. (2006). Opioid-induced hyperalgesia: A qualitative systematic review. *Anesthesiology 104*, 570–587.

Arnold-Reed, D. E., & Hulse, G. K. (2005). A comparison of rapid (opioid) detoxification with clonidine-assisted detoxification for heroin-dependent persons. *Journal of Opioid Management 1*(1), 17–23.

Askitopoulou, H., Ramoutsaki, I. A., & Konsolak, E. (2002). Archaeological evidence on the use of opium in the Minoan world. *International Congress Series 1242*, 23–29.

Aurin, M. (2000). Chasing the dragon: The cultural metamorphosis of opium in the United States, 1825–1935. *Medical Anthropology Quarterly 14*(3), 414–441.

Bailey, W., & Truong, L. (2001). Opium and empire: Some evidence from colonial-era Asian stock and commodity markets. *Journal of Southeast Asian Studies 32*, 173–193.

Baker, D. D., & Jenkins, A. J. (2008). A comparison of methadone, oxycodone, and hydrocodone related deaths in northeast Ohio. *Journal of Analytical Toxicology 32*, 185–171.

Baker, J., Rainey, P. M., Moody, D. E., Morse, G. D., Ma, Q., & McCance-Katz, E. F. (2010). Interactions buprenorphine and antiretrovirals: Nucleos(t)ide reverse transcriptase inhibitors (NRTI) didanosine, lamivudine, and tenofovir. *American Journal on Addictions 19*, 17–29.

Ballantyne, J. C. (2006). Opioids for chronic nonterminal pain. *Southern Medical Journal 99*, 1245–1255.

Barnett, P. G., & Hui, S. S. (2000). The cost-effectiveness of methadone maintenance. *Mount Sinai Journal of Medicine 67*, 365–374.

Baumler, A. (2007). *The Chinese and opium under the republic: Worse than floods and wild beasts*. Albany, NY: State University of New York Press.

Baumohl, J. (2004). Maintaining orthodoxy: The depression-era struggle over morphine maintenance in California. In S. W. Tracy & C. J. Acker (Eds.), *Altering American consciousness: The history of alcohol and drug use in the United States, 1800–2000* (pp. 225–266). Amherst, MA: University of Massachusetts Press.

Beg, M., Strathdee, S. A., & Kazatchkine, M. (2015). State of the art science addressing injecting drug use, HIV and harm reduction. *International Journal of Drug Policy 26*(Sup. 1), s1–s4.

Bentzley, B. S., Barth, K. S., Back, S. E., & Book, S. W. (2015). Discontinuation of buprenorphine maintenance therapy: Perspectives and outcomes. *Journal of Substance Abuse Treatment 52*, 48–57.

Berridge, V. (2003). History and twentieth-century drug policy: Telling true stories? *Medical History 47*, 518–524.

Bertol, E., Fineschi, V., Karch, S. B., Mari, F., & Riezzo, I. (2004). *Nymphaea* cults in ancient Egypt and the New World: A lesson in empirical pharmacology. *Journal of the Royal Society of Medicine 97*, 84–85.

Bird, J. (2003). Selection of pain measurement tools. *Nursing Standard 18*(13), 33–39.

Biruni, M. i. A. (1973). *al-Biruni's book on pharmacy and materia medica* (H. M. Said, Ed.). Karachi: Hamard National Foundation.

Bobo, L. D., & Thompson, V. (2006). Unfair by design: The war on drugs, race, and the legitimacy of the criminal justice system. *Social Research: An International Quarterly 73*, 445–472.

Boettcher, C., Fellermeier, M., Boettcher, C., Drager, B., & Zenk, M. H. (2005). How human neuroblastoma cells make morphine. *Proceedings of the National Academy of Sciences 102*, 8495–8500.

Booth, M. (1996). *Opium: A history*. London: Simon & Schuster.

Bourgois, P. (2000). Disciplining addictions: The bio-politics of methadone and heroin in the United States. *Culture, Medicine and Psychiatry 24*, 165–195.

Boys, A., Farrell, M., Bebbington, P., Brugha, T., Cold, J., Jenkins, R., Lewis, G., Marsden, J., Meltzer, H., Singleton, N., & Taylor, C. (2002). Drug use and initiation in prison: Results from a national prison survey in England and Wales. *Addiction 97*, 1551–1560.

Broussard, L. A., Preseley, L. C., Tanous, M., & Queen, C. (2001). Improved gas chromatography-mass spectrometry method for simultaneous identification and quantification of opiates in urine as propionyl and oxine derivatives. *Chemical Chemistry 47*(1), 127–129.

Burns, T. L., & Ineck, J. R. (2006). Cannabinoid analgesia as a potential new therapeutic option in the treatment of chronic pain. *Annals of Pharmacotherapy 40*, 251–260.

Buttner, A., Mall, G., Penning, R., & Weis, S. (2000). The neuropathology of heroin abuse. *Forensic Science International 113*(1), 435–442.

Buxton, J. (2006). *The political economy of narcotics: Production, consumption and global markets*. New York: Palgrave Macmillan/St. Martin's Press.

Calabresi, M. (2015). The price of relief: Why America can't kick its painkiller problem. *Time 185*(22), 26–33.

Calkins, A. (1871). *Opium and the opium-appetite: With notices of alcoholic beverages, Cannabis Indica, tobacco and coca, and tea and coffee, in their hygienic aspect*. Philadelphia: J. B. Lippincott & Co.

Carnwath, T. (2005). Prescribing heroin. *American Journal on Addictions 14*(4), 311–318.

Chein, I., Gerard, D. L., Lee, R. S., & Rosenfeld, E. (1964). *The road to H: Narcotics, delinquency, and social policy.* New York: Basic Books.

Chou, R., Fanciullo, G. J., Fine, P. G., Miaskowski, C., Passik, S. D., & Portenoy, R. K. (2009). Opioids for chronic noncancer pain: Prediction and identification of aberrant drug- related behaviors—a review of the evidence for an American Pain Society and American Academy of Pain Medicine clinical practice guideline. *Journal of Pain 10*(2), 131–146.

Cicero, T. J., Inciardi, J. A., & Munoz, A. (2005). Trends in abuse of OxyContin and other opioid analgesics in the United States: 2002–2004. *Journal of Pain 6*(10), 662–672.

Coid, J., Carvell, A., Kittler, Z., Healey, A., & Henderson, J. (2000). *Impact of methadone treatment on drug misuse and crime.* Research Findings, No. 120. London: Great Britain Home Office Research Development and Statistics Directorate.

Collins, E. D., & Kleber, H. D. (2004). Opioids: Detoxification. In M. Galanter & H. D. Kleber (Eds.), *Textbook of substance abuse treatment* (pp. 265–289). Arlington, VA: American Psychiatric Publishing.

Connock, M., Juarez-Garcia, A., Jowett, S., Frew, E., Liu, Z., Taylor, R. J., Fry-Smith, A., Day, E., Lintzeris, N., Roberts, T., Burls, A., & Taylor, R. S. (2007). Methadone and buprenorphine for the management of opioid dependence: A systematic review and economic analysis. *Health Technology Assessment 11*(9), 1–171.

Costello, J. J., & Van Vleck, E. (2009). National Institute on Drug Abuse. In G. L. Fisher & N. A. Roget (Eds.). *Encyclopedia of substance abuse prevention, treatment, and recovery.* (pp. 608–610). Thousand Oaks, CA: SAGE Publications.

Courtwright, D. T. (2002). *Forces of habit: Drugs and the making of the modern world.* Cambridge, MA: Harvard University Press.

Couto, J. E., Romney, M. C., Leider, H. L., Sharma, S., & Goldfarb, N. I. (2009). High rates of inappropriate drug use in the chronic pain population. *Population Health Management 12*(4), 185–190.

Crellin, J. K. (2004). *A social history of medicines in the twentieth century: To be taken three times a day.* New York: Routledge.

Crews, J. C. (2002). Multimodal pain management strategies for office-based and ambulatory procedures. *Journal of the American Medical Association 288,* 629–632.

Dalrymple, T. (2006). *Romancing opiates—pharmacological lies and the addiction bureaucracy.* New York: Encounter Books.

Dang, B. (2001). The royal touch. In W. A. Whitelaw (Ed.), *Proceedings of the 10th annual history of medicine days* (pp. 228–233). Calgary: University of Calgary.

Davenport-Hines, R. (2004). *The pursuit of oblivion: A global history of narcotics, 1500–2000.* New York: W. W. Norton & Company.

Davis, S. L. M., Triwulyuono, A., & Alexander, R. (2009). Survey of abuses against injecting drug users in Indonesia. *Harm Reduction Journal 6,* 28.

Dehue, T. (2004). Historiography taking issue: Analyzing an experiment with heroin abusers. *Journal of the History of the Behavioral Sciences 40*(3), 247–264.

De Loache, W. C., Russ, Z. N., Narcross, L., Gonzales, A. M., Martin, V. J. J., & Dueber, J. E. (2015). An enzyme-coupled biosensor enables (S)-reticuline production in yeast from glucose. *Nature Chemical Biology* (http://dx.doi.org/10.1038/nchembio.1816).

Devulder, J., Jacobs, A., Richarz, U., & Wiggert, H. (2009). Impact of opioid rescue medication for breakthrough pain on the efficacy and tolerability of long-acting opioids in patients with chronic non-malignant pain. *British Journal of Anaesthesia 103*(4), 576–585.

Dikotter, F., Laamann, L., & Zhou, X. (2004). *Narcotic culture: A history of drugs in China.* Chicago: University of Chicago Press.

Dilts, S. L., Jr., & Dilts, S. L. (2005). Opioids. In R. J. Frances, S. I. Miller, & A. H. Mack (Eds.), *Clinical textbook of addictive disorders* (pp. 138–156). New York: Guilford.

Dole, V. P., & Nyswander, M. (1965). A medical treatment for diacetylmorphine (heroin) addiction: A clinical trial with methadone hydrochloride. *Journal of the American Medical Association 193*(8), 646–650.

Downs, J. M. (1968). American merchants and the Chinese opium trade, 1800–1840. *Business History Review 42*, 432.

Dumchev, K., Soldyshev, R., Qian, H.-Z., Zezyulin, O. O., Chandler, S. D., Slobodyanyuk, P., Moroz, L. & Schumacher, J. E. (2009). HIV and hepatitis C virus infections among hanka injection drug users in central Ukraine: A cross-sectional survey. *Harm Reduction Journal 6*, 23.

Dunn, K. M., Saunders, K. W., Rutter, C. M., Banta-Green, C. J., Merrill, J. O., Sullivan, M. D., Weisner, C. M., Silverberg, M. J., Campbell, C. I., Psaty, B. M., & Von Korff, M. (2010). Opioid prescriptions for chronic pain and overdose: A cohort study. *Annals of Internal Medicine 152*(2), 85–92.

Eaton, V. G. (1888). How the opium habit is acquired. *Popular Science Monthly 33*, 665–666.

Emmanuel, F., Akhtar, S., & Rahbar, M. H. (2003). Factors associated with heroin addiction among male adults in Lahore, Pakistan. *Journal of Psychoactive Drugs 35*(2), 219–226.

Epstein, D. H., Preston, K. L., & Jasinski, D. R. (2006). Abuse liability, behavioral pharmacology, and physical-dependence potential of opioids in humans and laboratory animals: Lessons from tramadol. *Biological Psychology 73*(1), 90–99.

Evans, C. J. (2004). Secrets of the opium poppy revealed. *Neuropharmacology 47* (Sup. 1), 293–299.

Feroni, I., Peretti-Watel, P., Paraponaris, A., Masut, A., Ronfle, E., Mabriez, J. C., & Obadia, Y. (2005). French general practitioners' attitudes and prescription patterns towards buprenorphine maintenance treatment: Does doctor shopping reflect buprenorphine misuse? *Journal of Addictive Diseases 24*(3), 7–22.

Fiellin, D. A., & O'Connor, P. G. (2002). New federal initiatives to enhance the medical treatment of opioid dependence. *Annals of Internal Medicine 137*(8), 688–692.

Fiellin, D. A., Pantalon, M. V., Chawarski, M. C., Moore, B. A., Sullivan, L. E., O'Connor, P. G., & Schottenfeld, R. S. (2006). Counseling plus buprenorphine–naloxone maintenance therapy for opioid dependence. *New England Journal of Medicine 355*(4), 365–374.

Fishman, S. (2007). *Responsible opioid prescribing: A physician's guide.* Washington, DC: Waterford Life Sciences.

Foxcroft, L. (2007). *The making of addiction: The "use and abuse" of opium in nineteenth-century Britain.* Farnham, UK: Ashgate Publishing.

French, M. T., Salome, H. J., & Carney, M. (2002). Using the DATCAP and ASI to estimate the costs and benefits of residential addiction treatment in the state of Washington. *Social Science & Medicine 55*(12), 2267–2282.

Fries, D. S. (2008). Opioid analgesics. In T. L. Lemke, D. A. Williams, V. F. Roche, & S. W. Zito (Eds.), *Foye's principles of medicinal chemistry* (pp. 652–678). Baltimore, MD: Lippincott Williams & Wilkins/Wolters Kruwer.

Gallagher, J. R. (2015). The treatment of substance use disorders in criminal justice settings. *Alcoholism Treatment Quarterly 33*(1), 3–5.

Ganidagli, S., Cengiz, M., Aksoy, S., & Verit, A. (2004). Approach to painful disorders by Serefeddin Sabuncuoglu in the fifteenth century Ottoman period. *Anesthesiology 100*(1), 165–169.

Garty, C. C., Oviedo-Joekes, E., Laliberte, N., & Schechter, M. T. (2009). NAOMI: The trials and tribulations of implementing a heroin assisted treatment study in North America. *Harm Reduction Journal 6*, 2.

Gaston, R. L., Best, D., Manning, V., & Day, E. (2009). Can we prevent drug related deaths by training opioid users to recognize and manage overdoses? *Harm Reduction Journal 6*, 26.

Gilson, A. M., & Kreis, P. G. (2009). The burden of the nonmedical use of prescription opioid analgesics. *Pain Medicine 1*(Sup. 2), s89–s100.

Gloth, F. M., Scheve, A. A., Stober, C. V., Xhow, S., & Prosser, J. (2001). The Functional Pain Scale: Reliability, validity, and responsiveness in an elderly population. *Journal of Post-Acute and Long-Term Care Medicine 2*(3), 110–114.

Goldacre, B. (2012). *Bad pharma: How drug companies mislead doctors and harm patients.* London: Fourth Estate/HarperCollins Publishers.

Goodhand, J. (2005). Frontiers and wars: The opium economy in Afghanistan. *Journal of Agrarian Change 5*(2), 191–216.

Goodsell, D. S. (2005). The molecular perspective: Morphine. *Stem Cells 23*, 144–145.

Gossop, M., Marsden, J., Stewart, D., & Kidd, T. (2003). The National Treatment Outcome Research Study (NTORS): 4–5 year follow-up results. *Addiction 98* (3), 291–303.

Gossop, M., Stewart, D., Browne, N., & Marsden, J. (2003). Methadone treatment for opiate dependent patients in general practice and specialist clinic settings: Outcomes at 2-year follow-up. *Journal of Substance Abuse Treatment 24*(4), 313–321.

Gottschalk, A., & Smith, D. S. (2001). New concepts in acute pain therapy: Preemptive analgesia. *American Family Physician 63*(10), 1979–1984.

Grau, L. E., Dasgupta, N., Harvey, A. P., Irwin, K., Givens, A., Kinzly, M. L., & Heimer, R. (2007). Illicit use of opioids: Is OxyContin a "Gateway Drug"? *American Journal on Addictions 16*(3), 166–173.

Grau, L. E., Green, T. C., Torban, M., Blinnikova, K., Krupitsky, E., Ilyuk, R., Kozlov, A. P., & Heimer, R. (2009). Psychosocial and contextual correlates of opioid overdose risk among drug users in St. Petersburg, Russia. *Harm Reduction Journal 6*, 17.

Greenberg, B., Hall, D. H., & Sorensen, J. L. (2007). Methadone maintenance therapy in residential therapeutic community settings: Challenges and promise. *Journal of Psychoactive Drugs 39*(3), 203–210.

Greene, J. A. (2014). *Generic: The unbranding of modern medicine.* Baltimore, MD: Johns Hopkins University Press.

Grey-Wilson, C. (2000). *Poppies: The poppy family in the wild and in cultivation.* Portland, OR: Timber Press.

Griffin, J. P. (2004). Venetian treacle and the formulation of medicines regulation. *British Journal of Clinical Pharmacology 58*(3), 317–325.

Grim, R. (2009). *This is your country on drugs: A secret history of getting high in America.* New York: John Wiley & Sons.

Gschwend, P., Rehm, J., Blatter, R., Steffen, T., Seidenberg, A., Christen, S., Burki, C., & Gutzwiller, F. (2004). Dosage regimes in the prescription of heroin and other narcotics to chronic opioid addicts in Switzerland—Swiss National Cohort Study. *European Addiction Research 10*(1), 41–48.

Hamilton, G. R., & Baskett, T. F. (2000). In the arms of Morpheus, the development of morphine for postoperartive pain relief. *Canadian Journal of Anaesthesia 47*(4), 367–374.

Hari, J. (2015). *Chasing the scream: The first and last days of the war on drugs.* New York: Bloomsbury USA.

Harlow, B. L., & Stewart, E. G. (2003). A population-based assessment of chronic unexplained vulvar pain: Have we underestimated the prevalence of vulvodynia? *Journal of the American Medical Women's Association 58*, 82–88.

Hart, J. (2008). Complementary therapies for chronic pain management. *Alternative and Complementary Therapies 14*(2), 64–68.

Hays, L. R. (2004). A profile of OxyContin addiction. *Journal of Addictive Diseases 23*(4), 1–9.

Hodgson, B. (2001). *In the arms of Morpheus: The tragic history of morphine, laudanum and patent medicines.* Buffalo, NY: Firefly Books.

Hser, Y.-I., Hoffman, V., Grella, C., & Anglin, D. (2001). A 33-year follow-up of narcotic addicts. *Archives of General Psychiatry 58*, 503–508.

Hu, K., Connelly, N. R., & Viera, P. (2002). Withdrawal symptoms in a patient receiving intrathecal morphine via an infusion pump. *Journal of Clinical Anesthesia 14*(8), 595–597.

Hubbard, R. L., Craddock, S. G., Flynn, P. M., Anderson, J., & Etheridge, R. M. (1997). Overview of 1-year follow-up outcomes in Drug Abuse Treatment Outcome Study (DATOS). *Psychology of Addictive Behaviors 11*(4), 261–278.

Janzen, R. (2001). *The rise and fall of Synanon*. Baltimore, MD: Johns Hopkins University Press.

Jia, S., Wang, W., Liu, Y., & Wu, Z. (2005). Neuroimaging studies of brain corpus striatum changes among heroin-dependent patients treated with herbal medicine, U'finer™ capsule. *Addiction Biology 10*(3), 293–297.

Johnson, B., & Richert, T. (2015). Diversion of methadone and buprenorphine by patients in opioid substitution treatment in Sweden: Prevalence estimates and risk factors. *International Journal of Drug Policy 26*(2), 183–190.

Jones, C. M. (2013). Heroin use and heroin use risk behaviors among nonmedical users of prescription opioid pain relievers—United States, 2002–2004 and 2008–2010. *Drug and Alcohol Dependence 132*(1–2), 95–100.

Jones, H. E. (2009). Buprenorphine. In G. L. Fisher & N. A. Roget (Eds.). *Encyclopedia of substance abuse prevention, treatment, and recovery* (pp. 146–148). Thousand Oaks, CA: SAGE Publications.

Jones, J., Tomlinson, K., & Moore, L. (2002). The simultaneous determination of codeine, morphine, hydrocodone, hydromorphone, 6-acetylmorphine, and oxycodone in hair and oral fluid. *Journal of Analytical Toxicology 26*(3), 171–175.

Kabel, J. S., & van Puijenbroek, E. P. (2005). [Side effects of tramadol: 12 years experience in the Netherlands]. *Nederlands Tijdschrift voor Geneeskunde 149*(14), 754–757.

Kane, H. H. (1882). *Opium-smoking in America and China: A study of its prevalence, and effects, immediate and remote, on the individual and the nation*. New York: G. P. Putnam's Sons.

Kapoor, L. D. (1995). *Opium poppy: Botany, chemistry, and pharmacology*. Binghamton, NY: Haworth Press.

Katz, N., Fernandez, K., Chang, A., Benoit, C., & Butler, S. F. (2008). Internet-based survey of nonmedical prescription opioid use in the United States. *Clinical Journal of Pain 24*(6), 528–535.

Keast, S. L., Nesser, N., & Farmer, K. (2015). Strategies aimed at controlling misuse and abuse of opioid prescription medications in a state Medicaid program: A policymaker's perspective. *American Journal of Drug and Alcohol Abuse 41*(1), 1–6.

Keats, J., Micallef, M., Grebely, J., Hazelwood, S., Everingham, H., Shrestha, N., Jones, T., Bath, N., Treloar, C., Dore, G. J., & Dunlop, A. (2015). Assessment and delivery of treatment for hepatitis C virus infection in an opioid substitution treatment clinic with integrated peer-based support in Newcastle, Australia. *International Journal of Drug Policy 26*(10), 999–1006.

Khan, A. A., Awan, A. B., Qureshi, S. U., Razaque, A., & Zafar, S. T. (2009). Large sharing networks and unusual injection practices explain the rapid rise in HIV among IDUs in Sargodha, Pakistan. *Harm Reduction Journal 6*, 13.

Kirschmayer, U., Davoli, M., Verster, A. D., Amato, L., Ferri, M., & Peruci, C. A. (2002). A systematic review on the efficacy of naltrexone maintenance treatment in opioid dependence. *Addiction 97*, 1241–1249.

Kleber, H. D. (2008). Methadone maintenance 4 decades later: Thousands of lives saved but still controversial. *Journal of the American Medical Association 300* (19), 2303–2305.

Knisely, J. S., Campbell, E. D., Dawson, K. S., & Schnoll, S. H. (2002). Tramadol post-marketing surveillance in health care professionals. *Drug and Alcohol Dependence 68*(1), 15–22.

Kosten, T. R., & Gorelick, D. A. (2002). The Lexington narcotic farm. *American Journal of Psychiatry 159*(1), 22.

Kreek, M. J. (2000). Methadone-related opioid agonist pharmacotherapy for heroin addiction: History, recent molecular and neurochemical research and future in mainstream medicine. *Annals of the New York Academy of Sciences 909*, 186–216.

Kreutzmann, H. (2007). Afghanistan and the opium world market: Poppy production and trade. *Iranian Studies 40*(5), 605–621.

Krupitsky, E., Nunes, E. V., Ling, W., Illeperuma, A., Gastfriend, D. R., & Silverman, B. L. (2011). Injectable extended-release naltrexone for opioid dependence: A double-blind, placebo-controlled, multicenter randomized trial. *Lancet 377*(9776), 1506–1513.

Kupatadze, A. (2014). Kyrgystan—a virtual narco-state. *International Journal of Drug Policy 25*(6), 1178–1185.

Lanier, R. K., Umbricht, A., Harrison, J. A., Nuwayser, E. S., & Bigelow, G. E. (2008). Opioid detoxification via single 7-day application of buprenorphine transdermal patch: An open-label evaluation. *Psychopharmacology 198*(2), 149–158.

Leeman, R. F. (2009). Naltrexone. In G. L. Fisher & N. A. Roget (Eds.). *Encyclopedia of substance abuse prevention, treatment, and recovery* (pp. 586–589). Thousand Oaks, CA: SAGE Publications.

Lehmann, D. F., Roberts, G., & Moellentin, D. (2001). The search for a nonaddicting opioid. *Pharos of Alpha Omega Alpha-Honor Medical Society 64*(1), 24–27.

Leo, R. J., Narendran, R., & DeGuiseppe, B. (2000). Methadone detoxification of tramadol dependence. *Journal of Substance Abuse Treatment 19*(3), 297–299.

Leukefeld, C. G., & Stoops, W. W. (2009). OxyContin. In G. L. Fisher & N. A. Roget (Eds.), *Encyclopedia of substance abuse prevention, treatment, and recovery* (pp. 674–676). Thousand Oaks, CA: SAGE Publications.

Libby, R.T. (2006). Treating doctors as drug dealers: The Drug Enforcement Administration's war on prescription pain killers. *Independent Review 10*(4), 513–547.

Lin, C., Wu, Z., Rou, K., Pang, L., Cao, X., Shoptaw, S., & Detels, R. (2010). Challenges in providing services in methadone maintenance therapy clinics in China: Service providers' perceptions. *International Journal of Drug Policy 21* (3), 173–178.

Lind, J. T., Moene, K. O., & Willamsen, F. (2014). Opium for the masses? Conflict-induced narcotics production in Afghanistan. *Review of Economics and Statistics* *96*(5), 949–966.

Ling, W., Hillhouse, M., Ang, A., Jenkins, J., & Fahey, J. (2013). Comparison of behavioral treatment conditions in buprenorphine maintenance. *Addiction 108* (10), 1788–1798.

Lord, S., Downs, G., Furtaw, P., Chadhuri, A., Silverstein, A., Gammaitoni, A., & Budman, S. (2009). Nonmedical use of prescription opioids and stimulants among student pharmacists. *Journal of American Pharmacists Association 49*(4), 519–528.

Loudan, I. (1986). *Medical care and the general practitioner, 1750–1850*. Oxford: Oxford University Press.

Lu, L., & Wang, X. (2008). Drug addiction in China. *Annals of the New York Academy of Sciences 1141*, 304–317.

Ludwig, A. S., & Peters, R. H. (2014). Medication-assisted treatment for opioid use disorders in correctional settings: An ethics review. *International Journal of Drug Policy 25*(6), 1041–1046.

MacCoun, R. J., & Reuter, P. (2001). *Drug war heresies: Learning from other vices, times, and places*. Cambridge: Cambridge University Press.

Maher, L., & Ho, H. T. (2009). Overdose beliefs and management practices among ethnic Vietnamese heroin users in Sydney, Australia. *Harm Reduction Journal 6*, 6.

Manchikanti, L., Giordano, J., Boswell, M. V., Fellows, B., Manchukonda, R., & Pampati, V. (2007). Psychological factors as predictors of opioid abuse and illicit drug use in chronic pain patients. *Journal of Opioid Management 3*(2), 89–100.

Mani, D., & Dhawan, S. S. (2014). Scientific basis of therapeutic uses of opium poppy (*Papaver somniferum*) in Ayurveda. International Symposium on Papaver. *Acta Horticulturae 1036*, 175–180.

Mann, A. (2004). Successful trial caps 25-year buprenorphine development effort. *NIDA Notes 19*(3), 7–9.

March, J. C., Oviedo-Joekes, E., Perea-Milla, E., Carrasco, F., & PEPSA Team (2006). Controlled trial of prescribed heroin in the treatment of opioid addiction. *Journal of Substance Abuse Treatment 31*(2), 203–211.

Martin, M., Hurley, R. A., & Taber, K. H. (2007). Is opiate addiction associated with longstanding neurobiological change? *Journal of Neuropsychiatry and Clinical Neurosciences 19*, 242–248.

Masson, C. L., Barnett, P. G., Sees, K. L., Delucchi, K. L., Rosen, A., Wong, W., & Hall, S. M. (2004). Cost and cost-effectiveness of standard methadone maintenance treatment compared to enriched 180-day methadone. *Addiction 99*(6), 718–726.

McCabe, S. E., Boyd, C. J., Cranford, J. A., & Teter, C. J. (2009). Motives for non-medical use of prescription opioids among high school seniors in the United States: Self-treatment and beyond. *Archives of Pediatrics and Adolescent Medicine 163*(8), 739–744.

McCabe, S. E., Teter, C. J., Boyd, C. J., Knight, J. R., & Wechsler, H. (2005). Nonmedical use of prescription opioids among U.S. college students: Prevalence and correlates from a national survey. *Addictive Behaviors 30*(4), 789–805.

McCance-Katz, E. F., Jatlow, P., & Rainey, P. M. (2010). Effect of cocaine use on methadone pharmokinetics in humans. *American Journal on Addictions 19*(1), 47–52.

McCance-Katz, E. F., & Mandell, T. W. (2010). Drug interactions of clinical importance with methadone and buprenorphine. *American Journal on Addictions 19*(1), 2–3.

McCance-Katz, E. F., Rainey, P. M., & Moody, D. E. (2010). Effect of cocaine use on buprenorphine pharmacokinetics in humans. *American Journal on Addictions 19*(1), 38–46.

McLellan, A. T., & Turner, B. J. (2010). Chronic noncancer pain management and opioid overdose: Time to change prescribing practices. *Annals of Internal Medicine 152*(2), 123–124.

McMillin, G., & Urry, F. (2007). *Drug testing guide for chronic pain management services*. Salt Lake City, UT: ARUP Laboratories.

McNeil, D. G., Jr. (2015). A way to brew morphine raises concerns over regulation. *New York Times* (http://www.nytimes.com/2015/05/19/health/a-way-to-brew-morphine-raises-concerns-over-regulation.html).

Meier, B. (2015). *A world of hurt: Fixing pain medicine's biggest mistake*. New York: The New York Times Co.

Meinert, C. L. (2012). *Clinical Trials: Design, Conduct, and Analysis*. Oxford: Oxford University Press.

Mendelson, J., & Jones, R. T. (2003). Clinical and pharmacological evaluation of buprenorphine and naloxone combinations: Why the 4:1 ratio for treatment? *Drug and Alcohol Dependence 70*, s29–s37.

Merck & Co. (1899). *Merck's manual of the material medica*. New York: Merck & Company.

Merrill, J. O. (2007). Policy progress for physician treatment of opiate addiction. *Journal of General Internal Medicine 17*(5), 361–368.

Metha, V., & Langford, R. M. (2006). Acute pain management for opioid dependent patients. *Anaesthesia 61*(3), 269–276.

Miller, N. S., & Greenfeld, A. (2004). Patient characteristics and risk factors for development of dependence on hydrocodone and oxycodone. *American Journal of Therapeutics 11*(1), 26–32.

Milligan, B. (2005). Morphine-addicted doctors, the English opium-eater, and embattled medical authority. *Victorian Literature and Culture 33*(2), 541–553.

Mintzer, I. L., Eisenberg, M., Terra, M., MacVane, C., Himmelstein, D. U., & Woolhandler, S. (2007). Treating opioid addiction with buprenorphine-naloxone in community-based primary care settings. *Annals of Family Medicine 5*(2), 146–150.

Moallem, S.-A., Balali-Mood, K., & Balali-Mood, M. (2004). Opioids and opiates. In A. Mozayani & L. P. Raymon (Eds.), *Handbook of drug interactions: A clinical and forensic guide* (pp. 123–148). Totowa, NJ: Humana Press.

Mold, A. (2004). "British system" of heroin addiction treatment and the opening of drug dependence units, 1965–1970. *Social History of Medicine 17*(3), 501–517.

Moore, R. L. (2003). *The French connection: A true account of cops, narcotics, and international conspiracy.* Guilford, CT: Pequot Press.

Moraes, F., & Moraes, D. (2003). *Opium.* Berkeley, CA: Ronin Publishing.

Mott, J., & Bean, P. (2000). The development of drug control in Britain. In R. Coomber (Ed.), *The control of drugs and drug users: Reason or reaction* (pp. 31–48). Amsterdam: Harwood Academic Publishers/Gordon and Breach Publishing Group.

Myers, P. L., & Salt, N. R. (2013). *Becoming an addictions counselor: A comprehensive text.* Burlington, MA: Jones & Bartlett Learning.

Naliboff, B. D., Wu, S. M., & Pham, Q. (2006). Clinical considerations in the treatment of chronic pain with opiates. *Journal of Clinical Psychology 62*(11), 1397–1408.

National Institute on Drug Abuse. (2009). *Principles of addiction treatment.* NIH Publication No. 09-4180. Bethesda, MD: Author.

Neale, J., Robertson, M., & Saville, E., (2005). Understanding the treatment needs of drug users in prison. *Probation Journal 52*(3), 243–257.

Nemmani, K. V., & Mogil, J. S. (2003). Serotonin-GABA interactions in the modulation of mu- and kappa-opioid analgesia. *Neuropharmacology 44*(3), 304–310.

Nordt, C., & Stohler, R. (2006). Incidence of heroin use in Zurich, Switzerland: A treatment case register analysis. *Lancet 367*, 1830–1834.

Nunn, A., Zaller, N., Dickman, S., Tribur, C., Nijhawan, A., & Rich, J. D. (2009). Methadone and buprenorphine prescribing and referral practices in US prison systems: Results from a nationwide survey. *Drug and Alcohol Dependence 105* (1–2), 83–88.

O'Connor, P. G. (2005). Methods of detoxification and their role in treating patients with opioid dependence. *Journal of the American Medical Association 294*, 961–963.

Offiah, C., & Hall, E. (2008). Heroin-induced leukoencephalopathy: Characterization using MRI, diffusion-weighted imaging, and MR spectroscopy. *Clinical Radiology 63*(2), 146–152.

Office of National Drug Control Policy. (2014). *2013 Annual report, arrestees drug abuse monitoring program II.* Washington, DC: Executive Office of the President.

Olmedo, R., & Hoffman, R. S. (2000). Withdrawal symptoms. *Emergency Medicine Clinics of North America 18*(2), 273–288.

O'Neill, W. M., Hanks, G. W., Simpson, P., Fallon, M. T., Jenkins, E., & Wesnes, K. (2000). The cognitive and psychomotor effects of morphine in healthy subjects: A randomized controlled trial of repeated (four) oral doses of dextropropoxyphene, morphine, lorazepam and placebo. *Pain 85*(1–2), 209–215.

Otis-Green, S. (2006). Psychosocial Pain Assessment Form. In K. Dow (Ed.), *Nursing care of women with cancer* (pp. 556–561). St. Louis, MO: Elsevier Mosby.

Oviedo-Joekes, E., Nosyk, B., Marsh, D. C., Guh, D., Brissette, S., Garty, C., Kraus, M., Anis, A., & Schechter, M. T. (2009). Scientific and political challenges in North America's first randomized controlled trial of heroin-assisted treatment for severe heroin addiction: Rationale and design of the NAOMI study. *Clinical Trials* 6(3), 261–271.

Oye, K.A., Lawson, J. C. H., & Bubela, T. (2015). Drugs: Regulate "home-brew" opiates. *Nature* 521, 281–283.

Parsons, D., Burrows, D., & Bolotbaeva, A. (2014). Advocating for opioid substitution therapy in Central Asia: Much still to be done. *International Journal of Drug Policy* 25(6), 1174–1177.

Passik, S. D. (2001). Responding rationally to recent reports of abuse/diversion of Oxycontin. *Journal of Pain and Symptom Management* 21(5), 359–360.

Paulozzi, L. J., Budnitz, D., & Xi, Y. (2006). Increasing deaths from opioid analgesics in the United States. *Pharmacoepidemiology and Drug Safety* 15, 618–627.

Pezawas, L., Fischer, G., Podreka, I., Schindler, S., Brucke, T., Jassch, R., Thurnher, M., & Kasper, S. (2002). Opioid addiction changes cerebral blood flow symmetry. *Neuropsychobiology* 45(2), 67–73.

Pocock, S. J. (2009). *Clinical trials: A practical approach.* New York: John Wiley and Sons.

Poeaknapo, C., Schmidt, J., Brandsch, M., Drager, B., & Zenk, M. H. (2004). Endogenous formation of morphine in human cells. *Proceedings of the National Academy of Sciences* 101(39), 14091–14096.

Porter, P. (1884). "Regular" diagnosis. Laparotomy, cystosarcoma. *American Homoeopathist* 10(February), 42–43.

Poshyachinda, V. (1980). Thailand: Treatment at the Tam Kraborg Temple. In G. Edwards & A. Arif (Eds.), *Drug problems in the sociocultural context: A basis for policies and programme planning* (pp. 121–125). Geneva: World Health Organization.

Potter, J. S., Shiffman, S. J., & Weiss, R. D. (2008). Chronic pain severity in opioid-dependent patients. *American Journal of Drug and Alcohol Abuse* 34(1), 101–107.

Rashid, R. A., Kamali, K., Habil, M. H., Shaharom, M. H., Seghatolesam, T. & Looyeh, M. Y. (2014). A mosque-based methadone maintenance treatment strategy: Implementation and pilot results. *International Journal of Drug Policy* 25(6), 1071–1075.

Ratcliffe, G. E., Enns, M. W., Belik, S.-L., & Sareen, J. (2008). Chronic pain conditions and suicidal ideation and suicide attempts: An epidemiologic perspective. *Clinical Journal of Pain* 24, 204–210.

Reed, B. D. (2006). Vulvodynia: Diagnosis and management. *American Family Physician* 73(7), 1231–1238.

Rich, J. D., Boutwell, A. E., Shield, D. C., Key, R. G., McKenzie, M., Clarke, J. G., & Friedman, P. D. (2005). Attitudes and practices regarding the use of methadone in US state and federal prisons. *Journal of Urban Health* 82(3), 411–419.

Robbins, N. (2006). *The corporation that changed the world.* London: Pluto Press.

Robins, L. N., & Slobodyan, S. (2003). Post-Vietnam heroin use and injection by returning U.S. veterans: Clues to preventing injection today. *Addiction 98*(8), 1053–1060.

Robinson, M. B., & Scherien, R. G. (2007). *Lies, damned lies, and drug war statistics.* Albany, NY: State University of New York Press.

Roman, C. G., Ahn-Redding, H., & Simon, R. J. (2007). *Illicit drug policies, trafficking, and use the world over.* Lanham, MD: Lexington Books.

Rosenblum, D., Castrillo, F. M., Bourgois, P., Mars, S., Karandinos, G., Unick, G. J., & Ciccarone, D. (2014). Urban segregation and the US heroin market: A quantitative model of anthropological hypotheses from an inner-city drug market. *International Journal of Drug Policy 25*(3), 543–555.

Rowan-Szal, G. A., Bartholomew, N. G., Chatham, L. R., & Simpson, D. D. (2005). A combined cognitive and behavioral intervention for cocaine-using methadone clients. *Journal of Psychoactive Drugs 37*(1), 75–84.

Rowe, T. C. (2006). *Federal narcotics laws and the war on drugs: Money down a rat hole.* Binghamton, NY: Haworth Press.

Ruscheweyh, R., Verneuer, B., Dan, K., Marziniak, M., Wolowski, A., Colak-Enid, R., Schulte, T. L., Bullmann, V., Grewe, S., Gralow, I., Evers, S., & Knecht, S. (2012). Validation of the pain sensitivity questionnaire in chronic pain patients. *Pain 153*(6), 1210–1218.

Russo, E. (2004). History of cannabis as a medicine. In G. W. Gy, B. A. Whittle, & P. J. Robson (Eds.), *The medicinal uses of cannabis and cannabinoids* (pp. 1–16). London: Pharmaceutical Press.

Saffier, K., Colombo, C., Brown, D., Mundt, M., & Fleming, M. (2007). Addiction Severity Index in a chronic pain sample receiving opioid therapy. *Journal of Substance Abuse Treatment 33*, 303–311.

Sanchez-Rangel, D., Rivas-San Vincente, M., de la Torre-Hernandez, M. E., Najera-Martinez, M., & Plasencia, J. (2015). Deciphering the link between salicylic acid signaling and sphingolipid metabolism. *Frontiers in Plant Science 6*, 125.

Sangar, S. P. (1981). Intoxicants in Mughal India. *Indian Journal of History of Science 16*(2), 202–214.

Savage, S. R., Kirsh, K. L., & Passik, S. D. (2008). Challenges in using opioids to treat pain in persons with substance use disorders. *Addiction Science and Clinical Practice 4*(2), 4–25.

Schaub, M., Chtenguelov, V., Subata, E., Weiler, G., & Uchtenhagen, A. (2010). Feasibility of buprenorphine and methadone maintenance programmes among users of home made opioids in Ukraine. *International Journal of Drug Policy 21* (3), 229–233.

Seddon, T. (2008). Women, harm reduction and history: Gender perspectives on the emergence of the "British system" of drug control. *International Journal of Drug Policy 19*(2), 99–105.

Sees, K. L., DiMarino, M. E., Ruediger, N. K., Sweeney, C. T., & Shiffman, S. (2005). Non-medical use of OxyContin tablets in the United States. *Journal of Pain and Palliative Care Pharmacotherapy 19*(2), 13–23.

Shearing, C. (2004). *Opium: A journey through time.* London: Mercury Books.

Sherman, S. G., Gann, D. S., Scott, G., Carlberg, S., Bigg, D., & Heimer, R. (2008). A qualitative study of overdose responses among Chicago IDUs. *Harm Reduction Journal 5*(2) (http://doi:10.1186/1477-7517-5-2).

Siddiqi, A. (2005). Pathways of the poppy: India's opium trade in the nineteenth century. In M. Thampi (Ed.), *India and China in the colonial world* (pp. 21–32). Oxford: Berghahn Books.

Simpson, C. A. (2006). Complementary medicine in chronic pain treatment. *Physical Medicine and Rehabilitation Clinics of North America 17*(2), 451–472.

Singer, M. (2008). Drugs and development: The global impact of drug use and trafficking on social and economic development. *International Journal of Drug Policy 19*(6), 467–478.

Smith, M. Y., Haddox, J. D., & DiMarino, M. E. (2007). Correlates of nonmedical use of hydromorphone and hydrocodone: Results from a national household study. *Journal of Pain and Palliative Pharmacotherapy 21*(3), 5–17.

Sneader, W. (2005). *Drug discovery: A history.* Hoboken, NJ: Wiley.

Speaker, S. L. (2004). Demons for the twentieth century: The rhetoric of drug reform, 1920–1940. In S. W. Tracy & C. J. Acker (Eds.), *Altering American consciousness: The history of alcohol and drug use in the United States, 1800–2000* (pp. 203–224). Amherst, MA: University of Massachusetts Press.

Sporer, K. A. (2003). Strategies for preventing heroin overdose. *BMJ: British Medical Journal 326*, 442–444.

Stallwitz, A., & Stover, H. (2007). The impact of substitution treatment in prisons—a literature review. *International Journal of Drug Policy 18*(6), 464–474.

Stanley, L. L. (1915). Morphinism. *Journal of the American Institute of Criminal Law and Criminology 6*(4), 586–593.

Stevens, R. A., & Ghazi, S. M. (2000). Routes of opioid analgesic therapy in the management of cancer pain. *Cancer Control 7*(2), 132–141.

Stimson, G. V., & Metrebian, N. (2003). *Prescribing heroin: What is the evidence?* York: Joseph Rowntree Foundation.

Stolberg, V. B. (2006). A review of perspectives on alcohol and alcoholism in the history of American health and medicine. *Journal of Ethnicity in Substance Abuse 5* (4), 39–106.

Stolberg, V. B. (2007). A cross-cultural and historical survey of tobacco use among various ethnic groups. *Journal of Ethnicity in Substance Abuse 6*(3–4), 9–80.

Stolberg, V. B. (2009a). Comprehensive Drug Abuse Prevention and Control Act. In G. L. Fisher & N. A. Roget (Eds.). *Encyclopedia of substance abuse prevention, treatment, and recovery.* (pp. 224–225). Thousand Oaks, CA: SAGE Publications.

Stolberg, V. B. (2009b). Historical images and reviews of substance use and substance abuse in the teaching of addiction studies. *Journal of Teaching in the Addictions 8* (1–2), 65–83.

Stolberg, V. B. (2009c). Morphine. In G. L. Fisher & N. A. Roget (Eds.). *Encyclopedia of substance abuse prevention, treatment, and recovery* (pp. 563–565). Thousand Oaks, CA: SAGE Publications.

Stolberg, V. B. (2011a). "Comprehensive Drug Abuse Prevention and Control Act." In M. A. R. Kleiman & J. E. Hawdon (Eds.), *Encyclopedia of drug policy* (Vol. 1, pp. 155–158). Thousand Oaks, CA: SAGE Publications.

Stolberg, V. B. (2011b). "Morphine." In M. A. R. Kleiman & J. E. Hawdon (Eds.), *Encyclopedia of drug policy* (Vol. 2, pp. 534–538). Thousand Oaks, CA: SAGE Publications.

Stolberg, V. B. (2011c). "Narcotic Addict Rehabilitation Act." In M. A. R. Kleiman & J. E. Hawdon (Eds.), *Encyclopedia of drug policy* (Vol. 2, pp. 541–543). Thousand Oaks, CA: SAGE Publications.

Stolberg, V. B. (2011d). "Synthetic Narcotics." In M. A. R. Kleiman & J. E. Hawdon (Eds.), *Encyclopedia of drug policy* (Vol. 2, pp. 755–760). Thousand Oaks, CA: SAGE Publications.

Stolberg, V. B. (2011e). "United Nations Convention against the Illicit Traffic in Narcotic Drugs." In M. A. R. Kleiman & J. E. Hawdon, (Eds.), *Encyclopedia of drug policy* (Vol. 2, pp. 801–802). Thousand Oaks, CA: SAGE Publications.

Stolberg, V. B. (2011f). The use of coca: A mild stimulant through prehistory, history, and ethnography. *Journal of Ethnicity in Substance Abuse 10*(2), 126–146.

Stoller, K. B., Bigelow, G. E., Walsh, S. L., & Strain, E. C. (2001). Effects of buprenorphine/naloxone in opioid-dependent humans. *Psychopharmacology 154*(3), 230–242.

Storti, C. C. & De Grauwe, P. (2007). *Globalization and the price decline of illicit drugs*. CESifo Working Paper Series No. 1990. Munich: CESifo.

Strang, J., & Gossop, M. (2005). The "British System" of drug policy: Extraordinary individual freedom, but to what end? In J. Strang & M. Gossop (Eds.), *Heroin addiction and the British System: Treatment and policy responses* (pp. 206–219). London: Routledge.

Substance Abuse and Mental Health Services Administration. (2014). *Results from the 2013 National Survey on Drug Use and Health—summary of national findings*. NSDUAH Series H-48, HHS Pub. No. (SMA) 14-4863. Rockville, MD: Author.

Sullivan, M., & Ferrell, B. (2005). Ethical challenges in the management of chronic non-malignant pain: Negotiating through the cloud of doubt. *Journal of Pain 6*(1), 2–9.

Szalavitz, M. (2006). *Help at any cost*. New York: Penguin.

Tang, W.-M. (2015). Effects of transnational migration on drug use: An ethnographic study of Nepali female heroin users in Hong Kong. *International Journal of Drug Policy 26*(1), 8–14.

Tang, Y. L., Zhao, D., Zhao, C., & Cubells, J. F. (2006). Opiate addiction in China: Current situation and treatments. *Addiction 101*(5), 657–665.

Tibi, S. (2006). *The medicinal use of opium in ninth-century Baghdad*. Leiden: Brill.

Trescot, A. M., Datta, S., Lee, M., & Hansen, H. (2008). Opioid pharmacology. *Pain Physician 11*, S133–S153.

Trocki, C. A. (2005). A drug on the market: Opium and the Chinese in Southeast Asia, 1750–1880. *Journal of Chinese Overseas 1*(2), 147–168.

Tseng, W.-S. (2001). *Handbook of cultural psychiatry*. St. Louis, MO: Academic Press/Elsevier.

Tunis, S. R., Stryer, D. B., & Clancy, C. M. (2003). Practical clinical trials: Increasing the value of clinical research for decision making in clinical and health policy. *Journal of the American Medical Association 290*(12), 1624–1632.

Vandanyan, R., & Hruby, V. J. (2006). *Synthesis of essential drugs*. Amsterdam: Elsevier.

van Luijk, E. W. E., & van Ours, J. C. (2001). The effects of government policy on opium consumption: Java, 1875–1904. *Journal of Economic History 61*, 1–18.

Vigezzi, P., Guglielmino, L., Marzorati, P., Silenzio, R., De Chiara, M., Corrado, F., Coechi, L., & Cozzolino, E. (2006). Multimodal drug addiction treatment: A field comparison of methadone and buprenorphine among heroin- and cocaine-dependent patients. *Journal of Substance Abuse Treatment 31*(1), 3–7.

Virgil. (1982). *The Georgics* (L. P. Wilkinson, Trans.). London: Penguin Books.

Virk, M. S., Arttamangkul, S., Birdsong, W. T., & Williams, J. T. (2009). Buprenorphine is a weak partial agonist that inhibits opioid receptor desensitization. *Journal of Neuroscience 29*(22), 7341–7348.

Wadhwa, S. (2009). Pain management. In G. L. Fisher & N. A. Roget (Eds.). *Encyclopedia of substance abuse prevention, treatment, and recovery* (pp. 677–679). Thousand Oaks, CA: SAGE Publications.

Wailoo, K. (2014). *Pain: A political history*. Baltimore, MD: Johns Hopkins University Press.

Wang, J., & Christo, P. J. (2009). The influence of prescription monitoring programs on chronic pain management. *Pain Physician 12*(3), 507–515.

Webster, L. R., & Webster, R. M. (2005). Predicting aberrant behaviors in opioid-treated patients: Preliminary validation of the Opioid Risk Tool. *Pain Medicine 6*(6), 432–442.

Weinberg, M. (2014). Making the marketplace more patient focused. *American Journal of Pharmacy Benefits 6*(2), 89–91.

Wenger, L. D., Lopez, A. M., Comfort, M., & Kral, A. H. (2014). The phenomenon of low- frequency heroin injection among street-based urban poor: Drug user strategies and contexts of use. *International Journal of Drug Policy 25*(3), 471–479.

Weschules, D. J., Baib, K. T., & Richeimer, S. (2008). Actual and potential drug interactions associated with methadone. *Pain Medicine 9*(30), 315–344.

West, J. C., Kosten, T. R., Wilk, J., Svikis, D., Triffleman, E., Rae, D. S., Narrow, W. E., Duffy, F. F., & Regier, D. A. (2004). Challenges in increasing access to buprenorphine treatment for opiate addiction. *American Journal on Addictions 13*(S1), s8–s16.

West, S. L., O'Neal, K. K., & Graham, C. W. (2000). A meta-analysis comparing the effectiveness of buprenorphine and methadone. *Journal of Substance Abuse 12*(4), 405–414.

Wigal, D. (2004). *The mystique of opium*. New York: Parkstone Press.

Willoughby, W. W. (1925). *Opium as an international problem: The Geneva conferences*. Baltimore, MD: Johns Hopkins Press.

Winterburn, G. W. (1884). A seductive drug. *American Homoeopathist 10*(February), 46–47.

Winther, P. C. (2005). *Anglo-European science and the rhetoric of empire: Malaria, opium, and British rule in India, 1756–1895*. Lanham, MD: Lexington Books.

Witherspoon, J. (1900). Oration on medicine, a protest against some of the evils in the profession of medicine. *Journal of the American Medical Association 34*, 1591.

Wong, R. B. (2000). Opium and modern Chinese state-making. In T. Brook & B. T. Wakabayashi (Eds.), *Opium regimes: China, Britain, and Japan, 1839–1952* (pp. 189– 211). Berkeley, CA: University of California Press.

Wood, A. (1855). A new method of treating neuralgia by the direct application of opiates to the painful joints. *Edinburgh Medical and Surgical Journal 82*, 265–281.

Woodiwiss, M. (2000). Reform, racism and rackets: Alcohol and drug prohibition in the United States. In R. Coomber (Ed.), *The control of drugs and drug users: Reason or reaction* (pp. 13–30). Amsterdam: Harwood Academic Publishers/ Gordon and Breach Publishing Group.

Woody, G. E., Senay, E. C., Geller, A., Adams, E. H., Inciardi, J. A., Munoz, A., & Cicero, T. J. (2003). An independent assessment of MEDWatch reporting for abuse/dependence and withdrawal from Ultram (tramadol fydrochloride). *Drug and Alcohol Dependence 72*(2), 163–168.

World Health Organization. (2012) *WHO guidelines on the pharmacological treatment of persisting pain in children with medical illness* (http://apps.who.int/iris/bitstream/ 10665/44540/1/9789241548120_Guidelines.pdf; accessed September 2015).

Yangwen, Z. (2005). *The social life of opium in China: A history of consumption from the fifteenth to the twentieth century*. Cambridge: Cambridge University Press.

Zacny, J. P., & Lichtor, S. A. (2008). Nonmedical use of prescription opioids: Motive and ubiquity issues. *Journal of Pain 9*(6), 473–486.

Zador, D. (2005). Last call for injectable opiate maintenance: In pursuit of an evidence base for good clinical practice. In J. Strang & M. Gossop (Eds.), *Heroin addiction and the British System: Treatment and policy responses* (pp. 121–130). London: Routledge.

Zenghe, L. (2006). Conflicting viewpoints on opium prohibition: Radical changes to opium policy in the late Qing dynasty. *Frontiers of History in China 1*(4), 590–610.

Zhao, C., Liu, Z., Zhao, D., Liu, Y., Liang, J., Tang, Y., Liu, Z., & Zheng, J. (2004). Drug abuse in China. *Annals of the New York Academy of Sciences 1025*, 439–445.

Zieger, S. (2008). *Inventing the addict: Drugs, race, and sexuality in nineteenth-century British and American literature*. Amherst, MA: University of Massachusetts Press.

Index

About the Author

VICTOR B. STOLBERG is an Assistant Professor/Counselor at Essex County College in Newark, New Jersey, where he previously directed the Office of Disability Support Services and the Office of the Substance Abuse Coordinator. He has delivered hundreds of workshops and other presentations across the country. He has authored, or coauthored, 49 scholarly articles, 81 encyclopedia articles, 6 chapters and contributed papers, and 63 other miscellaneous publications. This amounts to a total of over 190 publications. He also has several publications currently in press; these include 6 entries for the upcoming *Encyclopedia of Pharmacology and Society*. Stolberg holds 9 master's degrees from Montclair State University, New Jersey Institute of Technology, Rutgers University, the State University of New York at Cortland, and the University of Buffalo.